Evaluation and Testing in Nursing Education

Second Edition

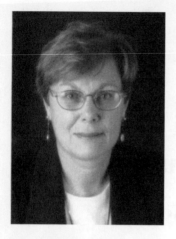

Marilyn H. Oermann, PhD, RN, FAAN, is a Professor in the College of Nursing, Wayne State University, Detroit, Michigan. She is author/co-author of 11 nursing education books and many articles on clinical evaluation, teaching in nursing, and writing for publication as a nurse educator. She is the Editor of the *Annual Review of Nursing Education* and *Journal of Nursing Care Quality.* Dr. Oermann lectures widely on teaching and evaluation in nursing.

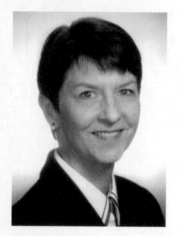

Kathleen B. Gaberson, PhD, RN, CNOR, is Professor, Chair of the Department of Nursing Education, and Director of Nursing at Shepherd University, Shepherdstown, WV. She has over 30 years of teaching experience in graduate and undergraduate nursing programs and has presented, written, and consulted extensively on evaluation and teaching in nursing education. She is Research Section Editor of the *AORN Journal.*

Evaluation and Testing in Nursing Education

Second Edition

Marilyn H. Oermann, PhD, RN, FAAN
Kathleen B. Gaberson, PhD, RN, CNOR

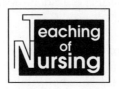

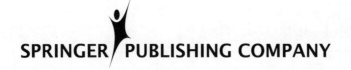

SPRINGER PUBLISHING COMPANY

Springer Publishing Company, Inc.
11 West 42nd Street
New York, NY 10036

Acquisitions Editor: Ruth Chasek
Production Editor: Pam Lankas
Cover design by Joanne Honigman
Typeset by International Graphic Services, Inc., Newtown, PA

07 08 09 10 / 5 4 3

Library of Congress Cataloging-in-Publication Data

Oermann, Marilyn H.
    Evaluation and testing in nursing education / Marilyn H. Oermann, Kathleen B. Gaberson. — 2nd ed.
        p. ; cm. — (Teaching of nursing series)
    Includes bibliographical references and index.
    ISBN 0-8261-9951-8
        1. Nursing—Examinations. 2. Nursing—Ability testing. 3. Nursing —Study and teaching—Evaluation. I. Gaberson, Kathleen B. II. Title. III. Series: Springer series on the teaching of nursing (unnumbered)
[DNLM: 1. Education, Nursing—standards—United States. 2. Educational Measurement—methods—United States. 3. Evaluation Studies—United States. WY 18 O29e 2006]
RT73.7.O47 2006
610.73'071'1—dc22   2005023071

To our parents:
Laurence and Dorothy Haag
Homer and Dorothy Bollen

and families:
David, Eric, and Ross Oermann
Paul Gaberson and Matthew Ammon

Contents

Preface

All teachers at some time or another need to measure and evaluate learning. The teacher may write test items, prepare tests and analyze their results, develop rating scales and clinical evaluation methods, and plan other strategies for assessing learning in the classroom, clinical practice, online and distance education courses, and other settings. Often teachers are not prepared to carry out these tasks as part of their instructional role. This second edition of *Evaluation and Testing in Nursing Education* is a resource for teachers in nursing education programs and health care agencies and a textbook for graduate students preparing for teaching roles, for nurses in clinical practice who teach others and are responsible for evaluating their learning and performance, and for other health professionals involved in evaluation, measurement, and testing. While the examples of test items and other types of evaluation methods provided in this book are nursing-oriented, they are easily adapted to assessment and evaluation in other health fields.

The purposes of the book are to describe concepts of evaluation, measurement, and testing in nursing education; qualities of effective measurement instruments; how to plan for classroom testing, assemble and administer tests, and analyze test results; how to write all types of test items and develop evaluation strategies; methods for evaluating higher level cognitive skills and critical thinking; how to evaluate written assignments in nursing; clinical evaluation and how to evaluate clinical performance; social, ethical, and legal issues associated with evaluation and testing; grading; and program evaluation. The content is useful for teachers in any setting who are involved in evaluating others, whether they are students, nurses, or other types of health personnel.

Chapter 1 addresses the purposes of evaluation and measurement in nursing education and provides a framework for evaluating students and other learners. Differences between formative and summative evaluation and between norm- and criterion-referenced measurement are explored. Since effective evaluation requires a clear description of *what* and *how* to evaluate, the chapter describes the use of objectives as a basis for developing test items and evaluation strategies, provides examples of objectives at different taxonomic levels, and describes how test items would be developed at each of these levels. Some teachers, however, do not use objectives as the basis for testing and evaluation but instead develop test items and other evaluation methods from the content of the course. For this reason chapter 1 also includes an explanation of how to develop test items using this process.

In chapter 2, qualities of effective measurement instruments are discussed. The concepts of validity and reliability and their effects on the interpretive quality of measurement results are described in the chapter. Teachers must gather evidence to support their inferences about scores obtained on a measure. Although this evidence traditionally has been classified as content, criterion-related, and construct validity, a newer understanding of validity centers on construct validity as a unitary concept. New ways of thinking about reliability and its relationship to validity are explained. Also discussed in chapter 2 are important practical considerations that might affect the choice or development of tests and other instruments.

Chapter 3 describes the steps involved in planning for test construction, enabling the teacher to make good decisions about what and when to test; test length; difficulty of test items; item formats; and scoring procedures. An important focus of the chapter is how to develop a test blueprint and then use it for writing test items; examples are provided to clarify this process for the reader. Broad principles important in developing test items regardless of the specific type are described in the chapter.

There are different ways of classifying test items. One way is to group them according to how they are scored—objectively or subjectively. Another way is to group them by the type of response required of the test-taker, which is how we organized the chapters. *Selected-response* items require the test-taker to select the correct or best answer from options provided by the teacher. These items include true-false, matching exercises, multiple-choice, and multiple-response. *Constructed-response* items ask the test-taker to supply an answer rather than choose from options already provided. Constructed-response items include completion and essay (short and extended). Chapters 4 through 6 discuss these test items.

A true-false item consists of a statement that the student judges as true or false. In some forms, students also correct the response or supply a rationale as to why the statement is true or false. True-false items are most effective for recall of facts and specific information but may also be used to test the student's comprehension of the content. Chapter 4 describes how to construct true-false items and different variations, for example, correcting false statements or providing a rationale for the response, which allows the teacher to evaluate if the learner understands the content. Chapter 4 also explains how to develop matching exercises. These consist of two parallel columns in which students match terms, phrases, sentences, or numbers from one column to the other.

Principles for writing each type of item are presented, accompanied by sample items.

In chapter 5 the focus is on writing multiple-choice and multiple-response items. Multiple-choice items, with one correct answer, are used widely in nursing and other fields. This format of test item includes an incomplete statement or question, followed by a list of options that complete the statement or answer the question. Multiple-response items are designed similarly, although more than one answer may be correct. Both of these formats of test items may be used for evaluating learning at the recall, comprehension, application, and analysis levels, making them adaptable for a wide range of content and learning outcomes. There are three parts in a multiple-choice item, each with its own set of principles for development: (a) stem, (b) answer, and (c) distractors. In chapter 5 we discuss how to write each of these parts and provide many examples. Multiple-response items are now included on the NCLEX® Examination as one of the types of alternate item formats; we have a section in chapter 5 on how to write these items.

With selected-response items the test-taker chooses the correct or best answer from the options provided by the teacher. In contrast, with constructed-response items, the test-taker supplies an answer rather than selecting from the options already provided. Constructed-response items include completion, also referred to as fill-in-the-blank, and essay. Completion items can be answered by a word, phrase, or number. These are some of the alternate item formats used on the NCLEX® Examination; candidates may be asked to perform a calculation and type in the number or to put a list of responses in proper order. In this chapter we describe how to write fill-in-the-blank and short-answer items. We also explain how to develop and score essay items. With essay items, students construct responses based on their understanding of the content. Essay items provide an opportunity for students to select content to discuss, present ideas in their own words, and develop an original and a creative response to a question. We provide an extensive discussion on scoring essay responses.

There is much discussion in nursing education about developing higher-level cognitive skills and critical thinking ability of students. With higher-level thinking, students apply concepts, theories, and other forms of knowledge to new situations; use that knowledge to solve patient and other types of problems; and arrive at rational and well thought-out decisions about actions to take. The main principle in evaluating higher-level learning is to develop test items and other evaluation strategies that require students to apply knowledge and skills in a *new* situation; the teacher can then assess if the students are able to use what they have learned in a different context. Chapter 7 presents strategies for evaluating higher levels of learning in nursing. Context-dependent item sets or interpretative exercises are discussed as one format of testing appropriate for assessing higher-level cognitive skills. Suggestions for developing them are presented in the chapter, including examples of different items. Other methods for evaluating cognitive skills in nursing also are presented in the chapter: case method and study, unfolding cases, discussions using higher-level and Socratic questioning, debate, multimedia, and short written assignments.

Chapter 8 focuses on developing test items that prepare students for licensure and certification examinations. The chapter begins with an explanation of the NCLEX® Examination test plans and implications for nurse educators. Examples are provided of items written at different cognitive levels, thereby avoiding tests that focus only on recall and memorization of facts. The chapter also describes how to write questions about the nursing process and provides sample stems for use with those items. The types of items presented in the chapter are similar to those found on the NCLEX® Examination and many certification tests. By incorporating these items on tests in nursing courses, students acquire experience with this type of testing as they progress through the program, preparing them for taking licensure and certification examinations as graduates.

Chapter 9 explains how to assemble and administer a test. In addition to preparing a test blueprint and skillful construction of test items, the final appearance of the test and the way in which it is administered can affect the validity of its results. In chapter 9, test design rules are described; suggestions for reproducing the test, maintaining test security, administering it, and preventing cheating are presented in the chapter as well. We also included a section on administering tests in an online environment. As more courses and programs are offered through distance education, teachers are faced with how to prevent cheating on an assessment when they cannot directly observe their students; we discuss different approaches that can be used for this purpose.

After administering the test, the teacher needs to score it, interpret the results, and then use the results to make varied decisions. Chapter 10 discusses the processes of obtaining scores and performing test and item analysis. It also suggests ways in which teachers can use posttest discussions to contribute to student learning and seek student feedback that can lead to test item improvement. The chapter begins with a discussion of scoring tests, including weighting items and correcting for guessing, then proceeds to item analysis. How to calculate the difficulty index and discrimination index and analyze each distractor are described; performing an item analysis by hand is explained with an illustration for teachers who do not have computer software for this purpose. Teachers often debate the merits of adjusting test scores by eliminating items or adding points to compensate for real or perceived deficiencies in test construction or performance. We discuss this in the chapter and provide guidelines for faculty in making these decisions. A section of the chapter also presents suggestions and examples of developing a test item bank. Many publishers also offer test item banks that relate to the content contained in their textbooks; we discuss why faculty need to be cautious about using these items for their own examinations.

Through papers and other written assignments, students develop an understanding of the content they are writing about and improve ability to communicate their ideas in writing. Written assignments with feedback from the teacher help students improve their writing ability, an important outcome in any nursing program from the beginning level through graduate study. Chapter 11 provides guidelines for developing and evaluating written assignments in nursing courses. The chapter includes criteria for evaluating papers, an example of a scoring rubric, and suggestions for assessing and grading written assignments.

Through clinical evaluation, the teacher arrives at judgments about learners' competencies—their performance in practice. Chapter 12 describes the process of clinical evaluation in nursing. It begins with a discussion on the outcomes of clinical practice in nursing programs and then presents essential concepts underlying clinical evaluation. In this chapter we discuss fairness in evaluation, the stress experienced by learners in clinical practice and the relationship of this stress to evaluation, how to build feedback into the evaluation process, and how to determine *what* to evaluate in clinical courses.

Chapter 13 builds on concepts of clinical evaluation examined in the preceding chapter. Many evaluation methods are available for assessing competencies in clinical practice. We discuss observation and recording observations in anecdotal notes, checklists, and rating scales; simulations including patient simulators, standardized patients, and structured clinical examinations; written assignments useful for clinical evaluation such as journals, nursing care plans, concept maps, case analyses, and short papers; portfolio assessment and how to set up a portfolio system for clinical evaluation, including an electronic portfolio; and other methods such as conference, group projects, and self-evaluation. The chapter includes a sample form for evaluating student participation in clinical conferences and a rubric for peer evaluation of participation in group projects. Because most nursing education programs use rating scales for clinical evaluation, we have collected a variety of clinical evaluation forms from associate degree, baccalaureate, and graduate nursing programs for review by readers; these are found in Appendix A.

Chapter 14 explores social, ethical, and legal issues associated with testing and evaluation. Social issues such as test bias, grade inflation, effects of testing on self-esteem, and test anxiety are discussed. Ethical issues include privacy and access to test results. By understanding and applying codes for the responsible and ethical use of tests, teachers can assure the proper use of assessment procedures and the valid interpretation of test results. We include several of these codes in the Appendices. We also discuss selected legal issues associated with testing.

In chapter 15, the discussion focuses on how to interpret the meaning of test scores. Basic statistical concepts are presented and used for criterion- and norm-referenced interpretations of teacher-made and standardized test results.

Grading is the use of symbols, such as the letters A through F or pass-fail, to report student achievement. Grading is for summative purposes, indicating how well the student met the outcomes of the course and clinical practicum. To represent valid judgments about student achievement, grades should be based on sound evaluation practices, reliable test results, and multiple evaluation measures. Chapter 16 examines the uses of grades in nursing programs, criticisms of grades, types of grading systems, assigning letter grades, selecting a grading framework, how to calculate grades with each of these frameworks, and how to use a spreadsheet application and course management system for calculating grades. We also discuss grading clinical practice, using pass-fail and other systems for grading, and provide guidelines for the teacher when students have the potential for failing a clinical practicum.

Program evaluation is the process of judging the worth or value of an educational program. With the demand for high quality programs, the development of newer models for the delivery of higher education, such as Web-based instruction, and public calls for accountability, there has been a greater emphasis on systematic and ongoing program evaluation. Thus, chapter 17 presents an overview of program evaluation models and discusses evaluation of selected program components, including curriculum, outcomes, and teaching.

The authors wish to acknowledge Ruth Chasek for her encouragement, patience, and editorial assistance; Pamela Lankas, for her assistance during production; and Nancy A. Wilmes, Librarian at the Science and Engineering Library, Wayne State University, who assisted us in locating information and checked many references for us. We also thank Springer Publishing Company for its continued support of nursing education.

Marilyn H. Oermann
Kathleen B. Gaberson

Chapter 1

Evaluation, Measurement, and the Educational Process

In all areas of nursing education and practice, evaluation is an important process to measure learning and other outcomes, judge performance, determine competence to practice, and arrive at other decisions about students and nurses. Evaluation is integral to monitoring the quality of educational and health care programs. By evaluating outcomes achieved by students, graduates, and clients, the effectiveness of programs can be measured and decisions can be made about needed improvements.

Evaluation provides a means of ensuring accountability for the quality of education and services provided. Nurses, similar to other health professionals, are accountable to their clients and society in general for meeting their health needs. Along the same line, nurse educators are accountable for the quality of teaching provided to learners, outcomes achieved, and overall effectiveness of programs that prepare graduates to meet the health needs of society. Educational institutions are also accountable to their governing bodies and society in terms of educating graduates for present and future roles. Through evaluation, nursing faculty and other health professionals can measure the quality of their teaching and programs as well as document outcomes for others to review. All educators, regardless of the setting, need to be knowledgeable about the evaluation process, measurement, testing, assessment, and other related concepts.

EVALUATION

Evaluation is the process of collecting and interpreting information for making judgments about student learning and achievement, clinical performance, employee competence, and educational programs, among others. In nursing educa-

1

tion, evaluation typically takes the form of judging student attainment of the educational objectives and goals in the classroom and the quality of student performance in the clinical setting. Educational experiences produce changes in the learner; evaluation provides the means to assess those changes. With this evaluation, learning outcomes are measured, further educational needs are identified, and additional instruction can be provided to assist students in their learning and in developing competencies for practice. Similarly, evaluation of employees provides information on their performance at varied points in time as a basis for judging their competence.

Evaluation extends beyond a test score or clinical rating. In evaluating learners, teachers judge the merits of the learning and performance based on the data. Evaluation involves making value judgments about learners; in fact, value is part of the word e*valu*ation. Questions such as "How *well* did the student perform?" and "Is the student *competent* in clinical practice?" are answered by the evaluation process. The teacher collects and analyzes data about the student's performance, then makes a value judgment about the quality of that performance.

In terms of educational programs, evaluation includes collecting information prior to developing the program, during the process of program development to provide a basis for ongoing revision, and after implementing the program to determine its effectiveness. With program evaluation, faculty collect data about their students, alumni, curriculum, and other dimensions of the program for the purpose of documenting the program outcomes and for making sound decisions about curriculum revision. As faculty measure outcomes for accreditation and evaluate their courses and curriculum, they are engaging in program evaluation. While many of the concepts described in this book are applicable to program evaluation, the focus instead is on evaluating learners, including students in all types and levels of nursing programs and nurses in health care settings. The term "students" is used broadly to reflect both of these groups of learners.

Evaluation and Instruction

Through evaluation the teacher determines the progress of students toward meeting the objectives and developing clinical practice competencies and their achievement of them. The data that the teacher collects, through classroom testing, observations in clinical practice, and other assessment strategies, provide the basis for further instruction. Figure 1.1 demonstrates the relationship between evaluation and instruction. The objectives specify the intended learning outcomes; these may be designated for attainment in the classroom, clinical setting, learning laboratory, online environment, or other setting. Following assessment of learner needs to determine gaps in learning and clinical competency, the

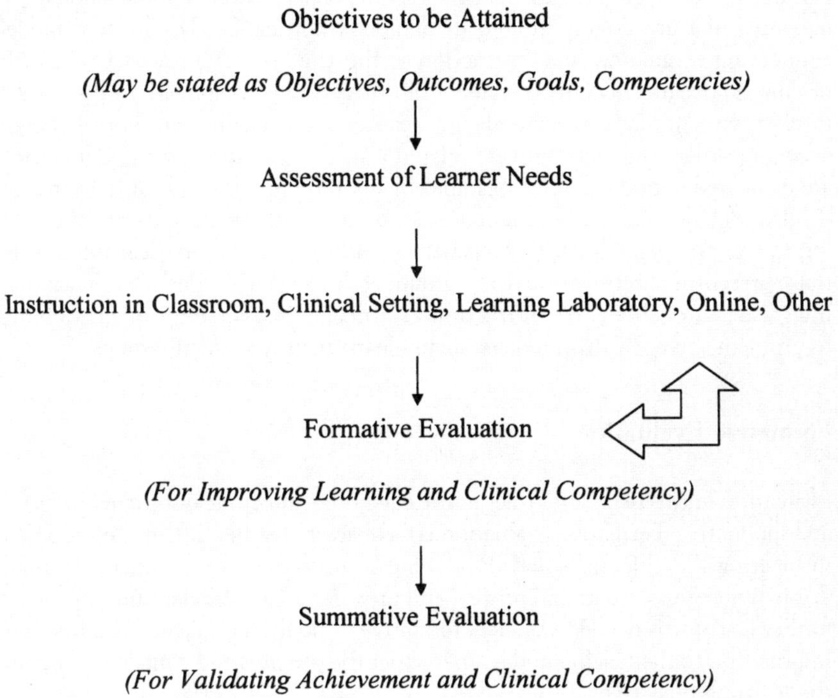

Objectives to be Attained

(May be stated as Objectives, Outcomes, Goals, Competencies)

↓

Assessment of Learner Needs

↓

Instruction in Classroom, Clinical Setting, Learning Laboratory, Online, Other

↓

Formative Evaluation

(For Improving Learning and Clinical Competency)

↓

Summative Evaluation

(For Validating Achievement and Clinical Competency)

FIGURE 1.1   Relationship of evaluation and instruction.

teacher selects teaching methods and plans clinical activities to meet those needs. This phase of the instructional process includes developing a plan for learning, selecting learning activities, and teaching learners in varied settings.

The remaining components of the instructional process relate to evaluation. With formative evaluation, during this process, the teacher assesses student progress toward meeting the objectives and demonstrating competency in clinical practice. This type of evaluation is displayed with a feedback loop to instruction. Formative evaluation provides information about further learning needs of students and where additional instruction is needed. This feedback to students reinforces successful learning and identifies learning errors that need correction (Linn & Gronlund, 2000). Summative evaluation, at the end of the instruction, determines if the objectives have been achieved and competencies developed.

This model of teaching has been called the continuous feedback model because it incorporates formative evaluation for providing feedback, focused instruction to fill gaps in learning so students achieve mastery, and summative measures that are usually limited in number (Mertler, 2003). Another model connecting evaluation and instruction is the time-restricted model in which evaluation occurs only after a segment of instruction is completed. In this model teachers present new content and guide learners in acquiring new clinical knowledge and skills, students complete related learning activities, and students then are evaluated periodically, for example, at midterm and the end of the term. A third model, integrated assessment, focuses on problem solving and critical thinking as the outcomes, with the teacher facilitating and guiding learning rather than presenting information to a group of learners (Mertler). Evaluation is integrated throughout the instruction as a means of assessing students' ability to problem solve. In this model students learn mainly in small groups.

Formative Evaluation

Evaluation fulfills two major roles in the classroom and clinical setting: formative and summative. Formative evaluation is feedback to learners about their progress in meeting the objectives and developing competencies for practice. It occurs throughout the instructional process and provides a basis for determining where further learning is needed. As such, formative evaluation is diagnostic, providing information to the teacher and learner about the progress being made in meeting the learning objectives.

In the classroom, formative information may be collected by teacher observation and questioning of students, diagnostic quizzes, small group activities, written assignments, and other activities that students complete in and out of class. In clinical practice, formative evaluation is an integral part of the instructional process. The teacher continually makes observations of students as they learn to provide patient care, questions them about their understanding and clinical decisions, discusses these observations and judgments with them, and guides them in how to improve performance. With formative evaluation the teacher gives feedback to learners about their progress in achieving the goals of clinical practice and how they can further develop their knowledge and skills. Anecdotal notes are commonly used to record the teacher's observations and judgments and to communicate them to the students.

Considering that the purpose of formative evaluation is to provide feedback, typically formative evaluation is not graded. Since formative evaluation is "directed toward improving learning and instruction, the results typically are not used for assigning course grades" (Linn & Gronlund, 2000, p. 41). Teachers should remember that the purpose of formative evaluation is to assess where further learning is needed and to guide continued teaching and learning.

Summative Evaluation

Summative evaluation, on the other hand, is end-of-instruction evaluation designed to determine what the student has learned in the classroom or clinical setting. Summative evaluation provides information on the extent to which objectives were achieved, not on the progress of the learner in meeting them. As such, summative evaluation occurs at the end of the learning process, for instance, the end of a course, to determine the student's grade and certify competence. Although formative evaluation occurs throughout the learning experience, for example, daily, summative evaluation is conducted on a periodic basis, for instance, every few weeks or at the midterm and final evaluation periods. This type of evaluation is "final" in nature and serves as a basis for grading and other high-stakes decisions.

Summative evaluation typically assesses broader content areas than formative evaluation, which tends to be more specific in terms of the content evaluated. Methods commonly used for summative evaluation in the classroom include tests, term papers, and other types of projects. In clinical practice, rating scales, written assignments, portfolios, projects completed about clinical experiences, and other performance measures may be used.

Both formative and summative evaluation are essential components of most nursing courses. However, because formative evaluation represents feedback to learners with the goal of improving learning, it should be a major part of any nursing course. By providing feedback on a continual basis and linking that feedback with further instruction, the teacher can assist students in developing the knowledge and skills they lack.

MEASUREMENT

Measurement is the process of assigning numbers to represent student achievement or performance according to certain rules, for instance, answering 85 out of 100 items correctly on a test. Measurement answers the question "how much?" (Linn & Gronlund, 2000). In contrast to evaluation, measurement does not imply value judgments about the quality of the results. Measurement is important for describing the achievement of learners on nursing and other tests, but not all outcomes important in nursing practice can be measured by testing. Many outcomes are evaluated qualitatively through other means, such as observations of performance.

While measurement involves assigning numbers to reflect learning, these numbers in and of themselves have no meaning. Scoring 15 on a test means nothing unless it is referenced or compared with other students' scores or to a predetermined standard. Perhaps 15 was the highest or lowest score on the test compared with other students. Or, the student might have set a personal goal of achieving 15 on the test; thus meeting this goal is more important than how others scored on the test. Another interpretation is that a score of 15 might reflect the standard expected of this particular group of learners. Having a reference point with which to compare a particular test score is essential to give it meaning and to interpret the score.

In clinical practice, how does a learner's performance compare with that of others in the group? Does the learner meet the clinical objectives and possess certain competencies regardless of how other students in the group perform in clinical practice? Answers to these questions depend on the basis used for interpreting clinical performance, similar to interpreting test scores.

Norm-Referenced Interpretation

There are two main ways of interpreting test scores and other types of evaluation conducted in the clinical setting, norm- and criterion-referenced. In norm-referenced interpretation, test scores and other evaluation data are referenced to a norm group. Norm-referenced interpretation compares a student's test scores with those of others in the class or with some other relevant group. The student's score may be described as below or above average or at a certain rank in the class. Norm-referenced interpretations are limited because they do not indicate what the student can and cannot do (Oosterhof, 2001).

In clinical settings, norm-referenced interpretations compare the student's clinical performance with those of a group of learners, indicating that the student has more or less clinical competence than others in the group. A clinical evaluation instrument in which student performance is rated on a scale of below- to above-average reflects a norm-referenced system.

Criterion-Referenced Interpretation

Criterion-referenced interpretation, on the other hand, involves interpreting scores based on preset criteria, not in relation to the group of learners. With this type of measurement, an individual score is compared to a preset standard or criterion. The concern is how well the student performed and what the student can do regardless of the performance of other learners. Criterion-referenced interpretations may (a) describe the specific learning tasks a student can perform, e.g., define medical terms; (b) indicate the percentage of tasks performed or items answered correctly, e.g., define correctly 80% of the terms, and (c) compare performance against a set standard and decide whether the student met that standard, e.g., met the medical terminology competency (Linn & Gronlund, 2000, p. 43). Criterion-referenced interpretation determines how well the student performed at the end of the instruction in comparison with the objectives and competencies to be achieved.

With criterion-referenced clinical evaluation, student performance is compared against preset criteria. In some nursing courses these criteria are the clinical objectives to be met in the course. Other courses indicate competencies to be demonstrated in clinical practice, which are then used as the standards for evaluation. Rather than comparing the performance of the student to others in the group, and indicating that the student was above or below the average of the group, in criterion-referenced clinical evaluation, performance is measured against the objectives or competencies to be demonstrated. The concern with criterion-referenced clinical evaluation is whether students achieved the clinical objectives or demonstrated the competencies, not how well they performed in comparison to the other students.

TESTING

Tests are one form of measurement. A test is a set of questions to which the student responds in written or oral form. With tests the questions are administered during a fixed period of time under comparable conditions for all students (Linn & Gronlund, 2000). While students often dread tests, information from tests enables faculty to make important decisions about students, the instruction, and programs.

First, test results provide a basis for grading. For some nursing courses, tests may be the only source of information for determining grades, but in most courses, other means for grading student performance also are used, such as papers, projects, and other assignments. Tests are typically the primary means for arriving at grades in nursing courses, particularly in undergraduate programs.

Second, tests may be used to identify the student's knowledge and skills prior to the instruction, which enables the teacher to gear the instruction to the learner's needs. Mertler (2003) referred to this pretesting as diagnostic assessment. The test results indicate gaps in learning that should be addressed first and knowledge and skills already acquired. With this information teachers can plan their instruction better. When teachers are working with large groups of students, it is difficult to gear the instruction to meet each student's needs. However, the teacher can use diagnostic tests to reveal content areas for which individual learners may be lacking and then suggest remedial learning activities.

Third, tests are used for selection and fourth, placement of students in nursing programs. In some nursing programs, students take tests for admission to the program, providing data for faculty to accept or reject applicants. For example, the National League for Nursing (NLN) offers pre-admission examinations for registered nurse (RN) and licensed practical nurse (LPN) programs. Test results provide norms that allow comparison of the applicant's performance with those of other applicants (National League for Nursing, 2003). Tests also may be used to place students into appropriate courses. Placement tests, taken after the individual has been admitted, provide data for determining which courses students should complete in their programs of study. For example, a diagnostic test of math skills may determine whether a nursing student is required to take a medication dosage calculation course.

Fifth, test results provide clues as to content areas that students learned or did not learn in a course. With this information, faculty can modify the instruction to better meet student learning needs. Student responses to higher-level test questions, such as ones measuring critical thinking, may suggest changes in teaching strategies to encourage development of cognitive skills rather than memorization of facts and principles.

Last, testing may be an integral part of the curriculum and program evaluation in a school of nursing. Students may complete tests to measure program outcomes rather than to document what was learned in a course. Test results for this purpose often suggest areas of the curriculum for revision.

ASSESSMENT

Even though a test is a one-time measure, educational assessment involves the collection of data about learners and programs over a period of time. Through assessment the teacher examines students' performance over time, for example, covering the length of a semester or a clinical rotation. Assessment includes a variety of techniques to obtain information about students' performance (Linn & Gronlund, 2000). These techniques include not only tests but also other strategies for evaluating learning such as papers, other types of written assignments, projects, portfolios, and conferences, among others.

Assessment is broader and more inclusive than measurement and testing. Assessment involves all of the strategies planned for determining student performance in a course. Through assessment teachers systemically collect data about performance in the classroom, learning laboratory, and clinical setting, providing information for making decisions about course grades and clinical competence.

OBJECTIVES FOR EVALUATION AND TESTING

Objectives play a role in teaching students in varied settings in nursing. They provide guidelines for student learning and instruction and a basis for evaluating learning. The objectives represent the outcomes of learning; these outcomes may include the acquisition of knowledge, development of values, and performance of psychomotor and technological skills. Evaluation serves to determine the extent and quality of the student's learning in relation to these outcomes. This does not mean that the teacher is unconcerned about learning that occurs and is not expressed as outcomes. Many students will acquire knowledge, values, and skills beyond those expressed in the objectives, but the evaluation methods planned by the teacher focus on the preset outcomes to be met by students.

To develop test items, clinical evaluation strategies, and other evaluation methods, teachers needs a clear description of *what* to evaluate. The knowledge, values, and skills to be evaluated are specified by the outcomes of the course and clinical practicum. These provide the basis for evaluating learning in the classroom, practice laboratories, and clinical setting.

Writing Objectives   (Learning outcomes)

In developing instructional objectives, there are two important dimensions. The first is the actual technique for writing objectives and the second is deciding on their complexity. The predominant format for writing objectives in past years was to develop a highly specific objective that included (a) a description of the learner, (b) behaviors the learner would exhibit at the end of the instruction, (c) conditions under which the behavior would be demonstrated, and (d) the standard of performance. An example of this format for an objective is: Given a written nursing assessment, the student identifies in writing two nursing diagnoses with supporting rationale. This objective includes the following components:

Learner:	Student
Behavior:	Identifies in writing nursing diagnoses
Conditions:	Given a written nursing assessment
Standard:	Two nursing diagnoses must be identified with supporting rationale.

It is clear from this example that specific instructional objectives are too prescriptive for use in nursing. The complexity of learning expected in a nursing program makes it difficult to use such a system for specifying the objectives. Linn and Gronlund (2000) also suggested that highly specific objectives are concerned mainly with simple knowledge and skills, making them inappropriate for nursing courses that require problem solving and critical thinking. In addition, they limit flexibility in planning instructional methods and in developing evaluation techniques. For these reasons, a general format for writing objectives is sufficient to express the learning outcomes and to provide a basis for evaluating learning in nursing courses.

General objectives include the behavior the learner will exhibit as a result of the instruction and content to which that behavior relates. A general objective similar to the earlier outcome is: The student identifies nursing diagnoses based on the assessment. With this example, the components would be:

Learner: Student
Behavior: Identifies
Content: Nursing diagnoses from the assessment.

This general objective, which is open-ended, provides flexibility for the teacher in developing instruction to meet it and for evaluating student learning. The outcome could be met and evaluated in the classroom through varied activities in which students analyze assessment data, presented as part of a lecture, in a written case study, or in a videotape, and identify nursing diagnoses. Students might work in groups in or out of class, reviewing various assessments and discussing possible diagnoses. Or, they might complete a simulated experience in which they collect data and identify nursing diagnoses. In the clinical setting, patient assignments, conferences, discussions with students, and reviews of patient records provide other strategies for developing an ability to derive nursing diagnoses and for evaluating student competency. Generally stated objectives, therefore, provide sufficient guidelines for instruction and evaluation of student learning.

Gronlund (2000) identified two criteria to be met when writing objectives. First, the objective should specify the behavior that the student should demonstrate at the end of the instruction, not what the teacher does. Second, the behavior should be objective and measurable so students can demonstrate what they have learned and teachers can measure their performance.

The objectives are important in developing evaluation methods that measure the behavior and content area intended by the objective. In evaluating the sample objective cited earlier, the method selected—for instance, a test—needs to examine student ability to identify nursing diagnoses from assessment data. The objective does not specify the number of nursing diagnoses, type of client problem, complexity of the assessment data, or other variables associated with the clinical situation; there is opportunity for the teacher to develop various types of test questions and evaluation measures as long as they ask the learner to identify nursing diagnoses based on the given assessment.

Clearly written objectives guide the teacher in selecting evaluation methods. The behavior indicated by the objective suggests evaluation methods, such as tests, observations in the clinical setting, written assignments, and others. When tests are chosen as the method, the objective in turn suggests the type of test question, for instance, true-false, multiple-choice, or essay. In addition to guiding decisions about evaluation methods, the objective gives clues to faculty about teaching methods and learning activities to assist students in meeting it. For the sample objective, teaching methods might include: readings, lecture, discussion, case study, simulation, role play, videotape, interactive video, clinical practice, post-clinical conference, and other methods that present assessment data and ask students to identify varied nursing diagnoses.

Objectives that are useful for test construction and for designing other evaluation methods meet three general principles. First, the behavior, or action verb, should be measurable. The behavior represents the outcome expected of the learner at the end of the instruction. Terms such as identify, describe, and analyze are specific and may be measured; words such as understand and know, in contrast, represent a wide variety of behaviors, some simple and others complex, making these terms difficult to evaluate. The student's knowledge might range from identifying and naming through synthesizing and evaluating. Sample behaviors are presented in Table 1.1.

Second, the objectives should be as general as possible to allow for their achievement with varied course content. For instance, instead of stating that the student identifies physiological nursing diagnoses from the assessment of acutely ill patients, indicating that the learner identifies nursing diagnoses from assessment data provides more flexibility for the teacher in designing evaluation strategies that reflect different types of diagnoses from varied data sets presented in the course.

Third, the teaching method should be omitted from the objective to provide greater flexibility in how the instruction is planned. For example, in the objective "Uses effective communication techniques in a simulated client-nurse interaction," the teacher is limited to evaluating communication techniques through simulations rather than through interactions the student might have in the clinical setting. The objective would be better if stated as "Uses effective communication techniques with clients."

In test construction and evaluation, both the behavior to be achieved, for example, lists and applies, and the content area to which that behavior relates, such as pain management, are important. With clear and measurable objectives, teachers have a sound framework for developing the evaluation strategies for the course. Airasian (2000) suggested an easy to use model for writing objectives:

Model: The student will [*measurable behavior*] [*content*].
Example: The student will [*describe*] [*classifications for asthma severity.*]

A model such as this facilitates the development of test items and other evaluation strategies.

TABLE 1.1 Sample Verbs for Taxonomic Levels

Cognitive Domain	Affective Domain	Psychomotor Domain
Knowledge Define Identify Label List Name Recall State	Receiving Acknowledge Ask Reply Show awareness of	Imitation Follow example of Imitate
Comprehension Defend Describe Differentiate Draw conclusions Explain Give examples Interpret Select Summarize	Responding Act willingly Assist Is willing to Support Respond Seek opportunities	Manipulation Assemble Carry out Follow procedure
Application Apply Demonstrate use of Modify Operate Predict Produce Relate Solve Use	Valuing Accept Assume responsibility Participate in Respect Support Value	Precision Demonstrate skill Is accurate in
Analysis Analyze Breaks down Compare Contrast Detect Differentiate Identify Relate Select	Organization of Values Argue Debate	Articulation Carry out accurately and in reasonable time frame Is skillful
		Naturalization Is competent Carry out competently Integrate skill within care

TABLE 1.1 (*continued*)

Cognitive Domain	Affective Domain	Psychomotor Domain
Synthesis		
Compile		
Construct		
Design	Declare	
Develop	Defend	
Devise	Take a stand	
Generate	Characterization by Value	
Plan	Act consistently	
Produce	Stand for	
Revise		
Synthesize		
Write		
Evaluation		
Appraise		
Assess		
Critique		
Discriminate		
Evaluate		
Judge		
Justify		
Support		

TAXONOMIES OF OBJECTIVES

The need for clearly stated objectives becomes evident when the teacher translates them into test items and other evaluation methods. Test items need to adequately measure the behavior in the objective, for instance, identify, describe, apply, and analyze, as it relates to the content area. Objectives may be written to reflect three domains of learning, each with its own classification or taxonomic system: cognitive, affective, and psychomotor. A taxonomy is a classification system that places an objective within a broader system or scheme. While learning in nursing ultimately represents an integration of these domains, it is valuable in planning instruction and particularly in developing evaluation measures, for the domains to be considered separately.

Cognitive Taxonomy

The cognitive domain deals with knowledge and intellectual skills. Learning within this domain includes the acquisition of facts and specific information underlying the practice of nursing; concepts, theories, and principles about nursing; and cognitive skills such as decision making, problem solving, and critical thinking. The most widely used cognitive taxonomy was developed years ago, in 1956, by Bloom and associates. It provides for six levels of cognitive learning, increasing in complexity: knowledge, comprehension, application, analysis, synthesis, and evaluation. This hierarchy suggests that knowledge, such as recall of specific facts, is less complex and demanding intellectually than the higher levels of learning. Evaluation, the most complex level, requires judgments based on varied criteria. For each of the levels, except for application, Bloom, Englehart, Furst, Hill, and Krathwohl (1956) identified sublevels.

One advantage in considering this taxonomy when writing objectives and test items is that it encourages the teacher to think about higher levels of learning expected as a result of the instruction. If the course goals reflect application of concepts in clinical practice, use of theories in patient care, and critical thinking outcomes, these higher levels of learning should be reflected in the objectives and evaluation rather than focusing only on the recall of facts and other information.

In using the taxonomy, the teacher decides first on the level of cognitive learning intended and then develops objectives and evaluation methods for that particular level. Decisions about the taxonomic level at which to gear instruction and evaluation depend on the teacher's judgment in considering the background of the learner; placement of the course and learning experiences within the curriculum to provide for the progressive development of knowledge, skills, and values; and complexity of the behavior and content in relation to the time allowed for teaching. If the time for teaching and evaluation is limited, the objectives may need to be written at a lower level. The taxonomy provides a continuum for educators to use in planning instruction and carrying out evaluation, beginning with recall of facts and information and progressing toward understanding, using concepts and theories in practice, analyzing situations, synthesizing from different sources to develop new products, and evaluating materials and situations based on internal and external criteria.

A description and sample objective for each of the six levels of learning in the cognitive taxonomy follow. While sublevels have been established for these levels, except for application, only the six major levels are essential to guide the teacher for instructional and evaluation purposes.

1. Knowledge: Recall of facts and specific information. Memorization of specifics.

   The student defines the term systole.

2. Comprehension: Understanding. Ability to describe and explain the material.

   The learner describes the circulation through the heart.

3. Application: Use of information in a new situation. Ability to use knowledge in a new situation.

   The student applies concepts of aging in developing interventions for the elderly.

4. Analysis: Ability to break down material into component parts and identify the relationships among them.

   The student analyzes the organizational structure of the community health agency and its impact on client services.

5. Synthesis: Ability to develop a new product. Combining elements to form a new product.

   The student develops a plan for delivering services to elderly persons who are home-bound.

6. Evaluation: Judgments about value based on internal and external criteria. Extent to which materials and objects meet criteria.

   The learner evaluates nursing research based on predetermined criteria.

This taxonomy is useful in developing test items because it helps the teacher gear the item to a particular cognitive level. For example, if the objective focuses on application, the test question should measure whether the student can use the concept in a new situation, which is the intent of learning at that level. However, the taxonomy alone does not always determine the level of complexity of the item because one other consideration is how the information was presented in the instruction. For example, a test item at the application level requires use of previously learned concepts and theories in a new situation. Whether or not the situation is new for each student, however, is not known. Some students may have had clinical experience with that situation or been exposed to it through another learning activity. As another example, a question written at the comprehension level may actually be at the knowledge level if the teacher used that specific explanation in class and students only need to recall it to answer the item.

Mertler (2003) suggested a modification of the six levels of the taxonomy into a two-category system: lower- and higher-level cognitive behaviors. Lower-level behaviors focus on memorization, recall of facts, and understanding of content; this level captures the knowledge and comprehension level of Bloom's taxonomy. Higher-level behaviors extend beyond comprehension to include development of thinking skills, from application through evaluation. A two-level system works well in nursing because it helps avoid teaching and evaluating lower-level behaviors only.

Affective Domain

The affective domain relates to the development of values, attitudes, and beliefs consistent with standards of professional nursing practice. Developed by Krath-wohl, Bloom, and Masia (1964), the taxonomy of the affective domain includes five levels organized hierarchically based on the principle of increasing involvement of the learner and internationalization of a value. Krathwohl et al. (1964) believed that objectives for learning could be specified in the affective domain and instruction provided to assist the learner in developing a value system that guides decisions and behaviors. The principle on which the affective taxonomy is based relates to the movement of learners from mere awareness of a value, for instance, confidentiality, to internalization of that value as a basis for their own behavior.

There are two important dimensions in evaluating affective outcomes. The first relates to the student's knowledge of the values, attitudes, and beliefs that are important in guiding decisions in nursing. Prior to internalizing a value and using it as a basis for decision making and behavior, the student needs to know what are important values in nursing. There is a cognitive base, therefore, to the development of a value system. Evaluation of this dimension focuses on acquisition of knowledge about the values, attitudes, and beliefs consistent with professional nursing practice. A variety of test items and evaluation methods are appropriate to assess this knowledge base.

The second dimension of affective evaluation focuses on whether or not students have accepted these values, attitudes, and beliefs and are internalizing them to form a system for their own decision making and behavior. Evaluation at these higher levels of the affective domain is more difficult because it requires observation of student behavior over time to determine if there is commitment to act according to professional values. Test items are not appropriate for these levels as the teacher is concerned with the use of values in practice and motivation to carry them out consistently in patient care.

A description and sample objective for each of the five levels of learning in the affective taxonomy follow. While sublevels have been established for each of these levels, only these five major categories are essential to guide the teacher for instructional and evaluation purposes:

1. Receiving: Awareness of values, attitudes, and beliefs important in nursing practice. Sensitivity to a client, clinical situation, problem.

    The student expresses an awareness of the need for maintaining confidentiality of patient information.

2. Responding: Reacting to a situation. Responding voluntarily to a given phenomenon reflecting a choice made by the learner.

    The student shares willingly feelings about caring for a dying patient.

3. Valuing: Internalization of a value. Acceptance of a value and commitment to using it as a basis for behavior.

    The learner supports the rights of clients to their own life styles and decisions about care.

4. Organization: Development of a complex system of values. Organization of a value system.

    The learner forms a position about issues surrounding cost and quality of care.

5. Characterization by a value: Internalization of a value system providing a philosophy for practice.

    The learner acts consistently to involve clients and families in decision making about care.

Psychomotor Domain

Psychomotor learning involves the development of skills and competency in the use of technology. This domain includes activities that are movement oriented, requiring some degree of physical coordination. Motor skills have a cognitive base, which are the principles underlying the skill. They also have an affective component reflecting the values of the nurse while carrying out the skill, for instance, respecting the client while performing the procedure (Oermann, 2004).

Different taxonomies have been developed for the evaluation of psychomotor skills. One taxonomy useful in nursing education specifies five levels in the development of psychomotor skills. The lowest level is imitation learning; here the learner observes a demonstration of the skill and imitates that performance. In the second level, the learner performs the skill following written guidelines. By practicing skills the learner refines the ability to perform them without errors (precision) and in a reasonable time frame (articulation) until they become a natural part of care (naturalization) (Dave, 1970; Gaberson & Oermann, 1999). A description of each of these levels and sample objectives follows.

1. Imitation: Performance of skill following demonstration by teacher or through multimedia. Imitative learning.

   The student follows the example for changing a dressing.

2. Manipulation: Ability to follow instructions rather than needing to observe the procedure or skill.

   The student suctions a patient according to the accepted procedure.

3. Precision: Ability to perform skill accurately, independently, and without using a model or set of directions.

   The student takes vital signs accurately.

4. Articulation: Coordinated performance of a skill within a reasonable time frame.

   The learner demonstrates skill in suctioning patients with varying health problems.

5. Naturalization: High degree of proficiency. Integration of skill within care.

   The learner competently carries out skills needed for care of technology-dependent children in their homes.

Evaluation methods for psychomotor skills provide data on knowledge of the principles underlying the skill and ability to carry out the procedure in simulated settings and with clients. Most of the evaluation of performance is done in the clinical setting and learning laboratory; however, test items may be used for evaluating principles associated with performing the skill.

Integrated Framework

One other framework that could be used to classify objectives was developed by Linn and Gronlund (2000). This framework integrates the cognitive, affective, and psychomotor domains into one list and can be easily adapted for nursing education:

1. Knowledge (knowledge of terms, facts, concepts, and methods)
2. Understanding (understanding concepts; methods; written materials, graphs, and data; and problems)
3. Application (of knowledge and problem-solving skills)
4. Thinking skills (critical thinking)
5. General skills (psychomotor, communication, and other skills), and
6. Attitudes (and values reflecting standards of nursing practice).

Linn and Gronlund include three other categories in their framework: interests, appreciations, and adjustments, but these are not as applicable to evaluation in nursing as are the other six areas.

USE OF OBJECTIVES FOR EVALUATION AND TESTING

As described earlier, the taxonomies provide a framework for the teacher to plan instruction and design evaluation at different levels of learning, from simple to complex in the cognitive domain, from awareness of a value to developing a philosophy of practice based on internalization of a value system in the affective domain, and increasing psychomotor competency, from imitation of the skill to performance as a natural part of care. These taxonomies are of value in designing the evaluation protocol to gear tests and other evaluation methods to the level of learning anticipated from the instruction. If the outcome of learning is application, then test items also need to be at the application level. If the outcome of learning is valuing, then the evaluation methods need to examine students' behaviors over time to determine if they are committed to practice reflecting these values. If the outcome of skill learning is precision, then evaluation strategies need to focus on accuracy in performance, not the speed with which the skill is performed. The taxonomies, therefore, provide a useful framework to assure that test items and evaluation methods are at the appropriate level for the intended learning outcomes.

In developing test items and other types of evaluation methods, the teacher identifies first the objective to be evaluated, then designs test items or other evaluation strategies to measure that objective. The objective specifies the behavior, at a particular taxonomic level, to be evaluated and the content area to which it relates. For the objective, *Identifies* characteristics of premature ventricular contractions, the test item would examine student ability to recall these characteristics. The behavior, *identifies*, at the knowledge level, indicates that recall of facts is needed to answer the question, not comprehension or use of this knowledge in new client situations. The content area, characteristics of premature ventricular contractions, indicates the content to be tested.

Some teachers choose not to use objectives as the basis for testing and evaluation and instead develop test items and other evaluation methods from the content of the course. With this process the teacher identifies explicit content areas to be evaluated; test items then sample knowledge of this content. If using this method, the teacher should refer to the course outcomes for decisions about the level of complexity of the test items and methods of evaluation.

Throughout this book, multiple types of test items and other evaluation strategies are presented. It is assumed that these items were developed from specific outcomes or objectives, or from explicit content areas. Regardless of whether the teacher uses objectives or content domains as the framework for testing and evaluation, test items and other strategies should evaluate the learning outcome intended from the instruction. This outcome specifies a behavior to be evaluated, at a particular level of complexity indicated by the taxonomic level, and a content area to which it relates. The behavior and content area provide the framework for developing test items and other evaluation methods.

SUMMARY

Evaluation is an integral part of the instructional process in nursing. Through evaluation, the teacher makes important decisions about the extent and quality of learning. Evaluation fulfills two major roles in the classroom and clinical setting: formative and summative.

Measurement is the process of assigning numbers to represent student achievement according to certain rules. It answers the question "How much?" There are two main ways of interpreting test scores and other types of evaluation conducted in the clinical setting: norm- and criterion-referenced. In norm-referenced interpretation, test scores and other evaluation data are referenced to a norm group. The scores are interpreted by comparing them to those of other individuals. Norm-referenced clinical evaluation compares students' clinical performance with those of a group of learners, indicating that the learner has more or less clinical competence than other students. Criterion-referenced interpretation, on the other hand, involves interpreting scores based on preset criteria, not in relation to a group of learners. With criterion-referenced clinical evaluation, student performance is compared with a set of criteria to be met. A test, which is one form of measurement, is a set of items each with a correct answer.

Objectives play a role in teaching and evaluating students in varied settings in nursing. They provide guidelines for student learning and instruction and serve as a basis for evaluating learning. The objectives represent the outcomes of learning; these outcomes may include the acquisition of knowledge, development of values, and performance of psychomotor and technological skills. Evaluation serves to determine the extent of the student's learning in relation to these outcomes. Each of the domains of learning has its own classification or taxonomic system, which is of value in gearing testing and evaluation to the level of learning anticipated from the instruction. While different methods have been proposed for developing test items and other evaluation strategies, the important principle is that they relate to the learning outcomes.

REFERENCES

Airasian, P. W. (2000). *Assessment in the classroom: A concise approach* (2nd ed.). Boston: McGraw-Hill.

Bloom, B. S., Englehart, M. D., Furst, E. J., Hill, W. H., & Krathwohl, D. R. (1956). *Taxonomy of educational objectives: The classification of educational goals. Handbook I: Cognitive domain.* White Plains, NY: Longman.

Dave, R. H. (1970). Psychomotor levels. In R. J. Armstrong (Ed.), *Developing and writing behavioral objectives.* Tucson, AZ: Educational Innovators.

Gaberson, K. B., & Oermann, M. H. (1999). *Clinical teaching strategies in nursing education.* New York: Springer.

Gronlund, N. E. (2000). *How to write and use instructional objectives* (6th ed.). Upper Saddle River, NJ: Prentice Hall.

Krathwohl, D., Bloom, B., & Masia, B. (1964). *Taxonomy of educational objectives, Handbook II: Affective domain.* New York: Longman.

Linn, R. L., & Gronlund, N. E. (2000). *Measurement and assessment in teaching* (8th ed.). Upper Saddle River, NJ: Prentice Hall.

Mertler, C. A. (2003). *Classroom assessment.* Los Angeles: Pyrczak.

Oermann, M. H. (2004). Basic skills for teaching and the advanced practice nurse. In L. Joel (Ed.), *Advanced practice nursing: Essentials for role development* (pp. 398–429). Philadelphia: F. A. Davis.

Oosterhof, A. (2001). *Classroom applications of educational measurement* (3rd ed.). Upper Saddle River, NJ: Prentice Hall.

Chapter 2

Qualities of Effective Measurement Instruments

How does a teacher know if a test or another measurement instrument is good? If the results of measurement procedures will be used to make important educational decisions, teachers must have confidence in their interpretations of test scores. Good measurement tools produce results that can be used to make appropriate inferences about learners' knowledge and abilities. In addition, measurement tools should be practical and easy to use.

Two important questions have been posed to guide the process of constructing or proposing tests:

1. To what extent will the interpretation of the scores be appropriate, meaningful, and useful for the intended application of the results, and

2. What are the consequences of the particular uses and interpretations that are made of the results? (Linn & Gronlund, 2000)

This chapter will explain the concept of measurement validity, the role of reliability, and their effects on the interpretive quality of measurement results. It will also discuss important practical considerations that might affect the choice or development of tests and other instruments.

MEASUREMENT VALIDITY

Definitions of validity have changed over time. Early definitions, in the 1940s and early 1950s, emphasized the validity of the test itself. Tests were characterized as valid or not, apart from a consideration of how they were used. It was common in that era to support a claim of validity with evidence that a test correlated well with another "true" criterion. The concept of validity changed, however, in the 1950s through the 1970s to focus on evidence that a test is valid for a specific purpose. Most measurement textbooks of that era classified validity by three types: content, criterion-related, and construct, and suggested that validation of a test should include more than one approach. In the 1980s, the understanding of validity shifted again, to an emphasis on providing evidence to support the particular inferences that teachers make from test scores. Validity was defined in terms of the appropriateness and usefulness of the inferences made from test scores, and test validation was seen as a process of collecting evidence to support those inferences. The usefulness of the validity "triad" was also questioned; increasingly, measurement experts recognized that construct validity was the key meaning and unifying concept of validity (Goodwin, 1997).

The current philosophy of validity, therefore, focuses not on tests themselves or on the appropriateness of using a test for a specific purpose, but on the meaningfulness of the interpretations that teachers make of the test scores. Tests and other measurement instruments yield scores that teachers use to make inferences about how much the test-takers know or what they can do. Validity refers to the extent to which these score-based inferences are sound. The emphasis is on the consequences of measurement: does the teacher make accurate interpretations about a test-taker's knowledge or ability based on his or her test scores?

Measurement experts increasingly suggest that in addition to collecting various types of evidence to support the validity of inferences made, evidence should also be collected about the intended and unintended consequences of the use of a test (Goodwin, 1997; Nitko, 2004). Validity is not an either/or judgment; there are degrees of validity depending on the purpose of the test and how the scores are to be used. A given test may be used for many different purposes, and inferences about the resulting test scores may have greater validity for one purpose than for another. For example, a test designed to measure knowledge of perioperative nursing standards may produce scores that have validity for the purpose of determining certification for perioperative staff nurses, but it may yield scores that are less valid for assigning grades to students in a perioperative nursing elective course. Additionally, the validity evidence may change over time, so that validation of inferences must not be considered a one-time event.

Although there may be different kinds of validity evidence, typically referred to as content, criterion-related, and construct, validity should be considered a unitary concept (Nitko, 2004). Construct validity is proposed as the "umbrella" under which all types of test validity evidence belong. All attempts to obtain validity evidence focus on what we can and cannot infer about the scores we obtain on a given test (Goodwin, 1997).

Inferences about the Content of a Test

Evidence of content validity demonstrates the degree to which the sample of test items or tasks represents the domain of content or abilities that the teacher wants to measure (American Psychological Association [APA], 1999; Goodwin, 1997). Tests and other measurement instruments usually contain only a sample of all possible items that could be used to measure the domain of interest. However, interpretations of test scores are based on what the teacher believes to be the universe of items that could have been generated. In other words, when a student correctly answers 83% of the items on a maternity nursing final examination, the teacher usually infers that the student probably would answer correctly 83% of all items in the universe of maternity nursing content. The test score thus serves as an indicator of the student's true standing in the larger domain (Goodwin).

A superficial conclusion could be made about the match between a test's appearance and its intended use by asking a panel of experts to judge whether the test appears to be based on appropriate content. This type of judgment, sometimes referred to as face validity, is not sufficient evidence of content representativeness. Content validity evidence should be obtained through test-development procedures designed to assure content representativeness, and *post facto* appraisals of the resulting content.

Efforts to include suitable content on the test can be made during test development. This process begins with defining the universe of content. The content definition should be related to the purpose for which the test will be used. For example, if a test is supposed to measure a new staff nurse's understanding of hospital safety policies and procedures presented during orientation, the teacher first defines the universe of content by outlining the knowledge about policies that the staff nurse needs in order to function satisfactorily. The teacher then uses professional judgment to write or select test items that satisfactorily represent this desired content domain. A system for documenting this process, the construction of a test blueprint or table of specifications, will be described in chapter 3.

After the test is constructed, inferences about the representativeness of its content can be made through the process of content validation. A panel of experts reviews the test, item by item, to determine if the items are relevant and satisfactorily represent the defined domain, represented by the table of specifications. Because these judgments admittedly are subjective, the trustworthiness of this evidence depends on clear instructions to the experts and estimation of interrater reliability. Some measurement experts have questioned whether content validation really produces evidence of validity, since it does not take into account the scores produced by the test and therefore excludes the inferences made from the scores. Content-related evidence therefore is not sufficient for validity judgments (Goodwin, 1997).

Inferences about Relationships Between Test Scores and Other Variables

This approach to obtaining validity evidence focuses on relationships between scores on the test of interest and one or more criterion measures or outcome criteria (APA, 1999; Goodwin, 1997). This type of evidence, previously known as criterion-related validity, is important if teachers wish to make inferences from a student's test score about his or her performance on an independent criterion variable. For example, graduate program admissions committees often use scores from an aptitude test such as the Graduate Record Examination or the Miller Analogies Test to predict whether applicants are likely to be successful in graduate school (the criterion measure).

If the inference to be made is in regard to a future performance, the validity evidence is predictive; if the inference is related to another performance at the same time, the evidence is concurrent. The type of evidence needed for a given test depends on how the test scores will be used. The example given above related to testing applicants for a graduate program calls for predictive validity evidence. In nursing education programs, teachers typically want to make predictions of future performance. On the other hand, concurrent validity evidence may be desirable for making a decision about whether one test or measurement instrument may be substituted for another. For example, a staff development educator may want to collect concurrent validity evidence to determine if a checklist with a rating scale can be substituted for a less efficient narrative appraisal of a staff nurse's competence.

Teachers rarely conduct formal studies of the extent to which the scores on achievement tests that they have constructed are correlated with criterion measures. In some cases, adequate criterion measures are not available; the test in use is considered to be the best instrument that has been devised to measure the ability in question. If better measures were available, they might be used instead of the test being validated. However, for tests with high-stakes outcomes, such as licensure, certification, and admissions tests, this type of validity evidence is crucial. Multiple criterion measures often are used so that the strengths of one measure may offset the weaknesses of others (Goodwin, 1997).

The relationship between test scores and those obtained on the criterion measure usually is expressed as a correlation coefficient. A desired level of correlation between the two measures cannot be recommended because the correlation may be influenced by a number of factors, including test length. The teacher who uses the test must use good professional judgment to determine what magnitude of correlation is considered adequate for the intended use of the test being validated.

Inferences about Differences Between Groups

One approach to collecting construct validity evidence is the *known groups* or *contrasted groups* technique. This approach is based on the assumption that mean test scores should be significantly different for members of groups that are known to possess different levels of the ability being measured.

For example, if the purpose of a test is to measure students' ability to think critically about pediatric clinical problems, the validity evidence must show that the test items require students to demonstrate critical thinking ability. Students who achieve high scores on this test would be assumed to be better critical thinkers than students who achieve low scores. To collect evidence in support of this assumption, the teacher might design a study to predict that students should obtain scores on the test based on their observed critical thinking behavior in clinical practice. The teacher could divide the sample of students into two groups based on their clinical evaluation ratings: those who were rated by their clinical instructors as good critical thinkers in clinical practice in one group, and those who were rated as weak critical thinkers in the other group. Then the teacher would compare the test scores of the students in both groups. If the teacher's hypothesis is confirmed (that is, if the students with good clinical ratings obtained high test scores), this evidence could be used to support the validity of using the test scores to make inferences about the students' critical thinking abilities.

Group-comparison techniques also have been used in studies of test bias or test fairness. Approaches to detection of test bias have looked for differential item functioning (DIF) related to test-takers' race, gender, or culture. If test items function differently for members of groups with characteristics that do not directly relate to the variable of interest, differential validity of inferences from the test scores may result. Issues related to test bias will be discussed more fully in chapter 14.

Inferences about the Consequences of Using Tests

The incorporation of concern about the social consequences of testing into the concept of validity is a relatively recent trend. The use of tests has both intended and unintended consequences. Validity evidence should address the anticipated positive consequences of measuring the performance of interest as well as potential negative consequences such as bias or unfairness. For example, many under-graduate nursing programs have adopted programs of achievement testing that are designed to assess student performance throughout the nursing curriculum. The intended positive consequence of such testing is to identify students at risk of failure on the NCLEX®, and to use this information to design remediation programs to increase student learning. Unintended negative consequences, how-ever, may include tailoring instruction to more closely match the content of the tests, increased student anxiety, and decreased time for instruction related to increased time needed for testing. Goodwin (1997) suggested "comparing the content of certification or licensing examinations with curricular emphases over time, to try determine if the content of the examinations has been driving (or worse, narrowing) the curriculum" (p. 106).

RELIABILITY

Reliability refers to the consistency of test scores. If a test produces reliable scores, the same group of students would achieve approximately the same scores if the test were given on another occasion. Similar to the changing conceptions of validity, definitions of reliability have also undergone change in recent years. Traditionally, reliability has been classified into several types: stability, equivalent forms, internal consistency, and interrater reliability. However, before discussing each type of reliability, it is important to examine the relationship between reliability and validity.

Most measurement experts have stressed that reliability is a necessary but not sufficient condition for validity. If reliability were viewed this way, teachers would be unable to make valid inferences from test results that are inconsistent. Likewise, a set of test scores could not be expected to correlate with a criterion measure if it does not correlate with itself. However, some measurement experts now view reliability as an integral part of construct validity rather than as a separate precondition. Approaches to collecting construct validity evidence increasingly include estimation of reliability (instead of considering reliability to be a precursor of validity). Although reliability has been defined in terms of generalizability from one testing occasion to others, generalizability is also related to content and predictive validity (Goodwin, 1997).

An example may help to illustrate the relationship between validity and reliability. Suppose that the author of this chapter was given a test of her knowledge of measurement principles. The author of a textbook on measurement and evaluation in nursing education might be expected to achieve a high score on such a test. However, if the test were written in the Mandarin language, the author's score might be very low, even if she were a remarkably good guesser, because she cannot read Mandarin. If the same test were administered the following week, and every week for a month, her scores would likely be consistently low. Therefore, these test scores would be considered reliable, because there would be a high correlation among scores obtained on the same test over a period of several administrations. But a valid score-based interpretation of the author's knowledge of measurement principles could not be drawn because the test was not appropriate for its intended use.

Test scores may be inconsistent because the behavior being measured is unstable, or because the sample of test items varies, or because the scoring procedures are inconsistent. Therefore, when teachers interpret test scores, they need to have some understanding of the factors that may cause their inconsistency. For purposes of understanding sources of inconsistency, it is helpful to view a test score as having two components, a true score and an error score, represented by the following equation:

$$X = T + E \qquad \text{[Equation 2.1]}$$

A student's actual test score (X) is also known as the observed score. That student's hypothetical true score (T) cannot be measured directly because it is the average of all scores the student would obtain if tested on many occasions with the same test. The observed score contains a certain amount of measurement error (E), which may be a positive or a negative value. This error of measurement, representing the difference between the observed score and the true score, results in a student's obtained score being higher or lower than his or her true score (Gaberson, 1996; Nitko, 2004). If it were possible to measure directly the amount of measurement error that occurred on each testing occasion, two of the values in this equation would be known (X and E), and we would be able to calculate the true score (T). However, we can only estimate indirectly the amount of measurement error, leaving us with a hypothetical true score. Therefore, teachers need to recognize that the obtained score on any test is only an estimate of what the student really knows about the domain being tested.

For example, Matt may obtain a higher score than Kelly on a community health nursing unit test because Matt truly knows more about the content than Kelly does. Test scores should reflect this kind of difference, and if the difference in knowledge is the only explanation for the score difference, no error is involved. However, there may be other potential explanations for the difference between Kelly's and Matt's test scores. Matt may have behaved dishonestly to obtain a copy of the test in advance; knowing which items would be included, he had the opportunity to use unauthorized resources to determine the correct answers to those items. In his case, measurement error would have increased Matt's obtained score. Kelly may have worked overtime the night before the test and may not have gotten enough sleep to allow her to feel alert during the test. Thus, her performance may have been affected by her fatigue and her decreased ability to concentrate, resulting in an obtained score lower than her true score. One goal of test designers therefore is to maximize the amount of score variance that explains real differences in ability and to minimize the amount of random error variance of scores.

Figure 2.1 uses a target-shooting analogy to illustrate these relationships. When they design and administer tests and other measurement instruments, teachers attempt to consistently (reliably) measure the true value of what students know and can do (hit the bull's eye); if they succeed, they can make valid inferences from test results. Diagram 1 in Figure 2.1 displays test scores that are widely scattered at a distance from the true score; these scores are not reliable, contributing to a lack of validity evidence. In Diagram 2, the test scores are reliable because they are closely grouped together, but they are still distant from the true score. The teacher would not be able to make valid score-based interpretations of such scores. Diagram 3 illustrates the reliability of scores that

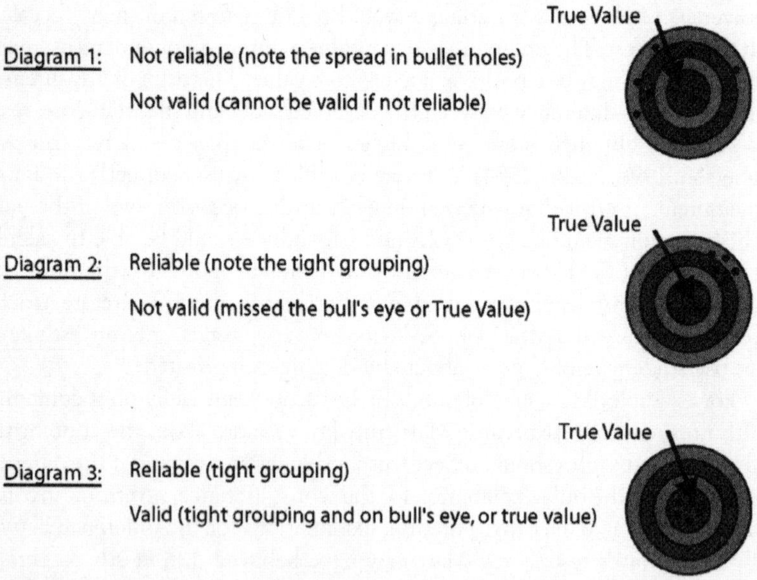

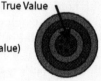

True Value

Diagram 1:   Not reliable (note the spread in bullet holes)

Not valid (cannot be valid if not reliable)

True Value

Diagram 2:   Reliable (note the tight grouping)

Not valid (missed the bull's eye or True Value)

True Value

Diagram 3:   Reliable (tight grouping)

Valid (tight grouping and on bull's eye, or true value)

FIGURE 2.1   True value, reliability, and validity.

From Gillis, A., & Jackson, W. (2002). *Research for nurses: Methods and interpretation.* Philadelphia: F. A. Davis, p. 443. Reprinted with permission from F. A. Davis Company, Philadelphia.

are closely grouped on the bull's eye, the true score, allowing the teacher to make valid inferences about them (Gillis & Jackson, 2002).

Stability Reliability

Most teachers think of reliability as consistency over time. That is, evidence of stability indicates whether students would achieve essentially the same scores if they took the same test at another time—a test-retest procedure. The correlation between the set of scores obtained on the first administration and the set obtained on the second yields a test-retest reliability coefficient. This type of reliability evidence is known as stability, and is appropriate for situations in which the trait being measured is expected to be stable over time. In general, the longer the period of time between administrations of the test, the lower the stability reliability estimate (Nitko, 2004). In nursing education settings, the test-retest method of obtaining reliability information may have limited usefulness. If the same test items are used on both tests, the students' answers on the retest are not independent of their answers on the first test. That is, their responses to the second test may be influenced to some extent by recall of their previous responses or by discussion or individual review of content after taking the first test. In addition, if there is a long interval between testing occasions, other factors such as real changes in student ability as a result of learning may affect the retest scores.

Alternate-Forms or Equivalent-Forms Reliability

Another type of reliability evidence, alternate- or equivalent-forms reliability, involves the use of two or more forms of the same test. Both forms of the test are administered to the same group of students, and the resulting scores are correlated. A high reliability coefficient indicates that the two forms sample the domain of content equally well. The major weakness of this form of reliability estimate is that most teachers do not find time to prepare two forms of the same test, let alone to assure that these forms indeed are equivalent (Nitko, 2004). Equivalent forms must be developed according to the same test blueprint so that the content domain sampling is essentially the same. Standardized tests typically do provide alternate forms so that test security is not compromised. When alternate forms are used, teachers assume that an individual who would take both forms of the test would likely obtain consistent scores.

Internal Consistency Reliability

Because most teachers cannot use alternate forms of the same test, another type of reliability evidence, internal consistency, may be more useful. The previously discussed types of estimating reliability involve two separate tests. Internal consistency methods can be used with a set of scores from only one administration of a single test. Sometimes referred to as split-half methods, estimates of internal consistency reveal the extent to which the test items are internally consistent or homogeneous.

The split-half technique consists of dividing the test into two equal subtests, usually by including odd-numbered items on one subtest and even-numbered items on the other. Then the subtests are scored separately, and the two subscores are correlated. The resulting correlation coefficient is an estimate of the extent to which the two halves consistently perform the same measurement. Longer tests tend to produce more reliable results than short tests, in part because they tend to sample the content domain more fully. Therefore, a split-half reliability estimate tends to underestimate the true reliability of the scores produced by the whole test (because each subtest includes only half of the total number of items). This underestimate can be corrected by using the Spearman-Brown prophecy formula, also called the Spearman-Brown double length formula, as represented by the following equation (Nitko, 2004, pp. 65–66):

$$\frac{2 \times \text{correlation between half-test scores}}{1 + \text{correlation between half-test scores}} \quad \text{[Equation 2.2]}$$

Another method of estimating the internal consistency of a test is to use one of the Kuder-Richardson formulae, which represent the average correlation obtained from all possible split-half reliability estimates. The computation of Formula 20 (K-R20) involves information about the difficulty (proportion of correct responses) of each test item, and therefore usually requires a computer. If the test items are not expected to vary much in difficulty, the simpler Formula 21 (K-R21) can be used to approximate the value of K-R20, although it will in most cases produce a slightly lower estimate of reliability. To use either formula, the test items must be scored dichotomously, that is, right or wrong (Nitko, 2004). If this condition cannot be met, coefficient alpha can be used to provide a reliability estimate for a test in which the items could receive a range of points.

Scorer Reliability

Depending on the type of test or other measurement instrument used, error may arise from the procedures or persons used to score a test. Teachers may need to collect evidence to answer the question, "Would this student have obtained the same score if a different person had scored the test or judged the performance?" The easiest method for collecting this evidence is to have two persons score each student's paper or rate each student's performance. The two scores then are compared to produce a percentage of agreement or correlated to produce an index of scorer consistency, depending on whether agreement in an absolute sense or a relative sense is required.

Factors that Influence the Reliability of Scores

From the previous discussion, it is obvious that various factors can influence the reliability of a set of test scores. These factors can be categorized into three main sources: the test, the student, and the test administration conditions.

Test-related factors include the length of the test, the homogeneity of test content, and the difficulty and discrimination ability of the individual items. In general, the greater the number of test items, the greater the score reliability. The Spearman-Brown reliability estimate formula can be used to estimate the effect on the reliability coefficient of adding test items. For example, if a 10-item test has a reliability coefficient of 0.40, adding 15 items (creating a test that is 2.5 times the length of the original test) would produce a reliability estimate of 0.625. Of course, adding test items to increase score reliability may be counterproductive after a certain point. After that point, adding items will increase the reliability only slightly, and student fatigue and boredom actually may introduce more measurement error. Score reliability also is enhanced by homogeneity of content covered by the test. Course content that is tightly organized and highly interrelated tends to make homogeneous test content easier to achieve. Finally, the technical quality of test items, their difficulty, and their ability to discriminate between students who know the content and students who don't also affects the reliability of scores. Moderately difficult items that discriminate well between high achievers and low achievers and that contain no technical errors contribute a great deal to score reliability.

Student-related factors include the heterogeneity of the student group, testwiseness, and motivation. In general, reliability tends to increase as the range of talent in the group of students increases. Therefore, in situations where students are very similar to one another in ability, such as in graduate school, tests are likely to produce scores with somewhat lower reliability than desired. A student's test-taking skill and experience may also influence score reliability to the extent that the student is able to obtain a higher score than true ability would predict. The effect of motivation on reliability relates to the extent to which it influences individual students differently. If some students are not motivated to put forth their best efforts on an exam, their actual achievement levels may not be accurately represented, and their relative achievement in comparison to other students will be difficult to judge.

Teachers need to control test administration conditions in order to enhance the reliability of test scores. Inadequate time to complete the test can lower the reliability of scores because some students who know the content well will be unable to respond to all of the items. Cheating also contributes random errors to test scores when students are able to respond correctly to items to which they actually do not know the answer. Cheating, therefore, has the effect of raising the offenders' observed scores above their true scores, contributing to inaccurate and less meaningful interpretations of test scores.

Because a reliability coefficient is an indication of the amount of measurement error associated with a set of scores, it is useful information for evaluating the meaning and usefulness of those scores. There is no absolute numerical value of a reliability coefficient that can be recommended as a cut-off for accepting this evidence; the usefulness of reliability information is a decision based on the purpose for which the test scores will be used. It also is important to remember that the numerical value of a reliability coefficient is not a stable property of a test; it will fluctuate from one sample of students to another each time the test is administered.

PRACTICALITY

While reliability and validity are used to describe the ways in which scores are interpreted and used, practicality is a quality of the instrument itself and its administration procedures. Measurement procedures should be efficient and economical. A test is practical or usable to the extent that it is easy to administer and score, does not take too much time away from other instructional activities, and has reasonable resource requirements. Whether they develop their own tests and other measurement tools or use published instruments, teachers should focus on the following questions to help guide the selection of appropriate assessment procedures (Nitko, 2004):

1. *Is the test easy to construct and use?* Essay test items may be written more quickly and easily than multiple-choice items, but they will take more time to score. Multiple-choice items that assess a student's ability to think critically about clinical problems are time-consuming to construct, but they may be machine-scored quickly and accurately. The teacher must decide what is the best use of the time available for test construction, administration, and scoring. If a published test is selected for confirmatory evaluation of students' competencies just prior to graduation, is it practical to use? Does proper administration of the test require special training? Are the test administration directions easy to understand?

2.   *Is the time needed to administer and score the test and interpret the results reasonable?* A teacher of a 15-week course wants to give a weekly 10-point quiz that would be reviewed immediately and self-scored by students; these procedures would take 30 minutes of class time. Is this the best use of instructional time? The teacher may decide that there is enormous value in the immediate feedback provided to students during the test review, and that the opportunity to obtain weekly information about the effectiveness of instruction is also beneficial; to that teacher, 30 minutes weekly is time well spent on evaluation. Another teacher, whose total instructional time is only four days, may find that administering more than one test consumes time that is needed for teaching. Evaluation is an important step in the instructional process, but it cannot replace teaching. While students often learn from the process of preparing for and taking tests, instruction is not the primary purpose of testing, and testing is not the most efficient or effective way to achieve instructional goals.

3.   *Are the costs associated with test construction, administration, and scoring reasonable?* While teacher-made tests may seem to be less expensive than published instruments, the cost of the instructor's time spent in test development must be taken into consideration. Additional costs associated with the scoring of teacher-made tests must also be calculated. What is the initial cost of purchasing test booklets for published instruments, and can test booklets be reused? What is the cost of answer sheets, and does that cost include scoring services? Sometimes test publishers offer volume discounts that may benefit larger educational programs; reduced prices for purchasing test materials and scoring services may also be available.

4.   *Can the test results be interpreted easily and accurately by those who will use them?* If teachers score their own tests, will they obtain results that will help them to interpret the test scores accurately? In other words, will they have test statistics that will help them make meaning out of the individual test scores? Scanners and software are available that will quickly score exams that use certain types of answer sheets, but the scope of the information produced in the score report varies considerably. Purchased tests that are scored by the publisher also yield reports of test results. Are these reports useful for their intended purpose? What information is needed or desired by the teachers who will make evaluation decisions, and is that information provided by the score-reporting service?

Examples of information on score reports include individual raw total scores, individual raw subtest scores, group mean and median scores, individual or group profiles, and individual standard scores. Will the teachers who receive the reports need special training in order to interpret this information accurately? Some test publishers restrict the purchase of instruments to users with certain educational and experience qualifications, in part so that the test results will be interpreted and used properly.

SUMMARY

Because test results are often used to make important educational decisions, teachers must have confidence in their interpretations of test scores. Good measurement tools produce results that teachers can use to make valid interpretations about what learners know and can do.

Test scores are valid if they permit the teacher to make accurate interpretations about a test-taker's knowledge or ability. Validity is not a static property of the test itself, but rather, it refers to the ways in which teachers interpret and use the test results. Validity is not an either/or judgment; there are degrees of validity depending on the purpose of the test and how the scores are to be used. A single test may be used for many different purposes, and the resulting test scores may have greater validity for one purpose than for another.

In order to make good judgments about the valid use of a set of scores, teachers must gather one or more types of validity evidence: content, criterion-related, and construct. Content validity evidence demonstrates the extent to which the sample of test items or tasks represents the domain of content or abilities that the teacher wants to measure. Content validity evidence may be obtained during the test development process as well as by appraising the resulting content. Criterion-related evidence illustrates that scores on the test of interest are related to one or more criterion measures or outcome criteria. Two forms of criterion-related evidence, concurrent and predictive, may be obtained. Concurrent evidence determines the student's present standing on a criterion measure, and predictive evidence gauges the student's probable future performance on an outcome criterion. Currently, construct validity is seen as the unifying concept of validity, representing the extent to which score-based inferences about the construct of interest are accurate and meaningful.

Reliability refers to the extent to which test scores are consistent. Stability reliability is appropriate for situations in which the trait being measured is expected to be stable over time. Evidence of stability indicates whether students would achieve essentially the same scores if they took the same test at another time. The correlation between the set of scores obtained on the first administration and the set obtained on the second yields a test-retest reliability coefficient. Another type of reliability evidence, alternate- or equivalent-forms reliability, involves the use of two or more forms of the same test. Both forms are administered to the same group of students, and the resulting scores are correlated. A high reliability coefficient indicates that the two forms sample the domain of content equally well. Because most teachers do not have alternate forms of the same test, another type of reliability evidence, internal consistency, may be more useful. Internal consistency methods can be used with a set of scores from only one administration of a single test. Sometimes referred to as split-half methods, estimates of internal consistency reveal the extent to which the test items are internally consistent or homogeneous.

Various factors can influence the reliability of a set of test scores. These factors can be categorized into three main sources: the test, the student, and the test administration conditions. Test-related factors include the length of the test, the homogeneity of test content, and the difficulty and discrimination ability of the individual items. Student-related factors include the heterogeneity of the student group, testwiseness, and motivation. Factors related to test administration include inadequate time to complete the test and cheating.

In addition, measurement tools should be practical and easy to use. While reliability and validity are used to describe the ways in which scores are interpreted and used, practicality is a quality of the instrument itself and its administration procedures. Measurement procedures should be efficient and economical. Teachers need to evaluate the following factors: ease of construction and use; time needed to administer and score the test and interpret the results; costs associated with test construction, administration, and scoring; and the ease with which test results can be interpreted easily and accurately by those who will use them.

REFERENCES

American Psychological Association. (1999). *Standards for educational and psychological testing.* Washington, DC: Author.

Gaberson, K. B. (1996). Test design: Putting all the pieces together. *Nurse Educator, 21*(4), 28–33.

Gillis, A., & Jackson, W. (2002). *Research for nurses: Methods and interpretation.* Philadelphia: F. A. Davis.

Goodwin, L. D. (1997). Changing conceptions of measurement validity. *Journal of Nursing Education, 36,* 102–107.

Linn, R. L., & Gronlund, N. E. (2000). *Measurement and assessment in teaching* (8th ed.). Upper Saddle River, NJ: Prentice Hall.

Nitko, A. J. (2004). *Educational assessment of students* (4th ed.). Upper Saddle River, NJ: Prentice Hall.

Chapter 3

Planning for Classroom Testing

P_{aul} Johnson was caught by surprise when he looked at his office calendar and realized that a test for the course he was teaching was only a week away, even though he was the person who had scheduled it! Thankful that he was not teaching this course for the first time, he searched his files for the test he had used last year. When he found it, his brief review showed that some of the content was outdated and that the test did not include items on the new content he had added this year. Because of a department policy that requires teachers to allow clerical staff one week to type a test, Paul realized that he would have to finish the necessary revisions of the test that night and submit it to be typed the next morning. Three days later when the department secretary was finished typing the test, Paul was out of town at a conference. When he returned to the office, there was no time for proofreading it because he had to administer the test the next day. He begged for an exemption from the two-day notice for photocopying, but when no one was available to do the job, Paul came in early on the morning of the test day and copied and stapled the test booklets himself.

With 5 minutes to spare, Paul rushed into the classroom and distributed the still-warm test booklets. He was still congratulating himself for meeting his deadline when the first student raised a hand with a question: "On item 1, is there a typo?" Then another student said, "I don't think that the correct answer for item 2 is there." A third student complained, "I'm missing page 2," and a fourth student stated, "There are 2 ds for item 5." Paul knew that it was going to be a long morning. But the worst was yet to come. As they were turning in their tests, students complained, "This test didn't cover the material that I thought it would cover," and "We spent a lot of class time analyzing case studies, but we were tested on memorization of facts." Needless to say, Paul did not look forward to the posttest discussion the following week.

Too often, teachers give little thought to the preparation of their tests until the last minute and then rush to get the job done. A test that is produced in this manner often contains items that are poorly chosen, ambiguous, and either too easy or too difficult, as well as grammatical, spelling, and other clerical errors. The solution lies in adequate planning for test construction before the item-writing phase begins, followed by careful critique of the completed test by other teachers. Table 3.1 lists the steps of the test construction process. This chapter discusses the steps involved in planning for test construction; subsequent chapters will focus on the techniques of writing test items of various formats, assembling and administering the test, and analyzing the test results.

PURPOSE AND POPULATION

All decisions involved in planning a test are based on a teacher's knowledge of the purpose of the test and the relevant characteristics of the population of learners to be tested. The *purpose* for the test involves why it is to be given, what it is supposed to measure, and how the test scores will be used. For example, if a test is to be used to measure the extent to which students have met learning

TABLE 3.1   Checklist for Test Construction

✓   Define the purpose of the test.
✓   Describe the population to be tested.
✓   Determine the optimum length of the test.
✓   Specify the difficulty and discrimination level of the test.
✓   Determine the scoring procedure or procedures to be used.
✓   Select item formats to be used.
✓   Construct a test blueprint or table of specifications.
✓   Write the test items.
✓   Have the test items critiqued.
✓   Determine the arrangement of items on the test.
✓   Write specific directions for each item format.
✓   Write general directions for the test and prepare a cover sheet.
✓   Print or type the test.
✓   Proofread the test.
✓   Reproduce the test.
✓   Prepare a scoring key.
✓   Prepare students for taking the test.

objectives in order to determine course grades, its primary purpose is summative. If the teacher expects the course grades to reflect real differences in the amount of knowledge among the students, the test must be sufficiently difficult to produce an acceptable range of scores. On the other hand, if a test is to be used primarily to provide feedback to staff nurses about their knowledge following a continuing education program, the purpose of the test is formative. If the results will not be used to make important personnel decisions, a large range of scores is not necessary, and the test items can be of moderate or low difficulty.

A teacher's knowledge of the population that will be tested will be useful in selecting the items formats to be used, determining the length of the test and the testing time required, and selecting the appropriate scoring procedures. The term *population* is not used here in its research sense, but rather to indicate the general group of learners that will be tested. The students' reading levels, English language literacy, visual acuity, health, and previous testing experience are examples of factors that might influence these decisions. For example, if the population to be tested is a group of five patients who have completed preoperative instruction for coronary bypass graft surgery, the teacher would probably not administer a test of 100 multiple-choice and matching items with a machine-scored answer sheet. However, this type of test might be most appropriate as a final course examination for a class of 75 senior nursing students.

TEST LENGTH

The length of the test is an important factor that is related to its purpose, the abilities of the students, the item formats to be used, the amount of testing time available, and the desired reliability of the test scores. As discussed in Chapter 2, the reliability of test scores generally improves as the length of the test increases, so the teacher should attempt to include as many items as possible in order to adequately sample the content. However, if the purpose of the test is to measure knowledge of a small content domain with a limited number of objectives, fewer items will be needed to achieve an adequate sampling of the content.

The test length probably is limited by the scheduled length of a testing period, so it is wise to construct the test so that the majority of the students working at their normal pace will be able to attempt to answer all items. This type of test is called a *power* test. A *speeded* test is one that does not provide sufficient time for all students to respond to all items. Although most standardized tests are speeded, this type of test generally is not appropriate for teacher-made tests in which accuracy rather than speed of response is important (Nitko, 2004).

The item formats used and the taxonomy level that the teachers are testing also will determine how many items should be included. Test items that require students to supply an answer, such as essay and completion items, generally require more testing time than items that require students to select an answer, such as multiple-choice and matching. Multiple-choice items with 5 options will require more reading and thinking time than items with 3 options.

DIFFICULTY AND DISCRIMINATION LEVEL

The desired difficulty of a test and its ability to differentiate among various levels of performance are related considerations. Both factors are affected by the purpose of the test and the way in which the scores will be interpreted and used. The difficulty of individual test items affects the average test score; the mean score of a group of students is equal to the sum of the difficulty levels of the test items. The difficulty level of each test item depends on the complexity of the task, the ability of the students who answer it, and the quality of the teaching. It also may be related to the perceived complexity of the item; if students perceive the task is too difficult, they may skip it, resulting in a lower percentage of students who answer the item correctly (Nitko, 2004).

If test results are to be used to determine the relative achievement of students (to rank them on the basis of their knowledge), the majority of items on the test should be moderately difficult. The recommended difficulty level for selection-type test items depends on the number of choices allowed. The percentage of students who answer each item correctly should be about midway between 100% and the chance of guessing correctly (e.g., 50% for true-false items, 25% correct for four-alternative multiple-choice items). For example, a moderately difficult true-false item should be answered correctly by 75–85% of students (Nitko, 2004). When the majority of items on a test are too easy or too difficulty, they will not discriminate well between students who vary in their levels of learning (Haladyna, 1997).

It is important to keep in mind that the difficulty level of test items can only be estimated in advance, depending on the teacher's experience in testing this content and knowledge of the abilities of the students to be tested. Procedures for determining how the test items actually perform are discussed in chapter 15.

ITEM FORMATS

Some students may be particularly adept at answering essay items; others may prefer multiple-choice items. However, tests should be designed to provide information about students' knowledge or abilities, not about their skill in taking certain types of tests. A test with a variety of item formats provides students with multiple ways to demonstrate their competence (Nitko, 2004). All item formats have their advantages and limitations, which are discussed in later chapters.

Selection Criteria for Item Formats

Teachers should select item formats for their tests based on a variety of factors, such as the learning outcomes to be evaluated, the specific skill to be measured, and the ability level of the students. Some objectives are better measured with certain item formats. For example, if the instructional objective specifies that the student will be able to "discuss the comparative advantages and disadvantages of breast and bottle feeding," a multiple-choice item would be inappropriate because it would not allow the teacher to evaluate the student's ability to organize and express ideas on this topic. An essay item would be a better choice for this purpose. Essay items provide opportunities for students to formulate their own responses, drawing on prior learning, and to express their ideas in writing; these often are desired outcomes of nursing education programs.

The teacher's time constraints for devising the test may affect the choice of item format. In general, essay items take less time to write than multiple-choice items, but they are more difficult and time-consuming to score. A teacher who has little time to prepare a test and therefore chooses an essay format, assuming that this choice is also appropriate for the objectives to be tested, must plan for considerable time after the test is given to score it.

In nursing programs, faculty often develop multiple-choice items as the predominant, if not exclusive, item format because for a number of years, licensure and certification examinations contained only multiple-choice items. While this provides essential practice for students in preparation for taking such high-stakes examinations, it negates the principle of selecting the most appropriate type of test item for the outcome and content to be evaluated. In addition, it limits variety in testing and creativity in evaluating student learning. Although practice with multiple-choice questions is critical, other types of test items and evaluation strategies also are appropriate for measuring student learning in nursing. In fact, while the majority of NCLEX® examination items currently are four-option multiple-choice, the item pools now contain other formats such as completion and multiple-response. It is clear from this example that nurse educators should not limit their selection of item formats based on the myth that learners must be tested exclusively with the item format most frequently used on a licensure or certification test.

On the other hand, each change of item format on a test requires a change of task for students. Therefore, the number of different item formats to include on a test also depends on the length of the test and the level of the learner. It is generally recommended that teachers use no more than three item formats on a test. Shorter assessments, such as a 10-item quiz, may be limited to a single item format.

Objectively and Subjectively Scored Items

Another powerful and persistent myth is that some item formats evaluate students more objectively than other formats. While it is common to describe true-false, matching, and multiple-choice items as "objective," objectivity refers to the way items are scored, not to the type of item or their content (Nitko, 2004). Objectivity means that once the scoring key is prepared, it is possible for multiple teachers on the same occasion or the same teacher on multiple occasions to arrive at the same score. Subjectively scored items, like essay items (and completion items, to a lesser extent) require the judgment of the scorer to determine the degree of correctness and therefore are subject to more variability in scoring.

Selected-Response and Constructed-Response Items

Another way of classifying test items is to identify them by the type of response required of the test-taker (Haladyna, 1997; Linn & Gronlund, 2000). *Selected-response* (or "choice") items require the test-taker to select the correct or best answer from among options provided by the teacher. In this category are item formats such as true-false, matching exercises, and multiple-choice. *Constructed-response* (or "supply") formats require the learner to supply an answer, and may be classified further as limited response (or short response) and extended response. These are the completion, short essay, and extended essay formats. Table 3.2

TABLE 3.2   Classification of Test Items by Type of Response

Selected-response Item Formats ("Choice" items)	Constructed-response Item Formats ("Supply" items)
True-false	Completion
Matching exercises	Fill-in-the-blank
Multiple-choice	Restricted response essay
Multiple-response	Extended essay

depicts this schema for classifying test item formats and the variations of each type.

SCORING PROCEDURES

Decisions about what scoring procedure or procedures to use are somewhat dependent on the choice of item formats. Student responses to short-answer, numerical calculation, and essay items, for instance, must be hand-scored, whether they are recorded directly on the test itself or on a separate answer sheet or in a booklet. Answers to objective test items such as multiple-choice, true-false, and matching also may be recorded on the test itself or on a separate answer sheet. Scannable answer sheets greatly increase the speed with which objective tests may be scored and have the additional advantage of allowing computer-generated item analysis reports to be produced. The teacher should decide if the time and resources available for scoring a test suggest that hand scoring or machine scoring would be preferable. In any case, this decision alone should not influence the choice of test item format.

TEST BLUEPRINT

Most people would not think of building a house without blueprints. In fact, the word "house" denotes diverse attributes to different individuals. For this reason, a potential homeowner would not purchase a lot, call a builder, and say only "Build a house for me on my lot." The builder might think that a proper house consists of a 2-story brick colonial with 4 bedrooms, 3 baths, and a formal dining room, while the homeowner had a 3-bedroom ranch with 2 baths, an eat-in kitchen, and a fireplace in mind. Similarly, the word "test" might mean different things to different teachers; students and their teacher might have widely varied expectations about what the test will contain. The best way to avoid misunderstanding regarding the nature of a test and to ensure that the teacher will be able to make valid judgments about the test scores is to develop a test blueprint, also known as a test plan or a table of specifications, before "building" the test itself.

The elements of a test blueprint include (a) a list of the major topics or instructional objectives that the test will cover, (b) the level of complexity of the task to be assessed, and (c) the emphasis each topic will have, indicated by number or percentage of items or points. Table 3.3 is an example of a test blueprint for a unit test on nursing care during normal pregnancy that illustrates each of these elements.

TABLE 3.3 Example of a Test Blueprint for a Unit Test on Normal Pregnancy (75 points)

	CONTENT	LEVEL OF COGNITIVE SKILL[a]				
		K	C	Ap	An	Total #[b]
I.	Conception and fetal development		2	3	3	8
II.	Maternal physiological changes in pregnancy	2	3	1	2	8
III.	Maternal psychological changes in pregnancy		2	2	3	7
IV.	Social, cultural, and economic factors affecting pregnancy outcome		3	2	3	8
V.	Signs and symptoms of pregnancy	2	2	2		6
VI.	Antepartal nursing care		8	10	12	30
VII.	Preparation for childbirth		4	1	3	8
	TOTAL #[b]	4	24	21	26	75

[a]According to Bloom et al. (1956) taxonomy of cognitive objectives. Selected levels are included in this test blueprint and are represented by the following key:
K = Knowledge
C = Comprehension
Ap = Application
An = Analysis
[b]Number of points. Test blueprints also may include the number or the percentage of items.

The row headings along the left margin of the example are the content areas that will be tested. In this case, the content is indicated by a general outline of topics. Teachers may find that a more detailed outline of content or a list of the relevant objectives is more useful for a given purpose and population. Some teachers combine a content outline and a list of objectives; in this case, an additional column of objectives would be inserted before or after the content list.

The column headings across the top of the example are taken from a taxonomy of cognitive objectives (Bloom, Englehart, Furst, Hill, & Krathwohl, 1956). Because the test blueprint is a tool to be used by the teacher, it can be modified in any way that makes sense to the user. Accordingly, the teacher who prepared this blueprint chose to use only selected levels of the taxonomy. Other teachers might include all levels or different levels of Bloom's taxonomy, or use a different taxonomy.

The body of the test blueprint is a grid formed by the intersections of content topics and cognitive levels. Each of the cells of the grid has the potential for representing one or more test items that might be developed. The numbers in the cells of the sample test blueprint represent the number of points on the test that will relate to it; some teachers prefer to indicate numbers of items or the percentage of points or items represented by each cell. It is not necessary to write test items for each cell; the teacher's judgment concerning the appropriate emphasis and balance of content governs the decision about which cells should be filled and how many items should be written for each. Rigorous classification of items into these cells also is unnecessary and, in fact, impossible (Nitko, 2004). The way in which the content is taught may affect whether the related test items will be written at the application or comprehension level. Minor adjustments in classification of items may be made after the content is taught, as long as the overall emphasis and balance of the test is preserved.

Once developed, the test blueprint serves several important functions. First, it is a useful tool for guiding the work of the item writer so that sufficient items are developed at the appropriate level to test important content areas and objectives. Using such a tool helps teachers to be accountable for the educational outcomes they produce. The test blueprint also can be used as evidence for judging the validity of the resulting test scores. The completed test and blueprint may be reviewed by content experts who can judge whether the test items adequately represent the specified content domain, as described in the procedures for collecting content-related evidence in chapter 2.

Another important use of the test blueprint is to inform students about the nature of the test and how they should prepare for it. Although the content covered in class and assigned readings should give students a general idea of the content areas to be tested, students often lack a clear sense of the cognitive levels at which they will be tested on this material. While it might be argued that the instructional objectives might give students a clue as to the level at which they will be tested, teachers often forget that students are not as sophisticated in interpreting objectives as teachers are. Also, some teachers are good at writing objectives that specify a reasonable expectation of performance, but their test items may in fact test higher or lower performance levels. Students need to know the level at which they will be tested because that knowledge will affect how they prepare for the test, not necessarily how much they prepare. They should prepare differently for items that test their ability to apply information than for items that test their ability to synthesize information.

Some teachers worry that if the test blueprint is shared with students, they will not study the content areas that would contribute less to their overall test scores, preferring to concentrate their time and energy on the more important areas of emphasis. If this indeed is the outcome, is it necessarily harmful? Lacking any guidance from the teacher, students may unwisely spend equal amounts of time reviewing all content areas. In fact, professional experience reveals that some knowledge is more important for use in practice than other knowledge. Even if they are good critical thinkers, students may be unable to discriminate more important content from that which is less important because they lack the practice experience to make this distinction. Withholding information about the content emphasis of the test from students might be perceived as an attempt to threaten or punish them for perceived shortcomings such as failure to attend class, failure to read what was assigned, or failure to discern the teacher's priorities. Such a use of testing would be considered unethical.

The best time to share the test blueprint with students is at the beginning of the course or unit of study. If students are unfamiliar with the use of a test blueprint, the teacher may need to explain the concept as well as to discuss how it might be useful to the students in planning their preparation for the test. Of course, if the teacher subsequently makes modifications in the blueprint after writing the test items, those changes also should be shared with the students (Nitko, 2004).

WRITING THE TEST ITEMS

After developing the test blueprint, the teacher begins to write the test items that correspond to each cell. Regardless of the selected item formats, the teacher should consider some general factors that contribute to the quality of the test items.

General Rules for Writing Test Items

1. *Every item should measure something important.* If a test blueprint is designed and used as described in the previous section, each test item will measure an important objective or content area. Without using a blueprint, teachers often write test items that test trivial or obscure knowledge. Sometimes the teacher's intent is to determine if the students have read assigned materials; however, if the content is not important information, it wastes the teacher's time to write the item and wastes the students' time to read it and respond to it. Similarly, it is not necessary to write "filler" items to meet a targeted number; a test with 98 well-written items that measure important objectives will work as well as or better than one with 98 good items and 2 meaningless ones. In fact, students who know the content well might regard a test item that measures trivial knowledge with annoyance or even suspicion, believing that it is meant to trick them into answering incorrectly.

2. *Every item should have a correct answer.* This may seem obvious, but this rule is violated frequently because of the teacher's failure to make a distinction

between fact and belief. In some cases, the correct or best answer to a test item might be a matter of opinion, and unless a particular authority is cited in the item, students might justifiably argue a different response than the one the teacher expected. For example, one answer to the question "When does life begin?" might be "When the kids leave home and the dog dies." If the intent of the question was to measure understanding of when a fetus becomes viable, this is not the correct answer, although if that was the teacher's intent, the question was poorly worded. There are a variety of opinions and beliefs about the concept of viability; a better way to word this question is, "According to the American College of Obstetricians and Gynecologists standards, at what gestational age does a fetus become viable?" If a test item asks the student to state an opinion about an issue and to support that position with evidence, that is a different matter. The item will not be scored as correct or incorrect, but with variable credit based on the completeness of the response, rationale given for the position taken, or the soundness of the student's reasoning.

3. *Use clear, concise, precise, grammatically correct language.* Students who read the test item need to know exactly what task is required of them. Wording a test item clearly is often difficult due to the inherent abstractness and imprecision of language. The teacher should include enough detail in the test item to communicate the intent of the item but without extraneous words that only serve to increase the reading time. Grammatical errors may provide unintentional clues to the correct response for the test-wise but unprepared student and, at best, annoy the well-prepared student.

4. *Avoid using jargon, slang, or unnecessary abbreviations.* Health care professionals frequently use jargon and abbreviations in their practice environment; in some ways, it allows them to communicate more quickly, if not more effectively, with others who understand the same language. Informal language in a test item, however, may fail to communicate the intent of the item accurately. Because most students are somewhat anxious when taking tests, they may fail to interpret an abbreviation correctly for the context in which it is used. For example, does MI mean myocardial infarction, mitral insufficiency, or Michigan? Of course, if the intent of the test item is to measure students' ability to define commonly used abbreviations, it would be appropriate to use the abbreviation in the item and ask for the definition, or give the definition and ask the student to supply the abbreviation. Slang almost always conveys the impression that the item-writer does not take the job seriously.

5. *Try to use positive wording.* It is difficult to explain this rule without using negative wording, but in general, avoid including words like *no, not,* and *except* in the test item. The use of negative wording is especially confusing in true-false items. If using a negative form is unavoidable, underline the negative word or phrase, or use bold text and all uppercase letters to draw the student's

attention to it. It is best to avoid asking students to identify the incorrect response, as in the following example:

Which of the following is **NOT** an indication that a skin lesion is a Stage IV pressure ulcer?

a.   Blistering*
b.   Sinus tracts
c.   Tissue necrosis
d.   Undermining

The structure of this item reinforces the wrong answer and may lead to confusion when a student attempts to recall the correct information at a later time. A better way to word the item is:

Which of the following is an indication that a skin lesion is a Stage II pressure ulcer?

a.   Blistering*
b.   Sinus tracts
c.   Tissue necrosis
d.   Undermining

6. *No item should contain irrelevant clues to the correct answer.* This is a common error among inexperienced test item writers. Students who are good test-takers can usually identify such an item and use its flaws to improve their chances of guessing the correct answer when they do not know it. Irrelevant clues include a multiple-choice stem that is grammatically inconsistent with one or more of the options, a word in the stem that is repeated in the correct option, using qualifiers such as "always" or "never" in incorrect responses, placing the correct response in a consistent position among a set of options, or consistently making true statements longer than false statements (Nitko, 2004). Such items contribute little to the validity of test results because they may not measure what students actually know, but how well they are able to guess the correct answers.

7. *No item should depend on another item for meaning or for the correct answer.* In other words, if a student answers one item incorrectly, he or she will likely answer the related item incorrectly. An example of such a relationship between two completion items follows:

1.   Which insulin should be used for emergency treatment of ketoacidosis?
2.   What is the onset of action for the insulin in Item 1?

---

* is correct answer.

In this example, Item 2 is dependent on Item 1 for its meaning. Students who supply the wrong answer to Item 1 are unlikely to supply a correct answer to Item 2. Items should be worded in such a way as to make them independent of each other. However, a series of test items can be developed to relate to a context such as a case study, database, diagram, graph, or other interpretive material. Items that are linked to this material are called context-dependent items (Nitko, 2004), and they do not violate this general rule for writing test items because they are linked to a common stimulus, not to each other.

8.   *Eliminate extraneous information unless the purpose of the item is to determine whether students can distinguish between relevant and irrelevant data.* Avoid the use of patient names in clinical scenarios; this information adds unnecessarily to reading time, it may distract from the purpose of the item, and it may introduce cultural bias (see Chapter 14). However, some items are designed to measure whether a student can evaluate the relevance of clinical data and use only pertinent information in arriving at the answer. In this case, extraneous data (but not patient names) may be included.

9.   *Arrange for a critique of the items.* The best source of this critique is a colleague who teaches the same content area or at least someone who is skilled in the technical aspects of item writing. If no one is available to critique the test items, the teacher who developed them should set them aside for a few days. This will allow the teacher to review the items with a fresh perspective in order to identify lack of clarity or faulty technical construction.

10.   *Prepare more items than the test blueprint specifies.* This will allow for replacement items for those discarded in the review process. The fortunate teacher who does not need to use many replacement items can use the remainder to begin an item bank for future tests.

PREPARING STUDENTS TO TAKE A TEST

A teacher-made test typically measures students' maximum performance rather than their typical performance. For this reason, teachers should create conditions under which students will be able to demonstrate their best possible performance. These conditions include adequate preparation of students to take the test (Nitko, 2004). Although this is the last point on the test construction checklist (Table 3.1), the teacher should begin preparing students to take the test at the time the test is scheduled. Adequate preparation includes information, skills, and attitudes that will facilitate students' maximum performance on the test.

Information Needs

Students need information about the test in order to plan for effective preparation. They need sufficient time to prepare for a test, and the date and time of a test should be announced well in advance. Although many teachers believe that unannounced or "pop" tests motivate students to study more, there is no evidence to support this position. In fact, surprise tests can be considered punitive or threatening and, as such, represent an unethical use of testing (Nitko, 2004). Adult learners with multiple responsibilities may need to make adjustments to their work and family responsibilities in order to have adequate study time, and generous notice of a planned test date will allow them to set their priorities.

In addition, students need to know about the conditions under which they are to be tested, such as how much time will be allotted, whether they will have access to resources such as textbooks, how many items will be included, the types of item formats that will be used, and if they need special tools or supplies to take the test, such as calculators, pencils, or black ink pens.

Of course, students also should know what content will be covered on the test, how many items will be devoted to each content area, and the cognitive level at which they will be expected to perform. As previously discussed, giving students a copy of the test blueprint and discussing it with them is an effective way for teachers to convey this information. Students should also have sufficient opportunity to practice the type of performance that will be tested. For example, if students will be expected to solve medication dose calculation problems without the use of a calculator, they should practice this type of calculation in class exercises or out-of-class assignments. Students also need to know if spelling, grammar, punctuation, or organization will be considered in scoring open-ended items so that they can prepare accordingly. Finally, teachers should tell students how their test results will be used, including the weight assigned to the test score in grading (Nitko, 2004).

Another way that teachers can assist students to study for a test is to have them prepare and use a "cheat sheet." Although this term can be expected to have negative connotations for most teachers, cheat sheets commonly are used in nursing practice in the form of memory aids or triggers such as procedure checklists, pocket guides, and reminder sheets. When legitimized for use in studying and test-taking, cheat sheets capitalize on the belief that while dishonest behavior should be discouraged, the skills associated with cheating can be powerful learning tools.

When students intend to cheat on a test, they usually try to guess potential test items and prepare cheat sheets with the correct answers to those anticipated items. Using this skill for a more honest purpose, the teacher can encourage all of the students to anticipate potential test items. In a test-preparation context, the teacher requires the students to develop a written cheat sheet that summarizes, prioritizes, condenses, and organizes content that they think is important and wish to remember during the test. The teacher may set parameters such as the length of the cheat sheet—for example, one side of one sheet of $8^1/2 \times 11$-inch paper. The students bring their cheat sheets on the day of the test and may use them during the test; they submit their cheat sheets along with their test papers. Students who do not submit cheat sheets may be penalized by deducting points from their test scores or may not be permitted to take the test at all.

Some students may not even consult their cheat sheets during the test, but they still derive benefit from the preparation that goes into developing them. The teacher also may review the cheat sheets with students whose test scores are low to identify weaknesses in thinking that may have contributed to their errors. When used for this purpose, the cheat sheet becomes a powerful diagnostic and feedback tool.

Test-Taking Skills

Because of an increasingly diverse population of learners in every educational setting, including growing numbers of students for whom English is a second language and whose testing experiences may be different from the teacher's expectations, teachers should determine if their students have adequate test-taking skills for the type of test to be given. If the students lack adequate test-taking skills, their test scores may be lower than their actual abilities. Skill in taking tests sometimes is called testwiseness. To be more precise, testwiseness is the ability to use test-taking skills, clues from poorly written test items, and test-taking experience to achieve a test score that is higher than the student's true knowledge would predict. Common errors made by item writers do allow some students to substitute testwiseness for knowledge. But, in general, all students should develop adequate test-taking skills so that they are not at a disadvantage when their scores are compared with those of more testwise individuals (Nitko, 2004).

Adequate test-taking skills include the following abilities:

1. Reading and listening to directions and following them accurately.
2. Recording answers to test items accurately and neatly.
3. Avoiding physical and mental fatigue by paced study and adequate rest before the test rather than late-night cram sessions supplemented by stimulants.
4. Using test time wisely and working at a pace that allows for careful reflection but also permits responding to all items that the student is likely to answer correctly.
5. Outlining and organizing responses to essay items before beginning to write.

6. Checking answers to test items for clerical errors and changing answers if a better response is indicated.

Many teachers advise students not to change their answers to test items, believing that the first response usually is the correct answer and that changing responses will not increase a student's score. Research findings, however, do not support this position. Studies of answer-changing and its effect on test performance have revealed that most students do change their answers to about 4% of test items and that approximately two-thirds of answer changes become correct responses. As item difficulty increases, however, this payoff diminishes; consequently, more knowledgeable students benefit more than less knowledgeable students from changing answers (Nitko, 2004).

Students should be encouraged to change their first response to any item when they have a good reason for making the change. For example, a student who has a clearer understanding of an item after re-reading it, who later recalls additional information needed to answer the item, or who receives a clue to the correct answer from another item should not hesitate to change the first answer. Improvement in test scores should not be expected, however, when students change answers without a clear rationale for making the change.

Test Anxiety

Finally, teachers should prepare students to approach a test with helpful attitudes. Although anxiety is a common response to situations in which performance is evaluated, high levels of anxiety are likely to interfere with maximum performance.

Whether some students can be characterized as test-anxious is a matter of frequent debate. Test anxiety can be viewed in several ways. Students who are motivated to do well often experience increased emotional tension in response to a test. Their perceptions of the testing situation affect their thoughts during test preparation and test taking. Students who perceive a test as a challenge usually have thoughts that are task-directed. They can focus on completing the task and easily manage any tension that is associated with it. Some students perceive tests as threats because they have poor test-taking skills, inadequate knowledge, or both. These students often have task-irrelevant thoughts about testing. They focus on what could happen if they fail a test, and their feelings of helplessness cause them to desire to escape the situation (Nitko, 2004).

Test anxiety often is characterized as a trait with two components: emotionality and worry. *Emotionality*, or autonomic arousal, refers to unpleasant feelings and nervousness, whereas the cognitive component of *worry* refers to thoughts or concerns related to performance and its consequences. Test anxiety research suggests that emotional responses to a test trigger worry, which functions as cognitive interference with performance (Nitko, 2004; Zeidner, 1998).

Indications of test anxiety may include physical symptoms such as sweaty palms and increased heart rate, although not all test-anxious individuals have physical symptoms. Cognitive and emotional indications of test anxiety include worries about other people performing better, impaired ability to concentrate and easy distractibility during the test, difficulty recalling information ("going blank"), misreading or misunderstanding directions or test items, exaggerated expectations of negative consequences (catastrophic fantasies), and feeling pressured to be perfect. Additionally, individuals with true test anxiety often have a history of poor performance on tests and other evaluative situations, particularly high-stakes tests. For example, these individuals may repeatedly fail a driver's license examination or achieve good scores on quizzes or unit tests but fail final examinations (Poorman, Mastorovich, Webb, & Molcan, 2003).

Students whose test anxiety interferes with their performance often benefit from treatment that addresses both emotionality and worry as well as training to improve their general test-taking skills. For example, the test-anxious student may learn techniques for stopping negative thoughts during study periods and testing situations, and behavioral techniques such as progressive relaxation and visual imagery (Poorman et al., 2003). A more comprehensive discussion of the diagnosis and treatment of test anxiety is beyond the scope of this textbook. However, teachers may be able to identify students whose performance suggests that test anxiety may be a factor, and to refer those students for treatment.

Students need to view tests and other assessment procedures as opportunities to demonstrate what they know and what they can do. To foster this attitude, the teacher should express confidence in the students' abilities to prepare for and perform well on an upcoming test. It may be helpful for the teacher to ask the students what would help them to feel more relaxed and less anxious before and during a test. Conducting a review session, giving practice items similar to those that will be used on the test, and not talking or interrupting students during a test are examples of strategies that are likely to reduce students' anxiety to manageable levels (Nitko, 2004).

SUMMARY

Teachers who leave little time for adequate preparation often produce tests that contain poorly chosen and poorly written test items. Sufficient planning for test construction before the item-writing phase begins, followed by a careful critique of the completed test by other teachers, is likely to produce a test that will yield more valid results.

All decisions involved in planning a test should be based on a teacher's knowledge of the purpose of the test and relevant characteristics of the population of learners to be tested. The purpose for the test involves why it is to be given, what it is supposed to measure, and how the test scores will be used. A teacher's knowledge of the population that will be tested will be useful in selecting the item formats to be used, determining the length of the test and the testing time required, and selecting the appropriate scoring procedures. The students' English language literacy, visual acuity, and previous testing experience are examples of factors that might influence these decisions.

The length of the test is an important factor that is related to its purpose, the abilities of the students, the item formats that will be used, the amount of testing time available, and the desired reliability of the test scores. The desired difficulty of the test and its ability to differentiate among various levels of performance are affected by the purpose of the test and the way in which the scores will be interpreted and used. If the test results are to be interpreted in a norm-referenced manner, the majority of the items should be of moderate difficulty and discriminate among students of various abilities.

A test with a variety of item formats usually provides students with more opportunity to demonstrate their competence than a test with only one item format. Test items may be classified as selected-response or constructed-response types, depending on the task required of the learner. All item formats have advantages and limitations. Teachers should select item formats based on a variety of factors, such as the objectives, specific skill to be measured, and the ability level of the students. Many objectives are better measured with certain item formats.

Decisions about what scoring procedure or procedures to use are somewhat dependent on the choice of item formats. Student responses to some item formats must be hand-scored, whether they are recorded directly on the test itself or on a separate answer sheet or in a booklet. The teacher should decide if the time and resources available for scoring a test suggest that hand-scoring or machine-scoring would be preferable.

The best way to ensure measurement validity of a teacher-constructed test is to develop a test blueprint, also known as a test plan or a table of specifications, before building the test itself. The elements of a test blueprint include (a) a list of the major topics or instructional objectives that the test will cover, (b) the level of complexity of the task to be assessed, and (c) the emphasis each topic will have, indicated by number or percentage of items or points. The test blueprint serves several important functions. It is a useful tool for guiding the work of the item writer so that sufficient items are developed at the appropriate level to test important content areas and objectives. It also should be used to inform students about the nature of the test and how they should prepare for it.

After developing the test blueprint, the teacher writes the test items that correspond to it. Regardless of the selected item formats, the teacher should follow some general rules that contribute to the development of high-quality test items.

Because teacher-made tests typically measure students' maximum performance rather than their typical performance, teachers should create conditions under which students will be able to demonstrate their best possible performance. These conditions include adequate preparation of the students to take the test. Adequate preparation includes information, skills, and attitudes that will facilitate students' maximum performance on the test.

REFERENCES

Bloom, B. S., Englehart, M. D., Furst, E. J., Hill, W. H., & Krathwohl, D. R. (1956). *Taxonomy of educational objectives: The classification of educational goals. Handbook I: Cognitive domain.* White Plains, NY: Longman.

Gaskins, S., Dunn, L., Forte, L., Wood, F., & Riley, P. (1996). Student perceptions of changing answers on multiple choice nursing examinations. *Journal of Nursing Education, 35,* 88–90.

Haladyna, T. M. (1997). *Writing test items to evaluate higher order thinking.* Boston: Allyn & Bacon.

Linn, R. L., & Gronlund, N. E. (2000). *Measurement and assessment in teaching* (8th ed.). Upper Saddle River, NJ: Prentice Hall.

Nitko, A. J. (2004). *Educational assessment of students* (4th ed.). Upper Saddle River, NJ: Prentice Hall.

Poorman, S. G., Mastorovich, M. L., Webb, C. A., & Molcan, K. L. (2003). *Good thinking: Test taking and study skills for nursing students* (2nd ed.). Pittsburgh, PA: STAT Nursing Consultants.

Zeidner, M. (1998). *Test anxiety: The state of the art.* New York: Plenum.

Chapter 4

Selected-Response Test Items:
True-False and Matching

There are different ways of classifying types of test items. One way is to group items according to how they are scored—objectively or subjectively. Another way is to group them by the type of response required of the test-taker. *Selected-response* items require the test-taker to select the correct or best answer from options provided by the teacher. These items include true-false, matching exercises, multiple-choice, and multiple-response. *Constructed-response* items ask the test-taker to supply an answer rather than choose from options already provided. Constructed-response items include completion and essay (short and extended). In this book, item formats are classified as selected-response (or "choice") and constructed-response (or "supply") items.

In addition to these test items, other evaluation strategies for classroom use are written assignments, case method and case studies, multimedia, and simulations. These strategies and methods for evaluating clinical performance are discussed in later chapters of the book.

SELECTED-RESPONSE ITEMS

Selected-response items can be used effectively to test a variety of student outcomes, as discussed in the previous chapter. The choice of the specific selected-response format should be guided by an understanding of the strengths and weaknesses of each item type. In general, selected-response items can be scored quickly and with a high degree of reliability, but each item format has specific limitations. In this chapter, two types of selected-response items are presented: true-false and matching exercises. Multiple-choice and multiple-response items are described in chapter 5.

For each of the item formats presented in this book, a number of principles should be considered when writing them. While important principles are discussed, the lists are not intended to be inclusive; other sources on test construction might include additional helpful suggestions for writing test items.

TRUE-FALSE

A true-false item consists of a statement that the student judges as true or false. In some forms, students also correct the response or supply a rationale as to why the statement is true or false. True-false items are most effective for recall of facts and specific information but also may be used to test the student's comprehension of an important principle or concept. Each item represents a declarative sentence stating a fact or principle and asking the learner to decide if it is true or false, right or wrong, correct or incorrect. Some authors refer to this type of test item as alternate response, allowing for these varied response formats. For affective outcomes, agree-disagree might be used, asking the learner to agree or disagree with a value-based statement.

There are different opinions as to the value of true-false items. While some authors express concern over the low level of testing, focusing on recall of facts, and the opportunity for guessing, others indicate that true-false items provide an efficient means of examining student acquisition of knowledge in a course. With true-false items, students can answer a large number of questions in a short time. Students often can answer twice as many true-false items as multiple-choice and completion items in the same amount of time (Oosterhof, 2001). For this reason, a large number of true-false items may be included in a test, which provides a way of testing a wide range of content.

While true-false items are relatively easy to construct, the teacher should avoid using them to test meaningless information. Designed to examine student recall and comprehension of *important* facts and principles, true-false items should not be used to evaluate memorization of irrelevant information. Prior to constructing these items, the teacher should ask: Is the content evaluated by the true-false item important considering the course objectives? Does the content represent knowledge taught in the class or through other methods of instruction? Do the students need an understanding of the content to progress through the course and for their further learning?

The main limitation to true-false items is guessing. Since one of the two responses has to be correct, the probability that a student will answer the item correctly is 50%. However, the issue with guessing is not as much of a problem as it seems. With no knowledge of the facts being tested, on a 10-point quiz, the student would only be expected to answer correctly 5 of the items or 50%.

In fact, Oosterhof (2001) emphasized that the problem with guessing is more "perceived than real" (p. 146). With blind guessing, fewer than 10% of the students would answer correctly more than 7 out of 10 items; the chances of blindly achieving 70% on a 100-item true-false test is less than 4 in 1 million (Oosterhof, p. 146).

Writing True-False Items

The following discussion includes some important principles for the teacher to consider when constructing true-false items.

1. *The true-false item should test recall of important facts and information.* Avoid constructing items that test trivia and meaningless information. The content should be worth knowing.

2. *The statement should be true or false without qualification*—unconditionally true or false. The teacher should be able to defend the answer without conditions.

3. *Avoid words such as usually, sometimes, often, and similar ones.* Linn and Gronlund (2000) indicated that these words typically occur in true statements, giving the student clues as to the correct response. Along the same line, avoid words such as never, always, all, and none, often indicating a false response.

4. *Avoid terms that indicate an infinite degree or amount* such as "large," which can be interpreted differently by each student (Chase, 1999).

5. *Each item should include one idea to be tested* rather than multiple ones. When there are different propositions to be tested, each should be designed as a single true-false item.

6. *Items should be worded precisely and clearly.* Avoid long statements with different qualifiers and focus the sentence instead on the main idea to be tested. Long statements take time for reading and do not contribute to testing student knowledge of an important fact or principle.

7. *Avoid the use of negatives*, particularly double negatives. They are confusing to read and may interfere with student ability to understand the statement. For instance, the item "It is not normal for a two-year-old to demonstrate hand-preference" (true) would be stated more clearly as, "It is normal for a two-year-old to demonstrate hand-preference" (false).

8. *With a series of true-false items, statements should be similar in length.* The teacher may be inclined to write longer true sentences than false ones in an attempt to state the concept clearly and precisely.

9. *Use an equal number, or close to it, of true and false items* on a test (Linn & Gronlund, 2000; Mertler, 2003). Some experts recommend including slightly more false than true statements because false statements tend to differen-

tiate better between most and least knowledgeable students. Higher discrimination power improves the reliability of test scores (Nitko, 2004).

10.   *Decide how to score true-false items prior to administering them* to students. In some variations of true-false items, students correct false statements; for this type, the teacher should award two points, one for identifying the statement as false and the second for correcting it. In another variation of true-false items, students supply a rationale for their answers, either true or false. A similar scoring principle might be used in which students receive one point for correctly identifying the answer as true or false and a second point for the rationale.

Sample items follow:

For each of the following statements, circle T if the statement is true and F if the statement is false:

T   F   Insulin-dependent diabetes mellitus also is known as Type
          I diabetes. (T)
T   F   Hypothyroidism is manifested by lethargy and fatigue. (T)
T   F   The most common form of congenital heart defect in children
          is Tetralogy of Fallot. (F)

Variations of True-False Items

There are many variations of true-false items that may be used for testing. One variation is to ask the students to correct false statements. Students may identify the words that make a statement false and insert words to make it true. In changing the false statement to a true one, students may write in their own corrections or choose words from a list supplied by the teacher. One other modification of true-false items is to have students include a rationale for their responses, whether they are true or false. This provides a means of testing their comprehension of the content.

For all of these variations, the directions should be clear and specific. Some examples follow:

If the statement is true, draw a circle around T and do no more. If the statement is false, draw a circle around F and underline the word or phrase that makes it false.

T   F   Tetany occurs with increased secretion of parathyroid hor-
          mones.

Since this statement is false, the student would circle F and underline the word "increased":

T   (F)   Tetany occurs with <u>increased</u> secretion of parathyroid hormones. (F)

If the statement is true, draw a circle around T and do no more. If the statement is false, draw a circle around F, underline the word or phrase that makes it false, and write in the blank the word or phrase that would make it true.

T   F   Canned soups are high in potassium.

_____

T   F   Fresh fruits and vegetables are low in sodium.

_____

In the first example, since the statement is false, the student would circle F, underline potassium, and write sodium in the blank to make the statement true. In the second example, since the statement is true, the student would only circle T:

T   (F)   Canned soups are high in <u>potassium</u>. (F)
           Sodium

(T) F   Fresh fruits and vegetables are low in sodium. (T)

_____

If the statement is true, draw a circle around T and do no more. If the statement is false, draw a circle around F and circle the *correct* word from the list that follows the item.

T   F   Bradycardia is a heart rate less than <u>80</u> beats per minute.
         40, 50, 60, 100

Since the statement is false, the student would circle both F and 60:

T   (F)   Bradycardia is a heart rate less than <u>80</u> beats per minute. (F)
           40, 50, (60), 100

If the statement is true, draw a circle around the T and explain why it is true. If the statement is false, draw a circle around F and explain why it is false.

T   F   Patients with emphysema should have low-flow oxygen. (T)

_____

_____

One other variation of true-false items is called multiple true-false. This is a cross between a multiple-choice and true-false item. Multiple true-false items have an incomplete statement followed by several phrases that complete it; learners indicate which of the phrases form true or false statements. This type of item clusters true-false statements under one stem. Directions for answering these items should be clear, and the phrases should be numbered consecutively since they represent individual true-false items. Consistent with any true-false, the phrases that complete the statement should be unequivocally true or false (Oosterhof, 2001).

Sample items follow:

The incomplete statements below are followed by several phrases. Each of the phrases completes the statement and makes it true or false. If the completed statement is true, draw a circle around T. If the completed statement is false, draw a circle around F.

A patient with a below-the-knee amputation should:

T   F   1.   Avoid walking until fitted with a prosthesis. (F)
T   F   2.   Keep the stump elevated at all times. (F)
T   F   3.   Lift weights to build up arm strength. (T)
T   F   4.   Wrap the stump in a figure-8 style. (T)

Bloom's taxonomy of the cognitive domain includes the:

T   F   5.   Application level. (T)
T   F   6.   Knowledge level. (T)
T   F   7.   Calculation level. (F)
T   F   8.   Recommended actions level. (F)
T   F   9.   Analysis level. (T)
T   F   10.   Manipulation level. (F)
T   F   11.   Synthesis level. (T)

MATCHING EXERCISES

Matching exercises consist of two parallel columns in which students match terms, phrases, sentences, or numbers from one column to the other. Students must identify the one-to-one correspondence between the columns (Mertler, 2003). One column includes a list of premises and the other column, from which the selection is made, is referred to as responses. The basis for matching responses to premises should be stated explicitly in the directions with the exercise. The student identifies pairs based on the principle specified in these directions. With some matching exercises, differences between the premises and responses are not apparent, such as matching a list of laboratory studies with their normal ranges, and the columns could be interchanged. In other exercises, however, the premises include descriptive phrases or sentences to which the student matches shorter responses.

Matching exercises lend themselves to testing categories, classifications, groupings, definitions, and other related facts. They are most appropriate for measuring facts based on simple associations (Linn & Gronlund, 2000). One advantage of a matching exercise is its ability to test a number of facts that can be grouped together rather than designing a series of individual questions. For instance, the teacher can develop one matching exercise on medications and related side effects rather than a series of individual items on each medication. This makes it possible to test a large number of related facts at one time (Nitko, 2004). A disadvantage, however, is the focus on recall of facts and specific information, although in many courses this reflects an important outcome of learning.

Writing Matching Exercises

Matching exercises are intended for categories, classifications, and information that can be grouped in some way. An effective matching exercise requires the use of homogeneous material with responses that are plausible for the premises. Responses that are not plausible for some premises provide clues to the correct match.

Principles for writing matching exercises include:

1. *Develop a matching exercise around homogeneous content.* All of the premises and responses to be matched should relate to that content, e.g., all laboratory tests and values, all terms and definitions, and all types of health insurance and characteristics. This is the most important principle in writing a matching exercise (Linn & Gronlund, 2000).

2. *Include an unequal number of premises and responses* to avoid giving a clue to the final match. Typically there are more responses than premises, but the number of responses may be limited by the maximum number of spaces per item allowed on a machine-scored answer sheet. In that case, the teacher may need to write more premises than responses.

3. *Use a short list of premises and responses.* This makes it easier for the teacher to identify ones from the same content area, and it saves students reading time. With a long list of items to be matched, it is difficult to review the choices and pair them with the premises. It also prohibits recording the answers on machine-scored answer sheets. Linn and Gronlund (2000) recommended using 4 to 7 items in each column. A longer list might be used for some exercises, but no more than 10 items should be included in either column.

4. *For matching exercises with a large number of responses, the teacher should develop two separate matching questions.* Otherwise students spend too much time reading through the options.

5. *Directions for the matching exercises should be clear and state explicitly the basis for matching the premises and responses.* This is an important principle in developing these items. Even if the basis for matching seems self-evident, the directions should include the rationale for matching the columns.

6. *Directions should specify if each response may be used once, more than once, or not at all.*

7. *Place the longer premises on the left and shorter responses on the right.* This enables the students to read the longer statement first, then search for the correct response, which often is a single word or a few words, on the right. This arrangement makes it more efficient for the students (Mertler, 2003).

8. *The order in which the premises and responses are listed should be alphabetical, numerical, or in some other logical order.* Alphabetical order eliminates clues from the arrangement of the responses (Linn & Gronlund, 2000). If the lists have a logical order, however, such as dates and other sequences, then they should be organized in that order. Numbers, quantities, and similar types of items should be arranged in decreasing or increasing order.

9. *The entire matching exercise should be typed on the same page and not divided across pages.*

Sample matching items follow:

Directions: For each definition in Column A, select the proper term in Column B. Use each letter only once or not at all.

Column A (Premises)

__b__	1.	Attaching a particular response to a specific stimulus
__f__	2.	Believing that one can respond effectively in a situation
__g__	3.	Changing behavioral patterns gradually
__d__	4.	Observing a behavior and its consequences and attempting to behave similarly
__a__	5.	Varying ways in which individuals process information

Column B (Responses)

a. Cognitive styles
b. Conditioning
c. Empowerment
d. Modeling
e. Self-care
f. Self-efficacy
g. Shaping

Directions: For each insulin in Column A, identify its peak action in Column B. Responses in Column B may be used once, more than once, or not at all.

Column A		Column B	
c	1. Humulin regular	a.	Long acting
b	2. NPH	b.	Intermediate acting
b	3. Lente	c.	Short acting
a	4. Ultralente		

SUMMARY

Test items may be categorized as selected- and constructed-response items. Selected-response formats, which are structured and ask the test-taker to choose an answer among alternatives, include true-false, matching exercises, multiple-choice, and multiple-response. Constructed-response items provide an opportunity for students to formulate their own ideas and express them in writing. In addition to these, many other types of evaluation methods are appropriate for assessing student learning in nursing courses and clinical practice.

This chapter described how to construct two types of test items: true-false and matching exercises, including variations of them. A true-false item consists of a statement that the student judges as true or false. In some forms, students correct a response or supply a rationale as to why the statement is true or false. True-false items are most effective for recall of facts and specific information but also may be used to test the student's comprehension of an important principle or concept.

Matching exercises consist of two parallel columns in which students match terms, phrases, sentences, or numbers from one column to the other. One column includes a list of premises and the other column, from which the selection is made, contains the responses. The student identifies pairs based on the principle specified in the directions. Matching exercises lend themselves to testing categories, classifications, groupings, definitions, and other related facts. Similar to true-false, they are most appropriate for recall of specific information.

In developing an evaluation protocol, the teacher has multiple types of test items and evaluation strategies from which to choose. Another important type of objective item in nursing, multiple-choice, is described in chapter 5.

REFERENCES

Chase, C. I. (1999). *Contemporary assessment for educators*. New York: Longman.

Linn, R. L., & Gronlund, N. E. (2000). *Measurement and assessment in teaching* (8th ed.). Upper Saddle River, NJ: Prentice-Hall.

Mertler, C. A. (2003). *Classroom assessment*. Los Angeles: Pyrczak.

Nitko, A. J. (2004). *Educational assessment of students* (4th ed.). Upper Saddle River, NJ: Prentice Hall.

Oosterhof, A. (2001). *Classroom applications of educational measurement* (3rd ed.). Upper Saddle River, NJ: Prentice Hall.

Trice, A. D. (2000). *A handbook of classroom assessment*. New York: Longman.

Chapter 5

Selected-Response Test Items: Multiple-Choice and Multiple-Response

This chapter focuses on two other kinds of selected-response items: multiple-choice and multiple-response items. Multiple-choice items, with one correct answer, are used widely in nursing and in other fields. This test-item format includes an incomplete statement or question, followed by a list of options that complete the statement or answer the question. Multiple-response items are designed similarly, although more than one answer may be correct. Both of these test-item formats may be used for evaluating learning at the recall, comprehension, application, and analysis levels, making them adaptable for a wide range of content and learning outcomes.

MULTIPLE-CHOICE ITEMS

Multiple-choice items can be used for measuring many types of learning outcomes. Some of these include:

- Knowledge of facts, specific information, and principles
- Definitions of terms
- Understanding of content
- Application of concepts, principles, and theories in clinical and other situations
- Analysis of data and clinical situations
- Comparison and selection of varied interventions
- Judgments and decisions about actions to take in clinical and other situations.

Multiple-choice items are particularly useful in nursing to measure application- and analysis-level outcomes. With multiple-choice items, the teacher can introduce *new* information requiring application of concepts and theories or analytical thinking in order to respond to the questions. Items at this level are effective for assessing critical thinking (McDonald, 2002). Experience with multiple-choice testing also provides essential practice for students who will later encounter this type of item on licensure, certification, and other commercially prepared examinations. Multiple-choice items also allow the teacher to sample the course content more easily than with items such as essay questions, which require more time for responding, and multiple-choice tests can be computer scored and analyzed.

While there are many advantages to multiple-choice testing, there are also certain disadvantages. First, these items are difficult to construct, particularly at the higher cognitive levels. Developing items to test memorization of facts is much easier than designing ones to measure use of knowledge in a new situation and skill in analysis. As such, many multiple-choice items are written at the lower cognitive levels, focusing only on recall and comprehension. Second, teachers often experience difficulty developing plausible distractors. These distractors—also spelled distracters—are the incorrect alternatives that seem plausible for test-takers who have not adequately learned the content. If a distractor is not plausible, it provides an unintended clue to the test-taker that it is not the correct response. Third, it is often difficult to identify only one correct answer. For these reasons, multiple-choice items are time-consuming to construct.

Some critics of multiple-choice testing suggest that essay and similar types of questions to which students develop a response provide a truer measure of learning than items in which students choose from available options. However, multiple-choice items written at the application and analysis levels require *use* of concepts and theories and analytical thinking to make a selection from the available options. For items at those levels, test-takers need to compare options and make a judgment about the correct or best response.

Writing Multiple-Choice Items

There are three parts to a multiple-choice item, each with its own set of principles for development: (a) stem, (b) answer, and (c) distractors. Figure 5.1 indicates each of these parts.

The stem is the lead-in phrase in the form of a question or an incomplete statement that relies on the alternatives for completion. Following the stem is a list of alternatives or options for the learner to consider and choose from. These alternatives are of two types: the answer, which is the correct or best response to answer the question or complete the statement, and distractors,

An early and common sign of pregnancy is:	STEM in form of incomplete statement
	OPTIONS OR ALTERNATIVES
a. amenorrhea. *	*Answer*
b. morning sickness.	*Distractor*
c. spotting.	*Distractor*
d. tenderness of the breasts.	*Distractor*

In which of the following groups does Raynaud's disease occur most frequently?	STEM in the form of question
	OPTIONS OR ALTERNATIVES
a. Men between 20–40 years old	*Distractor*
b. Men between 50–70 years old	*Distractor*
c. Women between 20–40 years old *	*Answer*
d. Women between 50–70 years old	*Distractor*

FIGURE 5.1   Example of parts of multiple-choice item.

which are the incorrect alternatives. The purpose of the distractors, as the word implies, is to *distract* students who are unsure of the correct answer. Suggestions for writing each of these parts are considered separately as follows.

Stem

The stem is the question or incomplete statement to which the alternatives relate. Whether the stem is written in a question form or as an incomplete statement, the most important quality is its clarity. The test-taker should be able to read the stem and know what to look for in the alternatives without having to read through them. Thus, the stem should stand alone (McDonald,

2002). One other important consideration in writing the stem is to ensure that it presents a problem or situation that relates to the learning outcome being evaluated.

Guidelines for writing the stem are:

1. *The stem should present clearly and explicitly the problem to be solved.* The student should not have to read the alternatives to understand the question or the intent of the incomplete statement. The stem should provide sufficient information for answering the question or completing the statement. An example of this principle follows:

Cataracts:

a.   are painful.
b.   may accompany coronary artery disease.
c.   occur with aging. *
d.   result in tunnel vision.

The stem of this question does not clearly present the problem associated with cataracts that the alternatives address. As such, it does not guide the learner in reviewing the alternatives. In addition, the options are dissimilar, which is possible because of the lack of clarity in the stem; alternatives should be similar. One possible revision of this stem is:

The causes of cataracts include:

a.   aging. *
b.   arteriosclerosis.
c.   hemorrhage.
d.   iritis.

After writing the item, the teacher can cover the alternatives and read the stem alone. Does it explain the problem and direct the learner to the alternatives? Is it complete? Could it stand alone as a short-answer item? In writing the stem, always include the nature of the response, such as, Which of the following *interventions, signs and symptoms, treatments, data,* and so forth. A stem that asks "Which of the following?" does not provide clear instructions as to what to look for in the options.

2. *Although the stem should be clear and explicit, it should not contain extraneous information unless the item is developed for the purpose of identifying significant versus insignificant data.* Otherwise, the stem should be brief, including only necessary

information. Long options that include irrelevant information take additional time for reading. This point can be illustrated as follows, using the previous cataract item:

You are caring for an elderly man who lives alone but has frequent visits from his daughter. He has congestive heart failure and some shortness of breath. Your patient was told recently that he has cataracts. The causes of cataracts include:

a.   aging. *
b.   arteriosclerosis.
c.   hemorrhage.
d.   iritis.

In this stem, the background information about the patient is irrelevant to the problem addressed. If subsequent items were to be written about the patient's other problems, related nursing interventions, the home setting, and so forth, then this background information might be presented as a scenario in a context-dependent item set (see chapter 7).

Stems also should not be humorous; laughing during the test can distract students who are concentrating. If one of the distractors is humorous, it will be recognized as implausible and eliminated as an option, increasing the chance of guessing the correct answer from among the remaining alternatives. Humorous content may be confusing to test-takers for whom English is a second language.

3.   *Avoid inserting information in the stem for instructional purposes.* In the example that follows, the definition of cataract has no relevance to the content tested, i.e., the causes of cataracts. The goal of testing is to evaluate outcomes of learning not to teach new information, as in this example:

Cataracts are an opacity of the lens or capsule of the eye leading to blurred and eventual loss of vision. The causes of cataracts include:

a.   aging. *
b.   arteriosclerosis.
c.   hemorrhage.
d.   iritis.

4.   *If words need to be repeated in each alternative to complete the statement, shift them to the stem.* This is illustrated as follows:

An early and common sign of pregnancy:

a.   *is* amenorrhea. *
b.   *is* morning sickness.
c.   *is* spotting.
d.   *is* tenderness of the breasts.

The word "is" may be moved to the stem:

An early and common sign of pregnancy *is*:

a.   amenorrhea. *
b.   morning sickness.
c.   spotting.
d.   tenderness of the breasts.

Similarly, a word or phrase repeated in each alternative does not test students' knowledge of it and should be included in the stem. An example follows:

Clinical manifestations of Parkinson's disease include:

a.   decreased perspiration, tremors at rest, and *muscle rigidity*. *
b.   increased salivation, *muscle rigidity*, and diplopia.
c.   *muscle rigidity*, decreased salivation, and nystagmus.
d.   tremors during activity, *muscle rigidity*, and increased perspiration.

This item does not test knowledge of muscle rigidity occurring with Parkinson's disease since it is included with each alternative. The stem could be revised as follows:

Clinical manifestations of Parkinson's disease include *muscle rigidity* and which of the following signs and symptoms?

a.   Decreased salivation and nystagmus
b.   Increased salivation and diplopia
c.   Tremors at rest and decreased perspiration *
d.   Tremors during activity and increased perspiration

5.   *Do not include key words in the stem that would clue the student to the correct answer.* This point may be demonstrated in the earlier question on cataracts.

You are caring for an *elderly* patient who was told recently that he has cataracts. The causes of cataracts include:

a.   *aging.* *
b.   arteriosclerosis.
c.   hemorrhage.
d.   iritis.

In this item, informing the student that the patient is elderly provides a clue to the correct response.

6.   *Avoid the use of negatively-stated stems, including words such as no, not, and except.* Negatively-stated stems are sometimes unclear; in addition, they require a change in thought pattern from selections that represent correct and best responses to ones reflecting incorrect and least likely responses. Most stems may be stated positively, asking for the correct or best response rather than the exception.

If there is no acceptable alternative to a negatively-stated stem, however, highlight this for the learner by underlining or capitalizing the negative word or by using bold text. Otherwise, words such as no, not, and except may be overlooked in reading the stem. A sample item follows:

You are working in an agency that cares for the chronically mentally ill in their homes. One of your patients is readmitted after refusing to take her medications. A highly structured routine is used with the goal of preparing her for discharge. All of the following outcomes suggest that this plan is effective EXCEPT:

a.   asking the nurse for assistance in dressing. *
b.   attending occupational therapy on the unit.
c.   going to the cafeteria for meals without prompting.
d.   telling another patient to move out of "her" chair.

7.   *The stem and alternatives that follow should be consistent grammatically.* If the stem is an incomplete statement, each option should complete it grammatically; if not, clues are provided as to the correct or incorrect responses. It is also important to check carefully that a consistent verb form is used with the alternatives. An example follows:

Your patient is undergoing a right carotid endarterectomy. Prior to surgery, which information would be most important to collect as a baseline for the early recovery period? Her ability to:

a.   follow movements with her eyes
b.   move all four extremities *
c.   rotat*ing* her head from side to side
d.   swallow and gag

Option 'c' provides a grammatical clue by not completing the statement "Her ability to." The item may be revised easily:

Your patient is undergoing a right carotid endarterectomy. Prior to surgery, which information would be most important to collect as a baseline for the early recovery period? Her ability to:

a.   follow movements with her eyes
b.   move all four extremities *
c.   rotate her head from side to side
d.   swallow and gag

8.   *Avoid ending stems with "a" or "an"* because these often provide grammatical clues as to the option to select. It is usually easy to rephrase the stem to eliminate the "a" or "an." For instance,

Narrowing of the aortic valve in children occurs with *an*:

a.   aortic stenosis. *
b.   atrial septal defect.
c.   coarctation of the aorta.
d.   patent ductus arteriosus.

Ending this stem with "an" eliminates alternatives "c" and "d" because of grammatical errors. The stem could be rewritten by deleting the "an":

Narrowing of the aortic valve in children occurs with:

a.   aortic stenosis. *
b.   atrial septal defect.
c.   coarctation of the aorta.
d.   patent ductus arteriosus.

9.   *If the stem is a statement completed by the alternatives, begin each alternative with a lower-case letter and place a period after it since it forms a sentence with the stem.* At the end of the stem, use a comma or colon as appropriate. Use upper-case letters to begin alternatives that do not form a sentence with the stem. If the stem is a question, place a question mark at the end.

10.   *Each multiple-choice item should be independent of the others.* This principle holds true except for multiple-choice items that are developed in a series, with a number of items that relate to a patient scenario, clinical situation, or common data set. In a series of items, the directions should indicate that questions ____ to ____ pertain to the scenario. A sample item follows illustrating questions that are not meant to stand alone.

Directions: Questions 1 and 2 relate to the following patient scenario. Select the best answer in each of these questions.

The patient is a 45-year old male who was treated in the ER for an asthma attack.

1.   You are the community health nurse developing his teaching plan. Which action should be implemented *FIRST?*

    a.   Assess other related health problems

    b.   Determine his level of understanding of asthma *

    c.   Review with him treatments for his asthma

    d.   Teach him actions of his medications

2.   On your second home visit, the patient is short of breath. Which of these statements indicates a need for further instruction?

    a.   "I checked my peak flow since I'm not feeling good."

    b.   "I have been turning on the air conditioner at times like this."

    c.   "I tried my Azmacort because my chest was feeling heavy." *

    d.   "I used my nebulizer mist treatment for my wheezing."

11.   *Write the stem so that the alternatives are placed at the end of the incomplete statement.* An incomplete statement with a blank in the middle, which the options then complete, interrupts the reading and may be confusing for the students to read and follow (McDonald, 2002).

Alternatives

Following the stem in a multiple-choice item is a list of alternatives or options, which include the (a) correct or best answer and (b) distractors. There are varying recommendations as to the number of alternatives to include, ranging from 3 to 5. The more options—as long as they are plausible—the more discriminating the item. Five options reduce the chance of guessing the correct answer to 1 in 5 (Linn & Gronlund, 2000). Unfortunately, it is usually difficult to develop four plausible distractors to accompany the correct answer when five options are included. For this reason, four options are typically used, allowing for one correct or best answer and three plausible distractors. Many standardized tests use four alternatives.

General principles for writing the alternatives follow:

1. *The alternatives should be similar in length, detail, and complexity.* It is important to check the number of words included in each option for consistency in length. Frequently the correct answer is the longest because the teacher attempts to write it clearly and specifically. Nitko (2004) suggested that the test-wise student may realize that the longest response is the correct answer without having the requisite knowledge to make this choice. In that case, the teacher should either shorten the correct response or add similar qualifiers to the distractors so that they are similar in length as well as in detail and complexity.

While there is no established number of words by which the alternatives may differ from each other without providing clues, one strategy is to count the words in each option and attempt to vary them by no more than a few words. This will provide a check that the options are consistent in length. In the sample item, the correct answer is longer than the distractors, which might provide a clue for selecting it.

> You are assessing a 14-year-old girl who appears emaciated. Her mother describes the following changes: resistance to eating and 20 lb. weight loss over the last 6 weeks. It is most likely that the patient resists eating for which of the following reasons?
>
> a.   Complains of recurring nausea
> b.   Describes herself as "fat all over" and fearful of gaining weight*
> c.   Has other GI problems
> d.   Seeks her mother's attention

The correct answer can be shortened to: Is fearful of gaining weight.

2. *In addition to consistency in length, detail, and complexity, the options should have the same number of parts.* The answer in the previous question is not only

longer than the other options but also includes two parts, providing another clue. In the example that follows, including two causes in option "a" provides a clue to the answer. Revising that option to only "aging" only avoids this.

Causes of cataracts include:

a.   aging and steroid therapy. *
b.   arteriosclerosis.
c.   hemorrhage.
d.   iritis.

3. *The alternatives should be consistent grammatically.* The answer and distractors should be similar in structure and terminology. Without this consistency in format, the test-taker may be clued to the correct response or to eliminate some of the options without knowing the content. In the sample item below, the student may be clued to the correct answer "a" because it differs grammatically from the others:

You are making a home visit with a new mother who is breastfeeding. She tells you that her nipples are cracked and painful. Which of the following instructions should be given to the mother?

a.   Put the entire areola in the baby's mouth during feeding.*
b.   The baby should be fed less frequently until the nipples are healed.
c.   There is less chance of cracking if the nipples are washed daily with soap.
d.   Wiping off the lotion on the nipples before feeding the baby may help.

4. *The alternatives should sample the same domain, for instance, all symptoms, all diagnostic tests, all nursing interventions, varying treatments, and so forth.* In the example that follows, option "b" is not a nursing diagnosis, which may clue the student to omit it as a possibility.

You are working in the Emergency Department, and your patient is having difficulty breathing. His respiratory rate is 40, heart rate 140, and oxygen saturation 90%. He also complains of a headache. Which of the following nursing diagnoses is of greatest priority?

a.   Activity intolerance
b.   COPD
c.   Impaired gas exchange *
d.   Pain

5. *Avoid including opposite responses among the options.* This is often a clue to choose between the opposites and not consider the others. A sample item follows:

The nurse should determine the correct placement of a nasogastric tube by:

a. asking the patient to swallow.

b. inserting water in the tube and auscultating in the epigastric area.

c. inserting air in the tube and auscultating in the epigastric area.*

d. taping the tube in place and checking it.

In this example, the correct response is opposite one of the distractors, which clues the student to select one of these alternatives. In addition, options "b" and "c" begin with "inserting," which may provide a visual clue to choose between them. Option "a" contains one part in contrast to the other alternatives, another possible clue.

6. *Arrange the options in a logical or meaningful order.* The order can be alphabetical, numerical, or chronological (Gaberson, 1996; Haladyna, 2004). Arranging the options in this way tends to randomly distribute the position of the correct response rather than the answer occurring most often in the same location, e.g., "b" or "c," throughout the test. It also helps students locate the correct response more easily when they have an answer in mind.

7. *Options with numbers, quantities, and other numerical values should be listed sequentially, either increasing or decreasing in value, and the values should not overlap.* When alternatives overlap, a portion of an option may be correct, or more than one answer may be possible. These problems are apparent in the sample item that follows:

Compressions for infant CPR should be:

a. $1^1/2$ to 2 inches.

b. $1/4$ to $1/2$ inch.

c. $1/2$ to 1 inch. *

d. 1 to 2 inches.

The values in these options overlap, such as with "a" and "d"; "b" and "c"; and "c" and "d." They would be easier to review if arranged sequentially from decreasing to increasing length. A revision follows:

Compressions for infant CPR should be:

a.   Less than $1/8$ inch.

b. $1/8$ to $1/4$ inch.

c. $1/2$ to 1 inch. *

d. $1^{1}/2$ to 2 inches.

Values such as laboratory values should be labeled appropriately, such as hemoglobin 14.0 g/dL.

8.   *Each option should be placed on a separate line for ease of student reading.* If answers are recorded on a separate answer sheet, the teacher should review the format of the sheet ahead of time so that responses are identified as "a" through "d" or 1 through 4 as appropriate.

9.   *Use the option of "call for assistance" sparingly.* Options that relate to getting assistance such as "notify the physician" or "call the supervisor" should be used sparingly because it is not known how they act as distractors in multiple-choice items. McDonald (2002) suggested that an option such as "call the physician" is not readily chosen by students and therefore may not be a good distractor unless it is the correct answer (p. 109). When it is the correct or best answer, the students would need to weigh that decision among the other options. However, some teacher-made tests may overuse this option as the correct answer, conditioning students to select it without considering the other alternatives.

Correct Answer. In a multiple-choice item there is one answer to be selected from among the alternatives. In some instances the best rather than the correct answer is chosen. Considering that judgments are needed to arrive at decisions about patient care, items can ask for the best or most appropriate response from those listed. Best answers are valuable for more complex and higher-level learning such as with questions written at the application and analysis levels. Even though best-answer items require a judgment to select the best option, there can be only one answer, and there should be consistency in the literature and among experts as to that response. A colleague can review the items, without knowing the answers in advance, to ensure that they are correct.

Listed below are suggestions for writing the correct answer. These suggestions are guided by the principle that the students should not be able to identify the correct response and eliminate distractors because of the way the stem or alternatives are written.

1.   *Review the alternatives carefully to ensure that there is only one correct response.* For example:

Symptoms of increased intracranial pressure include:

a.   blurred vision.*
b.   decreased blood pressure.
c.   disorientation.*
d.   increased pulse.

In this sample item, both "a" and "c" are correct; a possible revision follows:

Symptoms of increased intracranial pressure include:

a.   blurred vision and decreased blood pressure.
b.   decreased blood pressure and increased pulse.
c.   disorientation and blurred vision. *
d.   increased pulse and disorientation.

2.   *Review carefully terminology included in the stem to avoid giving a clue to the correct answer.* Key words in the stem, if also used in the correct response, may clue the student to select it. In the following example, "sudden weight loss" is in both the stem and the answer:

An elderly patient with *sudden weight loss,* thirst, and confusion is seen in the clinic. Which of the following signs would be indicative of dehydration?

a.   Below normal temperature
b.   Decreased urine specific gravity
c.   Increased blood pressure
d.   *Sudden weight loss**

The question could be revised by omitting "sudden weight loss" in the stem.

An elderly patient with dry skin, thirst, and confusion is seen in the clinic. Which of the following signs would also be indicative of dehydration?

a.   Below normal temperature
b.   Decreased urine specific gravity
c.   Increased blood pressure
d.   *Sudden weight loss**

3.   *The correct answer should be randomly assigned to a position among the alternatives to avoid favoring a particular response choice.* Some teachers may inadver-

tently assign the correct answer to the same option (e.g., "c"), or over a series of items, a pattern may develop from the placement of the correct answers (e.g., "a, b, c, d, a, b, c, d"). As indicated earlier in the discussion of how to write the options, this potential clue can be avoided by listing the alternatives in a logical or meaningful order such as alphabetical, numerical, or chronological. However, the teacher also should double check the position of the correct answers on a test to confirm that they are randomly distributed.

4. *The answers should not reflect the opinion of the teacher but instead be the ones with which experts agree or are the most probable responses.* The answers should be consistent with the literature and not be answers chosen arbitrarily by the teacher.

Distractors. Distractors are the incorrect but plausible options. Distractors should appeal to learners who lack the knowledge for responding to the question without confusing those who do know the content. If the option is obviously wrong, then there is no reason to include it as an alternative. Since the intent of the distractors is to distract the learners who have not mastered the content, at least some of the students should choose each option, or the distractors should be revised for the next administration of the test.

Each alternative should be appropriate for completing the stem. Hastily written distractors may be clearly incorrect, may differ in substance and format from the others, and may be inappropriate for the stem, providing clues as to how to respond. They also may result in a test item that does not measure the students' learning.

When writing a multiple-choice item, it is sometimes difficult to identify enough plausible distractors to have the same number of options for each item on the test. However, rather than using a filler, which is obviously incorrect or would not be seriously considered by the students, the teacher should use fewer options on that item. Nitko (2004) indicated that there is no rationale for using the same number of alternatives for each item on a test. The goal is to develop plausible and functional alternatives, ones that attract at least some of the students, rather than filler alternatives that no one chooses. Thus, for some items there may be only three alternatives, even though the majority of questions on that test use four. The goal, however, is to develop three plausible distractors so that most items have at least four responses from which to choose.

In writing distractors, it is helpful to think about common errors that students make, phrases that "sound correct," misperceptions students have about the content, and familiar responses not appropriate for the specific problem in the stem. Another way of developing distractors is to identify, before writing any of the options, the content area or domain to which all the responses must belong, e.g., all nursing interventions. If the stem asks about nursing measures for a patient with acute pneumonia, the distractors might be interventions for a patient with asthma that would not be appropriate for someone with pneumonia.

Terms used in the stem also give ideas for developing distractors. For example, if the stem asks about measures to avoid increasing anxiety in a patient who is delusional, the distractors may be interventions for a delusional patient that might inadvertently increase or have no effect on anxiety, or interventions useful for decreasing anxiety but not appropriate for a patient with a delusional disorder. Another strategy for developing distractors is to identify the category to which all alternative responses must belong. For a stem that asks about side effects of erythromycin, plausible distractors may be drawn from side effects of antibiotics as a group.

Suggestions for writing distractors include:

1. *The distractors should be consistent grammatically and should be similar in length, detail, and complexity with each other and the correct answer*. Examples were provided earlier in the chapter. The distractors should be written with the same specificity as the correct response. If the correct response is "quadratus plantae," distractors that are more general such as "motor" may be a clue not to choose that option.

2. *The distractors should sample the same content area as the correct answer*. When types of options vary, they may clue the student as to the correct response or to eliminate a particular distractor. In the following example, options "a", "b", and "c" pertain to factors in the work place. Because option "d" relates to diet, it may clue the student to omit it. A better alternative for "d" would be another factor to assess in the work setting such as how tiring the job is.

In planning teaching for a patient with a hiatal hernia, which of these factors should be assessed?

a.   Amount of lifting done at work *
b.   Number of breaks allowed
c.   Stress of the job
d.   Use of high-sodium foods

3. *Avoid using "all of the above" and "none of the above" in a multiple-choice item*. As distractors these are in contrast to the direction of selecting one correct or best response. With "all of the above" as a distractor, students aware of one incorrect response are clued to eliminate "all of the above" as an option. Similarly, knowledge of one correct alternative clues students to omit "none of the above" as an option. Often teachers resort to "all of the above" when unable to develop a fourth option, although it is better to rephrase the stem or to modify the options to provide fewer plausible alternatives.

McDonald (2002) suggested that the "none of the above" alternative was appropriate for multiple-choice items on calculations. By using "none of the above," the teacher avoids giving clues to students when their incorrect answer is not listed with the options (p. 113). In the following example the student would need to know the correct answer to identify that it is not among the alternatives:

> You are working in a pediatrician's office, and a mother calls and asks you how many drops of acetaminophen to give to her infant. The order is for 40 mg every 12 hours, but the container she has at home is 80 mg/0.8 mL. You should tell the mother to give:
>
> a.   1 dropperful
> b.   1 teaspoon
> c.   1.5 mL in a 3 mL syringe
> d.   None of the above *

4. *Omit terms such as always, never, sometimes, occasionally, and similar ones from the distractors.* These general terms often provide clues as to the correctness of the option. Mertler (2003) suggested that absolute terms such as always and never typically clue students that the options are incorrect because rarely does a situation occur always or never.

5. *Avoid using distractors that are essentially the same.* In the following example, alternatives "a" and "c" are essentially the same. If "rest" is eliminated as an option, the students are clued to omit both of these. In addition, the correct response in this item is more general than the others and is not specific to this particular student's health problems.

> A student comes to see the school nurse complaining of a severe headache and stiff neck. Which of the following actions would be most appropriate?
>
> a.   Ask the student to rest in the clinic for a few hours.
> b.   Collect additional data before deciding on interventions. *
> c.   Have a family member take the student home to rest.
> d.   Prepare to take the student to the emergency room.

The item could be revised as follows:

A student comes to see the school nurse complaining of a severe headache and stiff neck. Which of the following actions would be most appropriate?

a.   Ask the student to rest in the clinic for a few hours.
b.   Check the student's health record for identified health problems.*
c.   Prepare to take the student to the emergency room.
d.   Send the student back to class after medicating for pain.

Variation of Multiple-Choice Item

Mertler (2003) proposed a variation of the multiple-choice format that combined a multiple-choice item with short-answer or essay. In this format, after answering a multiple-choice item, students develop a rationale for why their answer is correct and the distractors are incorrect. For example:

Your patient is ordered 60 mg IM of morphine sulfate every 4 hours for pain. Which of the following actions should be taken?

a.   Administer 40 mg IM of morphine.
b.   Give the morphine as ordered.
c.   Have another RN review the order.
d.   Verify the order with the physician.*

In the space below, provide a rationale for why your answer is the best one and why the other options are not appropriate.

_____

_____

_____

MULTIPLE-RESPONSE

In multiple-response items several options may be correct, and students will choose the best combination of responses. Multiple-response items are now included on the NCLEX® Examination as one of the types of alternate item formats (National Council of State Boards of Nursing, 2004). The principles for writing multiple-response items are the same as for writing multiple-choice. Additional suggestions include:

1.   *The combination of alternatives should be plausible.* Options should be logically combined rather than grouped randomly.

2.   *The alternatives should be used a similar number of times in the combinations.*
If one of the alternatives is in every combination, it is obviously correct; this
information should be added to the stem as described earlier in the chapter.
Similarly, limited use of an option may provide a clue to the correct combination
of responses. After grouping responses, each letter should be counted to be sure
that it is used a similar number of times across combinations of responses and
that no letter is included in every combination.

3.   *The responses should be listed in a logical order, for instance, alphabetically
or sequentially, for ease in reviewing.* Alternatives are easier to review if shorter
combinations are listed before longer ones.

A sample item follows:

Causes of cataracts include:

1.   aging.
2.   arteriosclerosis.
3.   hemorrhage.
4.   iritis.
5.   steroid therapy.

    a.   1, 2
    b.   1, 5*
    c.   2, 4
    d.   1, 3, 4
    e.   2, 3, 5

On computerized tests, students may be asked to check off all of the responses
that apply. For example,

The preliminary diagnosis for your patient, a 20-year-old college student, is meningitis. Which signs and symptoms do you anticipate find-
ing? Select all that apply:

☐ 1.   Abdominal tenderness
☑ 2.   Fever
☐ 3.   Lack of pain with sudden head movements
☑ 4.   Nausea and vomiting
☑ 5.   Nuchal rigidity
☑ 6.   Sensitivity to light
☐ 7.   Sudden bruising in neck area

SUMMARY

This chapter has described the development of multiple-choice and multiple-response items. Multiple-choice questions, with one correct or best answer, are used widely in nursing and other fields. This test item format includes an incomplete statement or question, followed by a list of options that complete the statement or answer the question. Multiple-response items are designed similarly although more than one answer may be correct. Both of these item formats may be used for evaluating learning at the recall, comprehension, application, and analysis levels, making them adaptable for a wide range of content and learning outcomes.

Multiple-choice items are important for testing the application of nursing knowledge in simulated clinical situations and analytical thinking. Because of their versatility, they may be integrated easily within most testing situations.

There are three parts in a multiple-choice item, each with its own set of principles for development: (a) stem, (b) answer, and (c) distractors. The stem is the lead-in phrase in the form of a question or an incomplete statement that relies on the alternatives for completion. Following the stem is a list of alternatives, options for the learner to consider and choose from. These alternatives are of two types: the answer, which is the correct or best option to answer the question or complete the statement, and distractors, which are the incorrect yet plausible alternatives. Suggestions for writing each of these parts were presented in the chapter and were accompanied by sample items.

The ability to write multiple-choice items is an important skill for the teacher to develop. This is a situation in which "practice makes perfect." After writing an item, the teacher should have colleagues read it and make suggestions for revision. The teacher should also try out questions with students and maintain an electronic file of items for use in constructing tests. Although time-consuming to develop, multiple-choice items are an important means for evaluating learning in nursing.

REFERENCES

Gaberson, K. B. (1996). Test design: Putting all the pieces together. *Nurse Educator*, *21*(4), 28–33.

Haladyna, T. M. (2004). *Developing and validating multiple-choice test items* (3rd ed.). Mahwah, NJ: Lawrence Erlbaum.

Linn, R. L., & Gronlund, N. E. (2000). *Measurement and assessment in teaching* (8th ed.). Upper Saddle River, NJ: Prentice Hall.

McDonald, M. E. (2002). *Systematic assessment of learning outcomes: Developing multiple-choice exams*. Boston: Jones & Bartlett.

Mertler, C. A. (2003). *Classroom assessment*. Los Angeles: Pyrczak.

National Council of State Boards of Nursing. (2004). *Fast facts about alternate item formats and the NCLEX® examination*. Chicago: Author.

Nitko, A. J. (2004). *Educational assessment of students* (4th ed.). Upper Saddle River, NJ: Prentice Hall.

Chapter 6

Constructed-Response Test Items: Completion (Fill-in-the-Blank) and Essay

With constructed-response items, the test-taker supplies an answer rather than selecting from options already provided. Since students supply the answers, this type of item reduces the chance of guessing. Constructed-response items include completion and essay.

Completion items, or fill-in-the-blank, are test questions that can be answered by a word, phrase, or number. Short-answer items are similar to completion, but they typically ask a question that the student answer in a few words or phrases rather than by filling in the blank. In an essay item, the student develops a more extended response to a question. Essay tests and written assignments use writing as the means of expressing ideas although with essay items the focus of evaluation is the content of the answer rather than the writing ability. Completion, including the short-answer format, and essay items are described in this chapter.

COMPLETION

Completion, also referred to as fill-in-the-blank, and short-answer items can be answered by a word, phrase, or number. They are essentially the same type of test item except for format. Completion items consist of a statement with a key word or words missing; students fill in the blank to complete it. Other types of completion items ask students to perform a calculation and record the answer, or to order a list of responses.

Completion items are appropriate for recall of facts and specific information and for calculations. To complete the statement, the student recalls missing facts, such as a word or short phrase, or records the solution to a calculation problem. While completion items appear easy to construct, they should be designed in such a way that only one answer is possible. If students provide other correct answers, the teacher needs to accept them.

Fill-in-the-blank items are one of the alternate item formats used on the NCLEX® Examination. Items on the NCLEX may ask candidates to perform a calculation and type in the number or to put a list of responses in proper order (ordered response) (National Council of State Boards of Nursing, 2004). In ordered-response items, test-takers are given a list of words, phrases, and other alternatives and asked to place them in an appropriate order. For example, students might be given a list of Erikson's stages of development and asked to put them in the order they occur. On a computerized test, such as the NCLEX, candidates type in the order of responses. However, this same format can be used on a paper-and-pencil test with students writing the order on their test booklets or teacher-made answer sheets, or indicating it on a machine-scannable answer sheet.

The short-answer format includes a question that the student answers in a few words or phrases. Calculations may be included for the teacher to review the process that the student used to arrive at an answer. The questions or statements may stand alone and have no relationship to one another, or be a series of items in a similar content area.

Completion and short-answer items are useful for measuring student ability to interpret data, use formulas correctly, complete calculations, and solve mathematical-type problems. Items may ask students to label a diagram, name anatomical parts, identify various instruments, and label other types of drawings, photographs, and the like. Another type of short-answer item is called a list question that asks students to provide a complete or partial list of some content (Trice, 2000). For example, students might be asked to list Erikson's eight stages of psychosocial development in order.

Writing Completion and Short-Answer Items

Suggestions for developing completion and short-answer items are as follows:

1. *Questions and statements should not be taken verbatim from textbooks, other readings, and lecture notes.* These materials may be used as a basis for designing short-answer items, but taking exact wording from them may result in testing only recall of meaningless facts out of context. Such items measure memorization of content and may or may not be accompanied by student comprehension of it.

2. *Phrase the item so that a unique word, series of words, or number must be supplied to complete it.* Only one correct answer should be possible to complete the statement.

3.   *Write questions that are specific and can be answered in a few words, phrases, or short sentences.* The question "What is insulin?" does not provide sufficient direction as to how to respond; asking instead "What is the peak action time of NPH insulin?" results in a more specific answer.

4.   *Before writing the item, think of the correct answer first and then write a question or statement for that answer.* Although the goal is to develop an item with only one correct response, students may identify other correct answers. For this reason, develop a scoring sheet with all possible correct answers, and re-score student responses as needed if students provide additional correct answers that the teacher did not anticipate.

5.   *Fill-in-the-blank items requiring calculations and solving mathematical-type problems should include in the statement the type of answer and degree of specificity desired,* for instance, convert pounds to kilograms, rounding your answer to one decimal point.

6.   *For a statement with a key word or words missing, place the blank at the end of the statement.* This makes it easier for students to complete. It also is important to watch for grammatical clues in the statement, such as "a" versus "an" and singular versus plural, prior to the blank, which might give clues to the intended response. If more than one blank is included in the statement, they should be of equal lengths.

7.   *When students need to write longer answers, provide for sufficient space or use a separate answer sheet.* In some situations, longer responses might indicate that the item is actually an essay question, and the teacher then should follow principles for constructing and evaluating essay items.

8.   *Even though a blank space is placed at the end of the statement, the teacher may direct the student to record one-word answers in blanks arranged in a column to the left or right of the items, thereby facilitating scoring.* For example,

_____   1.   Streptococcus pneumoniae and Staphylococcus
                         aureus are examples of _____ bacteria.

Following are some examples of completion or fill-in-the-blank items:

Two types of metered-dose inhalers used for the treatment of bronchial asthma are:

_____

_____

List 3 methods of assessing patient satisfaction in an acute care setting.

1. _____
2. _____
3. _____

You are caring for a patient who weighs 128 lb. She is ordered 20 mcg/kg of an IV medication. What is the correct dose in micrograms?
Answer: _____

An example of a short-answer item, which differs slightly from the fill-in-the-blank by asking a question, is:

What congenital cardiac defect results in communication between the pulmonary artery and the aorta? _____

ESSAY ITEM

In an essay test, students construct responses to items based on their understanding of the content. With this type of test item, varied answers may be possible depending on the concepts selected by the student for discussion and the way in which they are presented. Essay items provide an opportunity for students to select content to discuss, present ideas in their own words, and develop an original and creative response to a question. This freedom of response makes essay items particularly useful for complex learning outcomes (Oermann, 1999). Higher-level responses, however, are more difficult to score than answers reflecting recall of facts.

Although some essay items are developed around recall of facts and specific information, they are more appropriate for higher levels of learning. Linn and Gronlund (2000) recommended that essay questions be used primarily for learning outcomes unable to be measured adequately through selected-response items. Essay items are effective for assessing students' ability to apply concepts, analyze theories, evaluate situations and ideas, and develop creative solutions to problems, drawing on multiple sources of information.

While essay items use writing as the medium for expression, the intent is to evaluate student understanding of specific content rather than judge writing ability in and of itself. Other types of assignments are better suited to evaluating the ability of students to write effectively; these are described in the next chapter. Low-level essay items are similar to short-answer and expect precise responses. An example of a low-level essay is "Describe three signs of increased intracranial pressure in children under 2 years old." Broader and higher-level essay items, however, do not limit responses in this way and differ clearly from short-answer items, such as "Defend the statement 'access to health care is a right.'"

Essay items may be written to evaluate a wide range of learning outcomes. These include:

- Comparing, such as comparing the side effects of two different medications

- Outlining steps to take and protocols to follow

- Explaining and summarizing in one's own words a situation or statement

- Discussing topics

- Applying concepts and principles to a clinical scenario and explaining their relevancy to it

- Analyzing patient data and clinical situations through use of relevant concepts and theories

- Critiquing different interventions and nursing management

- Developing plans and proposals drawing on multiple sources of information

- Analyzing nursing and health care trends

- Arriving at decisions about issues and actions to take accompanied by a rationale

- Analyzing ethical issues, possible decisions, and their consequences, and

- Developing arguments for and against a particular position or decision.

As with other types of test items, the objective or outcome to be evaluated provides the framework for developing the essay item. From the objective, the teacher develops a clear and specific question to elicit information about student achievement in terms of the content specified in the objective and the expected level of learning. If the outcome to be evaluated focuses on application of concepts to clinical practice, then the essay item should examine ability to apply knowledge to a clinical situation.

The question should be stated clearly so that the students know what they should write about. If it is ambiguous, the students will perceive the need to write all they know about a topic. The essay item, similar to other types of test items, should match the learning outcomes being assessed and be clearly phrased.

Issues with Essay Tests

Although essay items are valuable for examining the ability to select, organize, and present ideas and they provide an opportunity for creativity and originality in responding, they are limited by low reliability and other issues associated with their scoring. The teacher should have an understanding of these issues because they may influence the decision whether or not to use essay questions. Strategies are provided later in the chapter for addressing some of these issues.

Limited Ability to Sample Content

Essay items by their nature do not provide an efficient means of sampling course content in comparison with objective items. Considering the time it takes for students to formulate their thoughts and prepare an open-ended response, often only a few questions can be included on a test, particularly when the items are intended for assessing higher levels of learning. As a result, it is difficult to assess all of the different content areas in a nursing course using essay items. When the learning outcomes are memorization and recall of facts, essay items should not be used because there are more efficient means of measuring such outcomes. Instead, they should be developed for measuring complex outcomes requiring originality in responding (University of Illinois, 2002).

Unreliability in Scoring

The major limitation of essay items is the lack of consistency in evaluating responses. Scoring answers is a complex process, and teachers may be inconsistent in their evaluations of them (Airasian, 2000, 2001; Johnson & Johnson, 2002). Some teachers are more lenient or critical than others regardless of the criteria established for scoring. Even with preset criteria, teachers may evaluate answers differently, and scores may vary when the same teacher reads the paper again.

Factors such as misspelled words and grammar may affect scoring beyond the criteria to which they relate. Mertler (2003) suggested that there is a tendency to give lower scores for papers that have illegible writing, spelling errors, or poor grammar.

The unreliability with scoring, though, depends on the type of essay item. When the essay item is highly focused and structured, such as "List three side effects of bronchodilators," there is greater reliability in scoring. Of course, these lower-level items also could be classified as short-answer. Less restrictive essay items allowing for freedom and creativity in responding have lower rater reliability than more restricted ones. Questions asking students to analyze, defend, judge, evaluate, critique, and develop products are less reliable in terms of scoring the response. There are steps the teacher can take, though, to improve reliability, such as defining the content to be included in a "correct" answer and using a scoring rubric. These are presented later in the chapter.

Carryover Effects

Another issue in evaluating essay questions is a carryover effect where the teacher develops an impression of the quality of the answer from one item and carries it to the next. If the student answers one item well, the teacher may be influenced to score subsequent responses at a similarly high level; the same situation may occur with a poor response. For this reason, it is best to read all students' responses to one question before evaluating the next one. Oosterhof (2001) suggested that reading all the answers to one question at a time speeds up the evaluation, improves scoring accuracy by keeping the teacher focused on the standards, and reduces the chance of bias from scores of prior questions.

The same problem can occur with tests and written assignments. The teacher's impression of the student can carry over from one test to the next or from one paper to the next. When scoring essay tests and grading papers, the teacher should not know whose paper it is.

Halo Effect

There may be a tendency in evaluating essay questions to be influenced by a general impression of the student or feelings about the student, either positive or negative, that create a halo effect when judging the quality of the answers. For instance, the teacher may hold favorable opinions about the student from class or clinical practice and believe that this learner has made significant improvement in the course, which in turn might influence the scoring of responses. For this reason, essay tests should be scored anonymously by asking students to identify themselves by an assigned or selected number rather than by their names. Names can be matched with numbers after scoring is completed.

Effect of Writing Ability

It is difficult to evaluate student responses based on content alone even with clear and specific scoring guidelines. The teacher's judgment often is influenced by sentence structure, grammar, spelling, punctuation, and overall writing ability. Longer answers may be scored higher regardless of the content. Linn and Gronlund (2000) also noted that some students write well enough to bluff their answers. The teacher, therefore, needs to evaluate the *content* of the learner's response and not be influenced by the writing style. When writing also is evaluated, it should be scored separately.

Order-of-Scoring Effect

The order in which essay tests are read and scored influences the evaluation (Chase, 1999). Essay tests read early tend to be scored higher than those read near the end. As such, teachers should read papers in random order and read each response twice before computing a score. After reading and scoring all student answers to a question, the papers should be rearranged so that they are in a different order (Oosterhof, 2001).

Time

One other issue in using essay questions is the time it takes for students to answer them and for teachers to score them. In writing essay questions, the teacher should estimate how long it will take to answer each question, erring on allowing too much time rather than too little. Students should be told approximately how long to spend on each question so they can pace themselves (Linn & Gronlund, 2000).

Scoring essay items also can be a pressing issue for teachers, particularly if responsible for large numbers of students. Considering that responses should be read twice, in planning for essay tests consideration should be given to the time required by the teacher for scoring responses.

Scoring software is available that can scan an essay and, in a few seconds, identify what material the student has and has not learned (McCollum, 1998). One example is the Intelligent Essay Assessor™ that automatically evaluates and scores electronically submitted essays (Knowledge Analysis Technologies, 2002). It provides instant feedback on the content and quality of the essay using an algorithm called "latent semantic analysis." Nursing faculty need to assess, however, whether such software is appropriate for use in nursing courses and whether its use is cost effective.

Student Choice of Questions

Some essay tests allow students to choose a subset of questions to answer. This is often done because of limited time for testing and to provide options for students. For example, the teacher may include four questions on the care of patients with heart disease and ask students to answer two of them. However, Linn and Gronlund (2000) cautioned faculty against this because when students choose different items to answers, they are actually taking different tests; there is no guarantee that the same learning outcomes are being measured or that the complexity of the test is the same (p. 247).

Restricted-Response Essay Items

There are two types of essay items: restricted response and extended response. While the notion of freedom of response is inherent in essay items, there are varying degrees of this freedom in responding to the items. At one end of the continuum is the restricted-response item in which a few sentences are required for an answer. These are short-answer essays. At the other end is the extended-response item in which students have complete freedom of response, often requiring extensive writing (Oermann, 1999). Responses to essay items fall typically between these two extremes.

In a restricted-response item, the teacher limits the student's answer by indicating the content to be presented and frequently the amount of discussion allowed, for instance, limiting the response to one paragraph or page. With this type of essay item, the way in which the student responds is structured by the teacher. A restricted-response item may be developed by posing a specific problem to be addressed and asking questions about that problem (Linn & Gronlund, 2000). For example, specific material, such as patient data, a description of a clinical situation, research findings, a description of issues associated with clinical practice, and extracts from the literature, to cite a few, may be included with the essay item. Students read, analyze, and interpret this accompanying material, then answer questions about it (Nitko, 2004).

Examples of restricted response items follow:

- Define patient-focused care. Limit your definition to one paragraph.

- Select one environmental health problem and describe its potential effects on the community. Do not use an example presented in class. Limit your discussion to one page.

- Compare metabolic and respiratory acidosis. Include the following in your response: definitions, precipitating factors, clinical manifestations, diagnostic tests, and interventions.

- Your patient is 76 years old and 1 day postoperative following a femoral popliteal bypass graft. Name two complications the patient could experience at this time and discuss why they are potential problems. List four nursing interventions for this patient during the initial recovery period and supporting rationale for each.

- Describe five physiological changes associated with the aging process.

Along a similar line, Curran and Takata (2001) proposed the guided essay examination. With this format, students are given a basic outline to follow for answering the essay question. The outline includes key concepts with spaces to write in so that the students do not have to start out with a blank sheet of paper.

Extended-Response Essay Items

Extended-response essay items are less restrictive and as such provide an opportunity for students to choose concepts for responding, organize ideas in their own ways, arrive at judgments about the content, and demonstrate ability to communicate ideas effectively in writing. With these items, the teacher may evaluate students' ability to develop their own ideas and express them creatively, integrate learning from multiple sources in responding, and evaluate the ideas of others based on predetermined criteria. Since responses are not restricted by the teacher, evaluation is more difficult. This difficulty, however, is balanced by the opportunity students have to express their own ideas. As such, essay questions provide a means of evaluating more complex learning not possible with selected-response items. The teacher may decide to allow students to respond to these items outside of class.

Sample items include:

- Select an article describing a nursing research study. Critique the study, specifying the criteria used. Based on your evaluation, describe whether or not the research is of value to nursing practice.

- In the clinic you note that patients who are uninsured receive fewer diagnostic examinations and less comprehensive care than patients with similar health problems who are insured. Analyze these differences in care and related issues.

- Develop a plan for saving costs in the wound clinic.

- You receive a call in the allergy clinic from a mother who describes her son's problems as "having stomach pains" and "acting out in school." She asks you if these problems may be due to his allergies. How would you respond to this mother? How would you manage this call? Include a rationale for your response.

- You are caring for a child diagnosed recently with acute lymphocytic leukemia who lives with his parents and two teenage sisters. Describe how the family health and illness cycle would provide a framework for assessing this family and planning care.

Writing Essay Items

Essay items should be reserved for learning outcomes that cannot be measured effectively through multiple-choice and other selected-response formats. With essays, students can demonstrate their critical thinking, ability to integrate varied sources of information, and creativity. Suggestions for writing essay items follow.

1. *Develop essay items that require synthesis of the content.* Avoid items that students can answer by merely summarizing the readings and class discussions without thinking about the content and applying it to new situations. Evaluating students' recall of facts and specific information may be accomplished more easily using selected-response formats rather than essay.

2. *Phrase items clearly.* The item should direct learners in their responses and should not be ambiguous. Table 6.1 provides sample stems for essay questions based on varied types of learning outcomes. Framing the item to make it as specific as possible is accomplished more easily with restricted-response items. With extended-response items, directions as to the type of response intended may be provided without limiting the student's own thinking about the answer. In example 1, there is minimal guidance as to how to respond; the revised version, however, directs students more clearly as to the intended response without limiting their freedom of expression and originality.

Example 1: Evaluate an article describing a nursing research study.

Revised Version: Select an article describing a nursing research study. Critique the study, specifying the criteria you used to evaluate it. Based on your evaluation, describe whether or not the research provides evidence for nursing practice. Include a rationale supporting your decision.

3. *Prepare students for essay tests.* This can be done by asking thought-provoking questions in class; engaging students in critical discussions about the content; and teaching students how to apply concepts and theories to clinical situations, compare approaches, and arrive at decisions and judgments about patients and issues. Practice in synthesizing content from different sources, presenting ideas logically, and using creativity in responding to situations will help students prepare to respond to essay items in a testing situation. This practice may be through class and clinical discussions, written assignments, and small-group activities. For students lacking experience with essay tests, sample items may be used for formative purposes, providing feedback to students about the adequacy of their responses.

4. *Tell students about apportioning their time to allow sufficient time for answering each essay item.* In writing a series of essay questions, consider carefully the

TABLE 6.1   Sample Stems for Essay Items

Comparing

Compare the side effects of . . . methods for . . . interventions for . . .
Describe similarities and differences between . . .
What do . . . have in common?
Group these medications . . . signs and symptoms . . .

Outlining Steps

Describe the process for . . . procedure for . . . protocol to follow for . . .
List steps in order for . . .

Explaining and Summarizing

Explain the importance of . . . relevance of . . .
Identify and discuss . . .
Explain the patient's responses within the framework of . . .
Provide a rationale for . . .
Discuss the most significant points of . . .
Summarize the relevant data.
What are the major causes of . . . reasons for . . . problems associated with . . .
Describe the potential effects of . . . possible responses to . . . problems that might re-
    sult from . . .

Applying Concepts and Theories to a Situation

Analyze the situation using . . . theory/framework.
Using the theory of . . . , explain the patient's/family's responses.
Identify and discuss . . . using relevant concepts and theories.
Discuss actions to take in this situation and theoretical basis.
Describe a situation that demonstrates the concept of . . . principle of . . . theory of . . .

Analyzing

Discuss the significance of . . .
Identify relevant and irrelevant data with supporting rationale.
Identify and describe additional data needed for decision making.
Describe competing nursing diagnoses with rationale.
What hypotheses may be made?
Compare nursing interventions drawing upon research.
Describe multiple nursing interventions for this patient with supporting rationale.
Provide a rationale for . . .
Critique the nurse's responses to this patient.
Describe errors in assumptions made about . . . errors in reasoning . . .
Analyze the situation and describe alternate actions possible.
Identify all possible decisions, consequences of each, your decision, and supporting
    rationale.

TABLE 6.1   *(continued)*

Developing Plans and Proposals

Develop a plan for . . . discharge plan . . . teaching plan . . .
Develop a proposal for . . . protocol for . . .
Based on the theory of . . . , develop a plan for . . . proposal for . . .
Develop a new approach for . . . method for . . .
Design multiple interventions for . . .

Analyzing Trends and Issues

Identify one significant trend/issue in health care and describe implications for nursing
   practice.
Analyze this issue and implications for . . .
In light of these trends, what changes would you propose?
Critique the nurse's/physician's/patient's decisions in this situation. What other ap-
   proaches are possible? Why?
Analyze the ethical issue facing the nurse. Compare multiple decisions possible and
   consequences of each. Describe the decision you would make and why.
Identify issues for this patient/family/community and strategies for resolving them.

Stating Positions

What would you do and why?
Identify your position about . . . and defend it.
Develop an argument for . . . and against . . .
Develop a rationale for . . .
Do you support this position? Why or why not?
Do you agree or disagree with . . . Include a rationale.
Specify the alternative actions possible. Which of these alternatives would be most
   appropriate and why? What would you do and why?

time needed for students to answer them and inform students of the estimated
time before they begin the examination. In this way students may gauge their
time appropriately. Indicating the point value of each essay item also will guide
students to use their time appropriately, spending more time on and writing
longer responses to items that carry greater weight.

   5. *Score essay items that deal with the analysis of issues according to the rationale
that students develop rather than the position they take on the issue.* Students should
provide a sound rationale for their position, and the evaluation should focus on
the rationale rather than on the actual position.

   6. *Avoid the use of optional items and student choice of items to answer.*
As indicated previously, this results in different subsets of tests that may not
be comparable.

7. *In the process of developing the item, write an ideal answer to it.* This should be done while drafting the item to determine if it is appropriate, clearly stated, and reasonable to answer in the allotted time frame. Save this ideal answer for use later in scoring students' responses.

8. *If possible, have a colleague review the item and explain how he or she would respond to it.* Colleagues can assess the clarity of the question and whether it will elicit the intended response.

Scoring Essay Items: Holistic Versus Analytic

There are two methods of scoring essay items: holistic and analytic. The holistic method involves reading the entire answer to each question and evaluating its overall quality (Oosterhof, 2001, p. 110). With the analytic method of scoring, the teacher scores separately individual components of the answer.

Holistic Scoring

With holistic scoring, the teacher evaluates and scores the essay response as a whole without judging each part separately. There are different ways of scoring essays using the holistic method. One way is to compare each student's answer with the responses of others in the group, a relative standard. To score essay questions using this system, the teacher reads quickly the answers to each question to gain a sense of how the students responded overall, then re-reads the answers and scores them. Papers may be placed in a number of piles reflecting degrees of quality with each pile of papers receiving a particular score or grade.

Another way is to develop a model answer for each question and then compare each student's response to that model. This helps clarify the characteristics of the answers expected for each question (Oosterhof, 2001). Before using a model answer for scoring responses, teachers should read a few papers to confirm that students' answers are consistent with what was intended.

Holistic Scoring Rubric.   A third way of implementing holistic scoring is to use a scoring rubric, which is a guide for scoring essays, papers, written assignments, and other open-ended responses of students. Rubrics also can be used for grading posters, concept maps, presentations, and projects competed by students. The rubric consists of predetermined criteria used for evaluating the quality of the student's work (Mertler, 2003). With holistic scoring, the rubric includes descriptions for different levels of quality (Oosterhof, 2001; Trice, 2000). The student's answer is assigned the score associated with the one description within the rubric that best reflects its quality and therefore its score. The important concept in this method is that holistic scoring yields one overall score that considers the entire response to the question rather than scoring its component parts separately (Linn & Gronlund, 2000; Nitko, 2004).

Holistic rubrics are quicker to use for scoring because the teacher evaluates the overall response rather than each part of it. One disadvantage, though, is that they do not provide students with specific feedback about their answer. An example of a holistic scoring rubric for an essay item is in Table 6.2.

Analytic Scoring

In the analytic method of scoring, the teacher identifies the content that should be included in the answer and other characteristics of an ideal response. Each of these areas is evaluated and scored separately. Often a detailed scoring plan is used that lists content to be included in the answer and other characteristics of the response to be judged. The scoring plan is similar to a checklist (Oosterhof, 2001). Students accumulate points based on how well they address each content area and the other characteristics, not their overall response. This method of scoring is effective for essay items that require structured answers (Mertler, 2003).

Analytic Scoring Rubric.   A scoring rubric also can be developed with points assigned for each of the content areas that should be included in the response

TABLE 6.2   Example of Holistic Scoring Rubric for Essay Item on Health Care Issue

Score	Description
4	Presents thorough analysis of health care issue considering its complexities. Considers multiple perspectives in analysis. Analysis reflects use of theories and research. Discussion is well organized and supports analysis.
3	Analyzes health care issue. Considers different perspectives in analysis. Analysis reflects use of theories but not research. Discussion is organized and logical.
2	Describes health care issue but does not consider its complexities nor different perspectives. Basic analysis of issue with limited use of theory. Discussion accurate but limited.
1	Does not clearly describe health care issue. No alternate perspectives considered. Limited analysis with no relevant theory or literature to support ideas. Errors in answer.
0	Does not identify the health care issue. No application of theory to understand issue. Errors in answer. Off-topic.

and other characteristics to be evaluated. An analytic scoring rubric provides at least two benefits in evaluating essays and written work. First, it guides the teacher in judging the extent to which specified criteria have been met. Second, it provides feedback to students about how to improve their performance (Moskal, 2000). An example of an analytic scoring rubric for the same essay item is found in Table 6.3.

There are many Web sites to assist faculty in creating and using rubrics for evaluating student learning. Although most of these pertain to general education, the information can be adapted easily for assessment in nursing courses. Schrock (2003) has developed a valuable web site with many links on rubrics.

TABLE 6.3 Example of Analytic Scoring Rubric for Essay Item on Health Care Issue

Score	Analysis of Issue	Multiple Perspectives	Theory and Research	Presentation
4	Presents thorough analysis of health care issue considering its complexities	Considers multiple perspectives in analysis	Uses theories and research as basis for analysis	Discussion well organized and supports analysis. Logical
3	Analyzes health care issue	Considers a few varying perspectives	Uses theories in analysis but no research	Discussion organized and logical
2	Describes health care issue but does not consider its complexities	Describes one perspective without considering other points of view	Reports basic analysis of issue with limited use of theory	Discussion accurate but limited
1	Does not clearly describe health care issue	Considers no alternative perspectives	Presents limited analysis with no relevant theories nor literature to support ideas	Discussion has errors in content
0	Does not identify health care issue	Considers no alternative perspectives	Does not apply any theories in discussion	Discussion has errors in content. May be off-topic

Score

Mean Score _____

CRITERIA FOR EVALUATING ESSAY ITEMS

The criteria for evaluating essay items, regardless of the method, often address three areas: (a) content, (b) organization, and (c) process. Questions that guide evaluation of each of these areas are:

- Content: Is relevant content included? Is it accurate? Are significant concepts and theories presented? Are hypotheses, conclusions, and decisions supported? Is the answer comprehensive?

- Organization: Is the answer well organized? Are the ideas presented clearly? Is there a logical sequence of ideas?

- Process: Was the process used to arrive at conclusions, actions, approaches, and decisions logical? Were different possibilities and implications considered? Was a sound rationale developed using relevant literature and theories?

Suggestions for Scoring

1. *Identify the method of scoring to be used prior to the testing situation* and inform the students of it.

2. *Specify in advance an ideal answer.* In constructing this ideal answer, review readings, classroom discussions of the content, and other instructional activities completed by students. Identify content and characteristics required in the answer and assign points to them if using the analytic method of scoring.

3. *If using a scoring rubric, discuss it with the students ahead of time* so that they are aware of how their essay responses will be judged.

4. *Read a random sample of papers* to get a sense of how the students approached the items and an idea of the overall quality of the answers.

5. *Score the answers to one item at a time.* For example, read and score all of the students' answers to the first question before proceeding to the second question. This procedure enables the teacher to compare responses to an item across students, resulting in more accurate and fairer scoring, and saves time by only needing to keep in mind one ideal answer at a time (Linn & Gronlund, 2000).

6. *Read each answer twice before scoring.* In the first reading, note omissions of major points from the ideal answer, errors in content, problems with

organization, and problems with the process used for responding. Record corrections or comments on the students' paper. After reading through all the answers to the question, begin the second reading for scoring purposes.

7. *Read papers in random order.*

8. *Use the same scoring system for all papers.*

9. *Essay answers and other written assignments should be read anonymously.* Develop a system for implementing this in the nursing program, for instance, by asking the students to choose a code number.

10. *Cover the scores of the previous answers* to avoid being biased about the student's ability.

11. *For important decisions or if unsure about the evaluation, have a colleague read and score the answers* to improve reliability. A sample of answers might be independently scored rather than the complete set of student tests.

12. *Adopt a policy on writing* (sentence structure, spelling, punctuation, grammar, neatness, and writing style in general) and if it will be scored. Inform students of the policy in advance of the test. If writing is evaluated, then it should be scored separately, and the teacher should be cautious not to let the writing style bias the evaluation of content and other characteristics of the response.

SUMMARY

Completion items consist of a statement with a key word or words missing; students then fill in the blank to complete the statement. The short-answer format, which is similar, consists of a question that the student answers. These items are appropriate for recall of facts and specific information. With short-answer items, students can be asked to interpret data, use formulas, complete calculations, and solve mathematical-type problems.

In an essay test, students construct responses to items based on their understanding of the content. With this type of test item, varied answers may be possible depending on the concepts selected by the student for discussion and the way in which they are presented. Essay items provide an opportunity for students to select content to discuss, integrate concepts from various sources, present ideas in their own words, and develop original and creative responses to items. This freedom of response makes essay items particularly useful for complex learning outcomes.

There are two types of essay items: restricted response and extended response. In a restricted-response item, the teacher limits the student's answer by indicating the content to be presented and frequently the amount of discussion allowed, for instance, limiting the response to one paragraph or page. In an extended-response item, students have complete freedom of response, often requiring extensive writing. While essay items use writing as the medium for expression, the intent is to evaluate student understanding of specific content rather than judge the writing ability in and of itself. Other types of assignments are better suited to evaluating the ability of students to write effectively.

REFERENCES

Airasian, P. W. (2000). *Assessment in the classroom: A concise approach* (2nd ed.). Boston: McGraw-Hill.

Airasian, P. W. (2001). *Classroom assessment: Concepts and applications* (4th ed.). Boston: McGraw-Hill.

Chase, C. I. (1999). *Contemporary assessment for educators*. New York: Longman.

Curran, J., & Takata, S. R. (2001). *Review and teaching essay*. Retrieved January 17, 2003, from http://www.habermas.org/tchessay72.htm#guided

Johnson, D. W., & Johnson, R. T. (2002). *Meaningful assessment: A manageable and cooperative process*. Boston: Allyn & Bacon.

Knowledge Analysis Technologies. (2002). *Introducing the Intelligent Essay Assessor*™. Boulder, CO: Knowledge Analysis Technologies. Retrieved January 15, 2003, from http://www.knowledge-technologies.com/

Linn, R. L., & Gronlund, N. E. (2000). *Measurement and assessment in teaching* (8th ed.). Upper Saddle River, NJ: Prentice Hall.

McCollum, K. (1998). How a computer program learns to grade essays. *The Chronicle of Higher Education*. Retrieved January 15, 2003, from http://www.ou.edu/archives/it-fyi/0346.html

Mertler, C. A. (2003). *Classroom assessment*. Los Angeles: Pyrczak.

Moskal, B. M. (2000). Scoring rubrics: What, when and how? *Practical assessment, research and evaluation, 7*(3). Retrieved January 13, 2003, from http://ericae.net/pare/getvn.asp?v=7&n=3

National Council of State Boards of Nursing. (2004). *Fast facts about alternate item formats and the NCLEX® examination*. Chicago: Author.

Nitko, A. J. (2004). *Educational assessment of students* (4th ed.). Upper Saddle River, NJ: Prentice Hall.

Oermann, M. H. (1999). Developing and scoring essay tests. *Nurse Educator, 24*(2), 29–32.

Oosterhof, A. (2001). *Classroom applications of educational measurement* (3rd ed.). Upper Saddle River, NJ: Prentice Hall.

Schrock, K. (2003). *Assessment and rubric information*. DiscoverySchool.com. Retrieved January 20, 2003, from http://www.school.discovery.com/schrockguide/assess.html#web

Trice, A. D. (2000). *A handbook of classroom assessment*. New York: Longman.

University of Illinois. (2002). *Improving your test questions*. Division of Measurement and Evaluation, Office of Instructional Resources, University of Illinois at Urbana-Champaign. Retrieved January 24, 2003, from http://www.oir.uiuc.edu/dme/exams/itq.html#sec25

Chapter 7

Evaluation of Higher-Level Learning, Problem Solving, and Critical Thinking: Context-Dependent Item Sets and Other Evaluation Strategies

In preparing students to meet the needs of patients within the changing health care system, educators are faced with identifying essential content to teach in the nursing program. Mastery of this knowledge alone is not enough, however. Students also need to develop cognitive skills for processing and analyzing information, comparing different approaches, weighing alternatives, and arriving at sound conclusions and decisions. These cognitive skills include, among others, the ability to apply concepts and theories to new situations, problem solving, and critical thinking. The purpose of this chapter is to present strategies for evaluating these higher levels of learning in nursing.

HIGHER-LEVEL LEARNING

One of the concepts presented in Chapter 1 was that learning outcomes can be organized in a cognitive hierarchy or taxonomy, with each level representing more complex learning than the previous. Learning extends from simple recall and comprehension, which are lower-level cognitive behaviors, to higher-level thinking skills. Higher-level cognitive skills include application, analysis, synthesis, and evaluation. With higher-level thinking, students apply concepts, theories, and other forms of knowledge to new situations, use that knowledge to solve patient and other types of problems, and arrive at rational and well-thought-out decisions about actions to take.

The main principle in evaluating higher-level learning is to develop test items and other evaluation strategies that require students to apply knowledge and skills in a *new* situation (Nitko, 2004). Only then can the teacher assess if the students are able to use what they have learned in a different context. Considering that patients and treatments often do not match the textbook descriptions, and health status can change quickly, students need to develop their ability to think through clinical situations and arrive at the best possible decisions. By introducing novel materials into the evaluation process, the teacher can assess whether the students have developed these cognitive skills.

PROBLEM SOLVING

In the practice setting, students are continually faced with patient and other problems to be solved. Some of these problems relate to managing patient conditions and deciding what actions to take, while others involve problems associated with one's role and work environment. The ability to solve patient and setting-related problems is an essential skill to be developed and evaluated. Problem solving begins with recognizing and defining the problem, gathering data to clarify it further, developing solutions, and evaluating their effectiveness. Knowledge about the problem and potential solutions influences the problem-solving process. Students faced with patient problems for which they lack understanding and a relevant knowledge base will be impeded in their thinking. This is an important point in both teaching and evaluating problem solving. When students have an understanding of the problem and possible solutions, they can apply this knowledge and expertise to new situations they encounter in the clinical setting.

Past experience with similar problems, either real problems in the clinical setting or hypothetical ones used in teaching, also influences students' skill in problem solving. Experience with similar problems gives the student a perspective on what to expect in the clinical situation—typical problems the patient may experience and approaches that are usually effective for those problems. Expert nurses and beginners, such as students, approach patient problems differently (Benner, 2001). As a result of their extensive clinical experience, experts view the clinical situation as a whole and use their past experience with similar patients as a framework for approaching new problems.

Cognitive Development

Problem-solving skill is influenced in general by the student's level of cognitive development. Perry's (1970, 1981) theory of cognitive development suggests that students progress in their thinking through these four stages:

- *Dualism:* In this first stage, students view knowledge and values as absolutes. In terms of problem solving, they look for one problem with accepted solutions from their readings and prior learning. At this stage, students do not consider the possibility of different problems and varied solutions to them.

- *Multiplicity:* In the second stage, students are willing to acknowledge that the problems may be different from the first ones identified and that varied solutions may be possible. They begin to accept the notion that multiple points of view are possible in a given situation. In this stage, learners are able to see shades of gray rather than only "black and white."

- *Relativism:* In the third stage, which is relativism, students possess the cognitive ability and willingness to evaluate different points of views. At this stage in their cognitive development, students have progressed in their thinking to where they can evaluate varying perspectives and approaches relative to one another.

- *Commitment in Relativism:* Perry's final stage of cognitive development reflects a commitment to identify one's values and beliefs and to act on them in practice.

Perry's original studies were done with male students attending Harvard, and although further work by other researchers has broadened the sample, more study is indicated. Even so, his theory provides a way to view the development of cognitive skills among nursing students. Skill in problem solving and critical thinking may reflect the student's stage of cognitive development. Complexity of thinking and problem solving, acceptance of multiple perspectives, and ability to deal with ambiguity, which are important in critical thinking, occur at later stages of cognitive development.

Well-Structured and Ill-Structured Problems

Nitko (2004) defined two types of problems that students may be asked to solve: well-structured and ill-structured. Well-structured problems provide the information needed for problem solving, typically have one correct solution rather than multiple ones to consider, and in general are "clearly laid out" (p. 208). These are problems and solutions that the teacher may have presented in class and then asked students about in an evaluation. Well-structured problems provide practice in applying concepts and theories learned in class to hypothetical situations but do not require extensive critical thinking skills.

In contrast, ill-structured problems reflect real-life problems and clinical situations faced by students. With these situations, the problem may not be clear to the learner, different problems may be possible given the data, or there may be an incomplete data set to determine the problem. Along a similar line, the student may identify the problem but be unsure of the approaches to take; multiple solutions may also be possible. Some evaluation strategies for problem solving address well-structured problems, assessing understanding of typical problems and solutions. Other evaluation methods assess students' ability to analyze situations to identify different problems possible given the data, identify additional data needed to decide on a particular problem, compare and evaluate multiple approaches, and arrive at an informed decision as to actions to take in the situation.

Decision Making

Nurses continually make decisions about patient care—decisions about problems, solutions, other approaches that might be possible, and the best approach to use in a particular situation. Other decisions are needed for delivering care, managing the clinical environment, and carrying out other activities.

In decision making, the learner arrives at a decision after considering a number of alternatives and weighing the consequences of each. The decision reflects a choice after considering these different possibilities. In making this choice, the student collects and analyzes information relevant to identifying the problem and making a decision, compares the decisions possible in that situation, and then decides on the best strategy or approach to use. Critical thinking helps students compare alternatives and decide what actions to take.

CRITICAL THINKING

There has been extensive literature in nursing over the last decade about the importance of students developing the ability to think critically. The complexity of patient, family, and community needs; the amount of information the nurse needs to process in the practice setting; the types of decisions required for care and supervising of others in the delivery of care; and multiple ethical issues faced by the nurse require the ability to think critically. Critical thinking is needed to make reasoned and informed judgments in the practice setting; by using critical thinking, the nurse decides what to do or believe in a given situation. Critical thinking is particularly important when problems are unclear and have more than one possible solution. Ennis (1985) provided an early definition of critical thinking that remains valid today. He defined critical thinking as reflective and reasoned thinking that focuses on deciding what actions to take and what to believe in a situation.

There are eight elements of reasoning to be considered in the process of critical thinking:

1.   Purpose the thinking is to serve

2.   Question, issue, or problem to be resolved

3.   Assumptions on which thinking is based

4.   Analysis of own point of view and those of others

5.   Data, information, and evidence on which to base reasoning

6.   Concepts and theories for use in thinking

7.   Inferences and conclusions possible given the data, and

8.   Implications and consequences of reasoning (Paul, 2003; Paul & Elder, 2003).

These elements of reasoning may be used as a framework for evaluating students' critical thinking in nursing. Sample questions the teacher can use for assessing students' critical thinking are presented in Table 7.1.

In the clinical setting, critical thinking enables the student to arrive at sound and rational decisions to carry out patient care. Carrying out assessment; planning care; intervening with patients, families, and communities; and evaluating the effectiveness of interventions require critical thinking. In the assessment process, important cognitive skills include differentiating relevant from irrelevant data, identifying cues in the data and clustering them, identifying what additional data to collect prior to arriving at decisions about the problem, and specifying patient problems and nursing diagnoses based on these data. The ability to generate competing diagnoses and to evaluate each one is another important skill. Critical thinking also is reflected in the ability to compare different possible approaches, considering the consequences of each, and arrive at a decision as to nursing measures and approaches to use in a particular situation (Oermann, 1997, 1998). Judgments about the quality and effectiveness of care are influenced by the learner's critical thinking skill. It is through critical thinking that the student begins to consider and evaluate multiple perspectives to care.

Students who demonstrate critical thinking ability:

•   ask questions in class and clinical practice

•   are inquisitive and willing to search for answers

TABLE 7.1   Sample Questions for Evaluating Critical Thinking

---

Purpose of Critical Thinking

Is the student's purpose (e.g., in a discussion, a research paper, an essay, a care plan, and so forth) clear?

Can the student state the goals to be achieved as a result of the critical thinking?

Does the student use this purpose and these goals to stay focused?

Are the student's goals realistic and attainable?

Issue or Problem to Be Resolved

Does the student clarify the issue or problem to be resolved?

How does the student go about analyzing the issue or problem?

Does the student ask probing questions and focus on important issues and problems?

Are the questions relevant to resolving the issue or problem and unbiased?

Does the student recognize questions she or he is unable to answer and seek information independently for answering them?

Assumptions on Which Thinking Is Based

Does the student make assumptions that are clear? Reasonable? Consistent with one another?

Does the student question assumptions underlying own thinking?

Analysis of Own Point of View and Those of Others

Does the student keep in mind different points of view?

Does the student realize that people approach situations, questions, issues, and problems differently?

Does the student consider multiple perspectives?

Does the student have a broad point of view about issues and problems rather than a narrow perspective?

Is the student able to recognize own biases, values, and beliefs that influence thinking?

Does the student actively seek others' points of view?

Information and Evidence on Which to Base Reasoning

Does the student collect relevant data and evidence on which to base thinking?

Does the student search for information for and against own position and critically analyze both sets of data?

Can the student differentiate relevant and irrelevant information for the question, issue, or problem at hand?

Does the student avoid drawing conclusions beyond the information and evidence available to support them?

Does the student present clear and accurate data and evidence on which own thinking is based?

TABLE 7.1 *(continued)*

Concepts and Theories for Use in Thinking

Does the student apply relevant concepts and theories for understanding and analyzing the question, issue, or problem?
Is the student unbiased in presentation of ideas and thinking?
Does the student recognize implications of words used in presenting ideas?

Inferences and Conclusions

Does the student make clear and precise inferences?
Does the student clarify conclusions and make the reasoning easy to follow?
Does the student draw conclusions based on the evidence and reasons presented?
Are the conclusions consistent with one another?

Implications and Consequences of Reasoning

Does the student identify a number of significant implications of own thinking?
Does the student identify different courses of action and consequences of each?
Does the student consider both positive and negative consequences?

Adapted from: Paul, R. (2003). Using intellectual standards to assess student reasoning. Retrieved August 11, 2003, from http://www.criticalthinking.org/k12/k12class/using.html Adapted with permission of the Foundation for Critical Thinking www.criticalthinking.org, 2005.

- consider alternate ways of viewing information

- offer different perspectives to problems and solutions

- question current practices and express their own ideas about care

- extend their thinking beyond the readings, class instruction, clinical activities, and other requirements, and

- are open-minded.

These characteristics are important because they suggest behaviors to be developed by students as they progress through the nursing program. They also provide a framework for faculty to use when evaluating whether students have developed their critical thinking abilities.

CONTEXT-DEPENDENT ITEM SETS

In assessing students' cognitive skills, the test items and evaluation methods need to meet two criteria. They should (a) introduce *new* information not encountered by students at an earlier point in the instruction and (b) provide data on the thought process used by students to arrive at an answer, rather than the answer alone. Context-dependent item sets may be used for this purpose. Other evaluation methods include case method, case study, and unfolding case; discussion; debate; media clips; short written assignments; and varied clinical evaluation methods that are presented in chapter 13.

Writing Context-Dependent Item Sets

A basic principle in evaluating higher-level skills is that the test item or evaluation method has to introduce new or novel material for analysis. Without the introduction of new material as part of the evaluation, students may have memorized from prior discussion or their readings how to problem solve and arrive at decisions for the situation at hand; they may recall the typical problem and solutions without thinking through other possibilities themselves. In nursing education this principle is usually implemented through clinical scenarios that present a novel situation for students to apply concepts and theories, problem solve, arrive at decisions, and in general, engage in critical thinking. Nitko (2004) referred to these items as context-dependent item sets or interpretative exercises.

In a context-dependent item set, the teacher presents introductory material that students then analyze and answer questions about. The introductory material may be a description of a clinical situation, patient data, research findings, issues associated with clinical practice, and varied types of scenarios. The introductory material also may include diagrams, photographs, tables, figures, and excerpts from reading materials. Students read, analyze, and interpret the introductory material and then answer questions about it or complete other tasks. One advantage of a context-dependent item set is the opportunity to present new information for student analysis that is geared toward clinical practice. In addition, the introductory material provides the same context for problem solving, decision making, and critical thinking for all students (Nitko, 2004).

The questions asked about the introductory material may be selected- or constructed-response items. With selected-response items such as multiple-choice, however, the teacher is not able to assess the underlying thought process used by students in arriving at the answer; their responses reflect instead the outcomes of their thinking. If the intent is also to assess the thought process, then open-ended items such as short-answer and essay should be used.

Interpretive Items on the NCLEX®

On the NCLEX® Examination, candidates may be asked to interpret tables, figures, graphs, diagrams, and images, and to respond to questions about them using the standard multiple-choice format or alternate formats such as multiple-response or fill-in-the-blank (National Council of State Boards of Nursing, 2004). The NCLEX also has hot-spot items in which candidates identify an area on an image. Students should have experience answering these types of questions and other forms of context-dependent items as they progress through a nursing program. Items can be incorporated into quizzes and tests; can be developed for small group analysis and discussion in class, as out-of-class assignments, and as online activities; and can be analyzed and discussed by students in post-clinical conferences.

Layout

The layout of the context-dependent item set, i.e., the way it is arranged on the page, is important so that it is clear to the students which questions relate to the introductory material. Table 7.2 illustrates one way of arranging the material and related items on a page.

A heading should be used to indicate the items that pertain to the introductory material, for example, "Questions 1 through 3 refer to the scenario below." Nitko (2004) suggested that the material for interpretation be placed in the center of the page so that it is readily apparent to the students. If possible, the context and all items pertaining to it should be placed on the same page.

Strategies for Writing Context-Dependent Items

Suggestions follow for writing context-dependent item sets. The examples in this chapter are designed for paper-and-pencil testing; however, the scenarios and other types of introductory material for analysis may be presented through multimedia, computer-assisted instruction, interactive video, and other types of instructional technology.

TABLE 7.2   Layout of Context-Dependent Item Sets

Questions 1 through 3 relate to the scenario below.

Scenario (and other types of introductory material) here

1.   Item 1 here
2.   Item 2 here
3.   Item 3 here

If the intent is to evaluate students' skills in problem solving and critical thinking, the introductory material needs to provide sufficient information for analysis without directing the students' thinking in a particular direction. The first step is to draft the types of questions to be asked about the situation, then to develop a scenario to provide essential information for analysis. If the scenario is designed around clinical practice, students may be asked to analyze data, identify patient problems, decide on nursing interventions, evaluate outcomes of care, and examine ethical issues, among other tasks. The case method, discussed later in this chapter, uses a short clinical scenario followed by one or more open-ended questions.

The introductory material should be geared to the students' level of understanding and experience. The teacher should check the terminology used, particularly with beginning students. The situation should be a reasonable length without extending the students' reading time unnecessarily.

The questions should focus on the underlying thought process used to arrive at an answer, not on the answer alone. In some situations, however, the goal may be to assess students' ability to apply principles or procedures learned in class without any original thinking about them. In these instances, well-structured problems with one correct answer and situations that are clearly laid out for students are appropriate.

The teacher also should specify how the responses will be scored, if they are restricted in some way such as with page length, and the criteria used for evaluation. Context-dependent items may be incorporated within a test, completed individually or in small groups for formative evaluation, discussed in class for instructional purposes, completed during post-clinical conferences, or done as out-of-class assignments, either graded or ungraded. If group work is evaluated for summative purposes, students should have an opportunity to evaluate each other's participation. In chapter 13, a sample form (Figure 13.3) is provided for this purpose.

Item sets focusing on assessment of problem-solving ability may ask students to complete the following tasks:

- identify the problem and alternate problems possible
- develop questions for clarifying the problem further
- identify assumptions made about the problem and solutions
- identify additional data needed for decision making
- differentiate relevant and irrelevant information in the situation
- propose solutions, alternatives possible, advantages and disadvantages of each, and their choices

- identify obstacles to solving a problem

- relate information from different sources to the problem to be solved

- work backwards from the desired goal to develop a plan for solving the problem (Nitko, 2004), and

- evaluate the effectiveness of solutions and approaches to solving problems and the outcomes achieved.

The following item set evaluates students' skill in problem solving. After reading the introductory situation about the patient, students are asked to identify *all possible* problems and provide data to support them. Other questions ask students about additional data to be collected, again with a rationale for their answer.

Your eight-year-old patient had a closed head injury four weeks ago after falling off his bike. You visit him at home and find that he has weakness of his left leg. His mother reports that he is "getting his rest" and "sleeping a lot." The patient seems irritable during your visit. When you ask him how he is feeling, he tells you, "My head hurts where I hit it." The mother appears anxious, talking rapidly and changing position frequently.

1. List all possible problems in this situation. For each problem describe supporting assessment data.

2. What additional data are needed, if any, to decide on these problems? Provide a rationale for collecting this information.

3. What other assessment data would you collect at this time? Why is this information important to your decision making?

Context-dependent items may focus on actions to be taken in a situation. For this purpose, the teacher should briefly describe a critical event, then ask learners what they would do next. Because the rationale underlying the thinking is as important if not more important than the decision or outcome, students should also include an explanation of the thought process they used in their decision making. For example:

You are a new employee in a nursing home. At mealtime you find the patients sitting in chairs with their arms tied to the sides of the chair.

1. What would you do?

2. Why did you choose this action?

If the goal is to assess students' ability to think through different decisions possible in a situation, two approaches may be used with the item set. The introductory material (a) may present a situation up to the point of a decision, then ask students to make a decision or (b) may describe a situation and decision and ask whether they agree or disagree with it. For both of these approaches, the students need to provide a rationale for their responses. Examples of these strategies follow.

Your nurse manager on a busy surgery unit asks you to cover for her while she attends a meeting. You find out later that she left the hospital to run an errand instead of attending the meeting.

1.   Identify three alternate courses of action that could be taken in this situation.
2.   Describe the possible consequences of each course of action.
3.   What decision would you make? Why?

A patient calls the office to see if he can receive his flu shot today. He had a cold a few days ago but is feeling better and has returned to work. The nurse instructs the patient to come in for his flu shot.

1.   Do you agree or disagree with the nurse's decision?
2.   Why or why not?

Often context-dependent item sets are developed around clinical scenarios. However, they also are valuable techniques to assess student ability to analyze issues and describe how they would resolve them, articulate different points of view and the reasoning behind each one, evaluate evidence used to support a particular position, and draw inferences and conclusions that follow from the evidence. Students can be given articles and other material to read and analyze, presented with graphs and tables for interpretation, and given photographs and diagrams with questions to answer. Context-dependent items provide a way for teachers to examine how well students use information and think through situations. Examples of context-dependent items sets are found in Table 7.3.

EVALUATION STRATEGIES FOR HIGHER-LEVEL COGNITIVE SKILLS

While context-dependent item sets provide one means of testing higher-level cognitive skills, other evaluation methods are available for this purpose: case

TABLE 7.3   Sample Context-Dependent Item Sets

Questions 1 to 4 relate to the situation below.

A 36-year-old patient scheduled for a breast biopsy has been crying on and off for the last three hours during her diagnostic testing. When the nurse attempts to talk to the woman about her feelings, the patient says, "Everything is fine. I'm just tired."

1. What is the problem in this situation that needs to be solved?
2. What assumptions about the patient did you make in identifying this problem?
3. What additional information would you collect from the patient and her health records before intervening?
4. Why is this information important?

Questions 1 and 2 relate to the situation below.

You are unsure about a medication for one of your patients. When you call the pharmacy to learn more about the drug, you discover that the amount ordered is twice the acceptable dose. You contact the attending physician who tells you to "give it because your patient needs that high a dose."

1. What are your different options at this time? Describe advantages and disadvantages of each.
2. How would you solve this dilemma?

Items 1 to 3 relate to situation below.

The American Nurses Association (ANA) Code for Nurses states that "the nurse safeguards the patient's right to privacy by judiciously protecting information of a confidential nature." A 15-year-old girl is brought by her mother to the clinic with complaints of nausea and vomiting. When the mother leaves the room, the teenager confides in the nurse practitioner that she is pregnant.

1. What are different options for the nurse practitioner at this time? Describe advantages and disadvantages of each.
2. How would you solve this dilemma?
3. Include in your proposed solution how you used the ANA Code for Nurses.

Questions 1 to 4 relate to the scenario below.

A 1-month-old girl is brought to the pediatrician's office for a well-baby checkup. You notice that she has not gained much weight over the last month. Her mother explains that the baby is "colicky" and "spits up a lot of her feeding." There is no evidence of projectile vomiting and other GI symptoms. The baby has a macular-type rash on her stomach, her temperature is normal, and she appears well-hydrated.

1. Describe at least three different nursing interventions that could be used in this situation. Provide a rationale for each.

(continued)

TABLE 7.3 *(continued)*

2. What would you do in this situation? Why is the approach you selected better than the others?
3. Specify outcome criteria for evaluating the effectiveness of the interventions you selected.
4. What information presented in this situation is irrelevant to your decision making? Why?

Questions 1 to 3 relate to the scenario below.

A 68-year-old man who is receiving dialysis has been depressed lately and appears tired. He asks you if he can refuse further dialysis treatments.

1. How would you respond to him? Why is this an appropriate response?
2. What questions would you ask him?
3. What are issues to be resolved in this situation?

The following items are based on the readings you completed in preparation for this test.

Reading A   Reading B

1. From these readings on evidence-based practice, draw two conclusions supported by both readings.
2. What is the fundamental difference between the model presented in Reading A and the one presented in B? Identify issues in implementing each of these models in an acute care setting and describe how you would resolve those issues.

Read the short paragraph below and analyze the credibility of this statement. Respond to items 1 and 2.

The board of directors of a nursing organization in which you are actively involved announced at the annual meeting that membership had increased 30% over the last year. The board reported that this increase was the direct result of the continuing education programs offered to nurses.

1. Analyze the credibility of this statement. Indicate which parts are credible and which are not, including your reasons.

Credible Parts of Statement   Reasons Why Credible

2. What additional data would you obtain to understand the reasons for the membership increase?

TABLE 7.3   *(continued)*

Use this table to answer the question. Circle the letter of the correct answer.

	Men		Women		
Importance Ratings	M	(SD)	M	(SD)	T
Able to call RN with questions	4.23	(.93)	4.92	(.95)	2.76*
Have RN teach illness, medications, treatment options	4.47	(.79)	4.40	(.90)	.568
Have RN teach health promotion	4.35	(.90)	4.00	(1.1)	2.51*

*$p < .01$

Based on the data presented in the table, which of the following conclusions is accurate?

1. Health promoting activities were more important to men than to women.
2. It was more important to men to be able to call a registered nurse with questions after a visit.
3. Men valued teaching by the registered nurse more than women.
4. Teaching about health was more important to women than men.

Examples of Hot-Spot Items[1]

In the history it indicates that your patient has an aortic stenosis. Mark the spot where you would place the stethoscope to best hear the murmur.

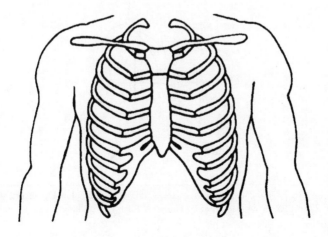

(continued)

TABLE 7.3   *(continued)*

In this fetal monitoring strip, identify the beginning of the contraction.

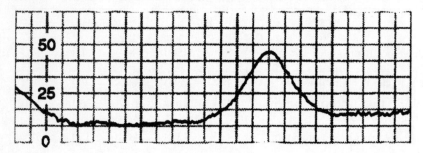

You are completing a physical examination of this infant. Mark the spot you would touch to assess plantar grasp reflex.

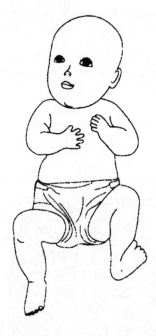

[1]Adapted from: *NCLEX-RN 250 new-format questions*. (2004). Philadelphia: Lippincott; Williams & Wilkins, pp. 22, 87, 95, by permission of Lippincott Williams & Wilkins.

method, case study, and unfolding cases; discussion; debate; media clips; short written assignments; and varied clinical evaluation methods presented in Chapter 13. Many of the evaluation strategies described in this section of the chapter also may be used for clinical evaluation.

Case Method, Case Study, and Unfolding Cases

With cases, students analyze a clinical scenario and answer related questions. The focus might be on identifying problems and possible approaches, making decisions after weighing the options, planning additional data to collect, applying concepts and theories from class and readings to the case, examining the case from different points of view, and identifying actions to take. When used in these ways, cases are effective for developing problem solving and critical thinking skills (Oermann, 2000; Tomey, 2003). In the case method, the cases tend to be short, providing only essential information about the scenario, in contrast to case studies that are longer and in more detail.

Cases work well for group analysis and discussion, either in class as small group activities or in post-clinical conference. In groups, students can critique each others' thinking; compare different perspectives of the problem, solutions, and decisions possible; and learn how to arrive at a group consensus. Used as a small group activity, the case method is more easily evaluated for formative purposes than summative. Table 7.4 presents an example of case method, case study, and unfolding case.

A case study provides a hypothetical or real-life situation for students to analyze and arrive at varied decisions. Case studies are more comprehensive than the introductory material presented with the case method (Table 7.4). With case studies, students are able to provide detailed and in-depth analyses and describe the evidence on which their conclusions are based. The case study also provides a means for students to apply relevant concepts and theories from class and from their readings. A case study may be completed as an individual assignment and evaluated similarly to other written assignments as long as the students provide a rationale for their decisions. The results of the case analysis may be presented orally for group critique and feedback.

One other method for assessing higher-level learning is unfolding cases, which provide a means of simulating a patient situation that changes over time. Rather than writing one short case, as in a case method, or a more comprehensive one with background information, as in a case study, unfolding cases describe changes in a patient's condition or a setting of care similar to what might occur with an actual patient (Table 7.4).

Ulrich and Glendon (1999) developed a model for writing unfolding cases, which can then be evaluated. This strategy includes at least three paragraphs

TABLE 7.4   Sample Case Method, Case Study, and Unfolding Case

---

Case Method

A 92-year-old man is brought to the Emergency Department clinic by his son. The patient seems to be dragging his right leg and has slurred speech. His blood pressure is 220/110.

1. What are possible diagnoses for this patient?
2. What additional data will you collect from the son, and why is this information important to confirming the patient's diagnosis?

Case Study

A 20-year-old woman has had abdominal pain for the last two weeks. Some mornings she has vomiting, but today she complains mainly of severe abdominal cramps and nausea. She has lost eight pounds since last week and has no appetite. She reports having diarrhea for the last few days. She has no masses that you can feel although she complains of increased pain with even a slight touching of her abdominal area. Her vital signs are normal.

Her mother, who brought her to the office today, reports that the patient has always been healthy and has had no prior illnesses except for colds and an occasional flu. She lives with both parents and her younger brother, and she is a student at the local college.

1. What are possible problems that this patient might have? What data would you collect to narrow down your list of problems?
2. What laboratory tests would you expect to be ordered? Why?
3. As you talk with the patient's mother, you learn that the family was on a cruise a few weeks ago, but no one "got sick on the cruise." How might this new information influence your thinking about the patient's possible problems?
4. Considering only the data presented in the case, develop a care plan to meet the patient's current needs. Provide a rationale for each intervention in your plan.

Unfolding Case

You are making a home visit to see a 71-year-old woman who has a leg ulcer that began after she fell. The patient is coughing and wheezing; she tells you she "feels terrible."

1. What additional data would you collect in the initial assessment? Why?
2. What actions would you take during this home visit? Provide a rationale.

In 3 days you visit this patient again. She has increased shortness of breath, more fatigue, and a pale color, and she seems cyanotic around her mouth.

1. Does this new information change your impression of her problems? Why or why not?
2. List priority problems for this patient with a brief rationale.
3. What will you report to the physician when you call?

The patient recovers from that episode, and you are able to visit her one more time. At this last visit, she is still short of breath but otherwise seems improved. Using the form from your agency, write your final report on this patient.

---

for analysis and discussion by students. The case is presented in the first paragraph followed by questions for problem solving and critical thinking. The case unfolds by the teacher's presenting new information about the patient or clinical situation in a second paragraph, again accompanied by higher-level questions for students to answer. By introducing new data in subsequent paragraphs, the teacher presents a changing patient scenario. In Ulrich and Glendon's model, at the end of the unfolding case, students complete a short writing exercise to identify where further learning is needed and to reflect on the case and their responses.

Discussion

Discussions with students individually and in small groups are an important strategy for evaluating problem solving, decision making, and critical thinking abilities. In a discussion, the teacher has an opportunity to ask careful questions about students' thinking and the rationale they used for arriving at decisions and positions on issues. Discussions may be impromptu, for formative evaluation, or structured by the teacher who provides the context and questions to which students respond. Use of discussion for evaluating cognitive skills, however, requires careful questioning with a focus on the critical thinking used by students to arrive at answers. In these discussions, the teacher can ask students about possible decisions, reasons underlying each decision, consequences and implications of options they considered as part of their decision making, and different points of view in the situation.

The level of questions asked is significant to avoid a predominance of factual questions and to focus instead on clarifying and higher level questions. With factual questions, students recall facts and specific information about the problem and issue being discussed. For example, factual questions are: "What is a nursing diagnosis?" and "What are subjective data?" Clarifying and explanatory questions require further thought and discussion. For instance, a clarifying question is: "Tell me the relationship between assessment and nursing diagnosis." For these questions, students explain their answers using their own terminology. Higher-level questions, geared toward critical thinking, cannot be answered by memory alone and require an evaluation or a judgment of the situation (Oermann, 2004a, 2004b; Oermann, Truesdell, & Ziolkowski, 2000). Examples of higher level questions are: "What are similarities and differences between the assessment and diagnoses for Mrs. S and the patient you had last week?" and "Which pain interventions would you propose for this patient? Why did you decide on these interventions compared with the others?"

Questions for discussions should be sequenced from a low to a high level, beginning with factual questions to evaluate students' knowledge of relevant concepts and theories and their ability to apply them to the situation, problem, and issue, and progressing to questions that evaluate students' critical thinking. Bloom's taxonomy can be used as a framework for developing questions for discussions focusing on critical thinking (Oermann, 2004b; Sedlak & Doheny, 2004). With this schema, low-level questions would ask for recall of facts and comprehension. Higher-level questions would focus on application, analysis, synthesis, and evaluation. This taxonomy of the cognitive domain was described and examples of each level were provided in chapter 1.

This discussion of the level of questions asked by the teacher is important because research suggests that teachers by nature do not ask higher-level questions of students. Questions asked of nursing students tend to focus on recall and comprehension rather than on higher levels of thinking (Gaberson & Oermann, 1999; Oermann, 2004a; Wink, 1995). If discussions are to be geared toward evaluation of problem solving and critical thinking, the teacher needs an awareness of the level of questions asked for this purpose. When a student answers a question correctly, the teacher should explore alternate possibilities and proceed to a higher-level question.

The questions presented in Table 7.1 for evaluating critical thinking may be used to guide discussions. In a discussion, ask students about:

- questions, issues, and problems to be resolved

- assumptions on which their thinking is based

- their own points of view and those of others

- the information and evidence on which they are basing their thinking

- concepts and theories applicable to the question, issue, or problem being discussed

- inferences and conclusions possible, and

- implications and consequences of their reasoning.

Socratic Method

The Socratic method may also be used for developing questions to evaluate students' critical thinking in a discussion. There are two phases in the Socratic method: systematic questioning and drawing comparisons. In systematic questioning, the initial phase, the teacher designs a series of questions that lead students along predetermined paths to rational thinking (Gaberson & Oermann, 1999; Overholser, 1992). Questions are open-ended, have multiple possibilities for responding, and ask students to defend their views and positions. In the

Socratic method, the teacher avoids asking questions with one correct answer. In the second phase of questioning, the teacher asks the students to draw comparisons and generalizations from the situation being analyzed to others.

Sedlak and Doheny (2004) suggested that Socratic questions arouse curiosity, encourage students to think on their own, and provide a logical, step-wise guide to assist students in understanding a complex topic or issue. Socratic questioning works well for formative evaluation and can be used in the classroom with the teacher leading the discussion with the class, in post-clinical conferences, and in the form of written questions that students answer in small groups. With this logical sequence of questions, students can analyze complex issues, examine alternate points of view, and draw generalizations across different content areas. However, these outcomes will not be achieved without carefully thought-out questions by the teacher.

Debate

Debate provides an effective mechanism for evaluating students' ability to analyze problems and issues in depth, consider alternative points of view, and formulate a position. The process of analyzing the issue for the debate, considering alternative viewpoints, developing a sound position, and preparing arguments for the position taken provide opportunities for an assessment of students' critical thinking skills. Bradshaw and Lowenstein (2001) also suggested that the debate itself allows students to gain experience in speaking to a group and to develop their oral communication skills.

The focus in evaluating a debate should be on the strength of the argument developed and presented to the group. Areas to consider in evaluating debates include:

1. Clarity and comprehensiveness of the analysis of the issue
2. Rationale developed for the position taken, including use of the literature and available research
3. Consideration of alternative positions
4. Clarity of responses to the opposing side
5. Organization and development of the argument
6. Degree of persuasiveness in presenting the argument, and
7. Presentation skills including keeping the audience interested and focused, presenting the information logically and clearly, and keeping within the allotted time frame.

Depending on the size of the class, not all students may be able to participate in the debate, but they can all learn from it. Debates expand students' understanding of an issue, develop their awareness of opposing views, encourage them to critically analyze issues that do not have a clear-cut answer, and help them learn how to persuade others (Bradshaw & Lowenstein, 2001).

Multimedia

Multimedia may be used to present a scenario for evaluating higher-level learning. Multimedia add to the reality of the situation in comparison with presenting the scenario in print form. Any type of media may be used for this purpose. For example, video and audio clips, interactive videodisks, CD-ROMs, Web animation, images, DVDs, and many other educational and computer technologies can be used to develop real-life scenarios for students to analyze and discuss. There is a wealth of resources on the World Wide Web for presenting scenarios and other situations for teaching and evaluating higher-level cognitive skills. These can be integrated easily within an online learning environment, and students can work individually or in groups to analyze them.

Short Written Assignments

Evaluation of written assignments is presented in chapter 11. For the purposes of assessing critical thinking and other cognitive skills, however, these assignments should reflect additional principles. Assignments for this purpose should be short and require students to think critically about the topic. With term papers and other long assignments, students often summarize the literature and report on the ideas of others, rather than thinking about the topic themselves. Short written assignments, in contrast, provide an opportunity for students to express their thinking in writing and for teachers to give prompt feedback to them on their reasoning.

Students should have clear directions as to what to write about and the length of the assignment. Assignments can be planned throughout a course and level in a nursing program so that they build on one another and students gradually develop their thinking and writing skills. Beginning assignments can ask students to describe a problem or an issue and how they would solve that problem or issue. In later assignments students can critique arguments and develop their own positions about issues with a rationale.

Examples of written assignments for assessing critical thinking, appropriate for either formative or summative evaluation, include short papers (one to two pages):

- Comparing different data sets

- Comparing problems and alternative approaches that could be used

- Analyzing issues

- Analyzing different points of view, perspectives, and positions on an issue

- Comparing a student's own and others' positions on an issue or topic

- Presenting evidence on which their reasoning is based

- Analyzing conclusions drawn, evidence to support these conclusions, and alternative ones possible given the same evidence

- Presenting an argument to support a position.

SUMMARY

This chapter provided a framework for evaluating higher-level learning skills among nursing students. The ability to solve patient and setting-related problems is an essential skill to be developed and evaluated. The nurse continually makes decisions about problems, solutions, possible alternative approaches, and the best approach to use in a particular situation, after weighing the consequences of each. Critical thinking is reflective and reasoned thinking about nursing problems without one solution focuses on decisions about what to believe and do.

In evaluating these cognitive skills, the teacher as a basic principle introduces new or novel material for analysis. Without the introduction of new material as part of the evaluation, students may have memorized from prior discussion or their readings how to problem solve and arrive at decisions for the situation at hand; they may recall the typical problem and solutions without thinking through alternative possibilities themselves. As a result, an essential component of this type of evaluation is the introduction of new information not encountered by the student at an earlier point in the instruction. In nursing this is frequently accomplished by developing scenarios that present a novel situation for students to apply concepts and theories, problem solve, arrive at decisions, and in general engage in critical thinking. These items are referred to as context-dependent item sets or interpretive exercises. In a context-dependent item set, the teacher presents introductory material that students then analyze and answer questions about. The introductory material may be a description of a clinical situation, patient data, research findings, issues associated with clinical practice, and tables, among other types. Students read, analyze, and interpret this material and then answer questions about it or complete other tasks.

Other methods for evaluating cognitive skills in nursing were presented in the chapter: case method and study, unfolding cases, discussions using higher-level and Socratic questioning, debate, multimedia, and short written assignments. In addition to these strategies, clinical evaluation methods that provide for an assessment of cognitive skills are presented in chapter 13.

REFERENCES

Benner, P. E. (2001). *From novice to expert: Excellence and power in clinical nursing practice.* Upper Saddle River, NJ: Prentice Hall.

Bradshaw, M. J., & Lowenstein, A. J. (2001). Debate as a teaching strategy. In A. J. Lowenstein & M. J. Bradshaw (Eds.), *Fuszard's innovative teaching strategies in nursing* (3rd ed., pp. 159–165). Gaithersburg, MD: Aspen.

Ennis, R. H. (1985). A logical basis for measuring critical thinking skills. *Educational Leadership, 43,* 44–48.

Gaberson, K. B., & Oermann, M. H. (1999). *Clinical teaching strategies in nursing education.* New York: Springer.

National Council of State Boards of Nursing. (2004). *Fast facts about alternate item formats and the NCLEX® examination.* Chicago: Author.

Nitko, A. J. (2004). *Educational assessment of students* (4th ed.). Upper Saddle River, NJ: Prentice Hall.

Oermann, M. H. (1997). Evaluating critical thinking in clinical practice. *Nurse Educator, 22*(5), 25–28.

Oermann, M. H. (1998). How to assess critical thinking in clinical practice. *Dimensions of Critical Care Nursing, 17,* 322–327.

Oermann, M. H. (2000). Clinical scenarios for critical thinking. *Academic Exchange Quarterly, 4*(3), 85–91.

Oermann, M. H. (2004a). Basic skills for teaching and the advanced practice nurse. In L. Joel (Ed.), *Advanced practice nursing: Essentials for role development* (pp. 398–429). Philadelphia: F. A. Davis.

Oermann, M. H. (2004b). Using active learning in lecture: Best of "both worlds." *Journal of Nursing Education Scholarship, 1*(1), 1–11. Available at http://www.bepress.com/ijnes/vol1/iss1/art1

Oermann, M. H., Truesdell, S., & Ziolkowski, L. (2000). Strategy to assess, develop, and evaluate critical thinking. *Journal of Continuing Education in Nursing, 31,* 155–160.

Overholser, J. C. (1992). Socrates in the classroom. *College Teaching, 40*(1), 14–19.

Paul, R. (2003). Using intellectual standards to assess student reasoning. Retrieved August 11, 2003, from http://www.criticalthinking.org/k12/k12class/using.html

Paul, R., & Elder, L. (2003). The elements of critical thinking. Foundation for Critical Thinking. Retrieved November 15, 2003, from http://www.criticalthinking.org/University/helps.html

Perry, W. G., Jr. (1970). *Forms of intellectual and ethical development in the college years.* New York: Holt, Rinehart, & Winston.

Perry, W. G., Jr. (1981). Cognitive and ethical growth: The making of meaning. In A. W. Chickering, *The modern American college: Responding to the new realities of diverse students and a changing society* (pp. 66–116). San Francisco: Jossey-Bass.

Sedlak, C. A., & Doheny, M. O. (2004). Critical thinking: What's new and how to foster thinking among nursing students. In M. H. Oermann & K. A. Heinrich (Eds.), *Annual review of nursing education* (Vol. 2, pp. 185–204). New York: Springer.

Tomey, A. M. (2003). Learning with cases. *Journal of Continuing Education in Nursing, 34*, 34–38.

Ulrich, D. L., & Glendon, K. J. (1999). *Interactive group learning: Strategies for nurse educators*. New York: Springer.

Wink, D. M. (1995). The effective clinical conference. *Nursing Outlook, 43*, 29–32.

Chapter 8

Test Construction and Preparation of Students for Licensure and Certification Examinations

One of the outcomes of prelicensure nursing programs is for graduates to pass an examination that measures their knowledge and competencies to engage in safe and effective nursing practice. At the entry level for professional nursing, graduates take the National Council Licensure Examination for Registered Nurses (NCLEX-RN® Examination), or if graduating from a practical or vocational nursing program, they take the National Council Licensure Examination for Practical/Vocational Nurses (NCLEX-PN® Examination). Certification validates knowledge and competencies for professional practice in a specialized area of nursing. As part of this process nurses take certification examinations, which evaluate their knowledge and skills in a nursing specialty such as acute care. There are certification examinations for graduates of associate/diploma, baccalaureate, and master's/doctoral nursing programs. At the master's and doctoral levels, the certification examinations measure knowledge and competencies for advanced practice in a variety of clinical and other areas. As students progress through a nursing program, they should have experience with tests that are similar to and prepare them for taking licensure and certification examinations when they graduate.

Because the focus of the NCLEX® and certification examinations is on nursing practice, the other advantage to incorporating items of these types in teacher-made tests is that it provides a way of measuring if students can apply their theoretical learning to clinical situations. Teachers can develop items that present new and complex clinical situations for students to critically analyze using relevant concepts and theories. Items can focus on collecting and analyzing data, setting priorities, selecting interventions, and evaluating outcomes as related to the content taught in the course. This type of testing is a means of evaluating higher and more complex levels of learning and provides essential practice before students encounter similar questions on licensure and certification examinations.

The chapter begins with an explanation of the NCLEX Examination test plans and implications for nurse educators. Examples are provided of items written at different cognitive levels, thereby avoiding tests that focus only on recall and memorization of facts. The chapter also describes how to write questions about the nursing process and provides sample stems for use with those items. The types of items presented in the chapter are similar to those found on the NCLEX Examination and many certification tests. By incorporating these items on tests in nursing courses, students acquire experience with this type of testing as they progress through the program, preparing them for taking licensure and certification examinations as graduates. The reader should keep in mind that chapter 7 presented other ways of evaluating higher-level learning such as context-dependent testing, case method, and other strategies for evaluating critical thinking.

NCLEX EXAMINATION TEST PLANS

In the United States and its territories, graduates of nursing programs cannot practice as professional nurses or as practical or vocational nurses until they have passed a licensure examination. These examinations are developed by the National Council of State Boards of Nursing, Inc. (NCSBN) based on extensive analyses of the practice requirements of registered nurses (RNs) and licensed practical nurses (LPNs) or vocational nurses (LVNs). The licensure examinations then are used by the state boards of nursing as one of the requirements for practice in that state or territory.

NCLEX-RN EXAMINATION TEST PLAN

In developing the NCLEX-RN, the NCSBN conducts an analysis of the current practice of newly licensed RNs across clinical areas and settings. This is a continuous process in order for the licensure examination to keep current with the knowledge and competencies needed by entry level nurses. To ensure that the NCLEX-RN measures the essential competencies for practice by a newly licensed RN, the NCSBN reviews the test plan or blueprint every 3 years (Wendt, 2003). For the most recent revision of the test plan, more than 4,000 newly licensed RNs were asked how frequently they performed 130 nursing activities and the priority of these (NCSBN, 2003). The NCSBN then analyzes these activities in terms of impact on patient safety and settings where they are implemented. A test plan is developed from this analysis, guiding the selection of content and behaviors to be tested and the percentage of items for each of the categories of the test. Each candidate's examination is based on this test plan (NCSBN, 2003).

Client-Needs Framework

Test items on the NCLEX-RN are categorized by client needs: (a) safe and effective care environment, (b) health promotion and maintenance, (c) psychosocial integrity, and (d) physiological integrity. Two of the categories, safe and effective care environment and physiological integrity, also have subgroups. The client needs represent the content tested on the examination. Table 8.1 lists the percentage of items on the examination from each of the categories or subcategories.

Safe and Effective Care Environment

In the safe and effective care environment category, two subcategories of content are tested on the NCLEX-RN: (a) management of care and (b) safety and

TABLE 8.1   Percentage of Items in NCLEX-RN Examination Test Plan

Client Needs	Percentage of Items from each Category or Subcategory
Safe Effective Care Environment	
Management of Care	13–19
Safety and Infection Control	8–14
Health Promotion and Maintenance	6–12
Psychosocial Integrity	6–12
Physiological Integrity	
Basic Care and Comfort	6–12
Pharmacological and Parenteral Therapies	13–19
Reduction of Risk Potential	13–19
Physiological Adaptation	11–17

Source: National Council of State Boards of Nursing, Inc. (2003). NCLEX-RN® Examination: Test plan for the National Council Licensure Examination for Registered Nurses. Chicago: Author, p. 4.

infection control. In the management of care subcategory, the questions focus on nursing care and delivery of care that protect patients, families, significant others, and health care providers. Examples of content tested in this category include advance directives, advocacy, case management, concepts of management, delegation, ethics of practice, legal responsibilities, multidisciplinary collaboration, patient rights, priority setting, source management, and staff education, among others (NCSBN, 2003, p. 5). In the safety and infection control subcategory, test items focus on prevention of accidents, errors, and injuries; disaster planning and emergency response plans; handling infectious and hazardous materials; medical and surgical asepsis; reporting incidences and irregular occurrences; safe use of equipment; and use of restraints, among others (NCSBN, 2003, p. 6).

Health Promotion and Maintenance

The second category of client needs is health promotion and maintenance. There are no subcategories of needs. Examples of content tested in this category are developmental stages and growth and development, disease prevention, health and wellness, health promotion and screening, physical assessment techniques, sexuality, and teaching and learning principles.

Psychosocial Integrity

The third category of client needs, psychosocial integrity, also has no subgroups. This category focuses on nursing care that promotes the emotional, mental, and social well-being of patients, families, and others, and the care of patients with acute and chronic mental illnesses. Examples of content tested include abuse, behavioral interventions, chemical dependency, cultural diversity, grief and loss, mental health, psychopathology, sensory and perceptual alterations, and therapeutic communication and environment (NCSBN, 2003, p. 6).

Physiological Integrity

The last client needs category, physiological integrity, is a significant content area tested on the NCLEX-RN. Questions in this category focus on nursing care that promotes physical health and comfort, reduces risk potential, and manages health alterations of patients. Four subcategories of content are examined by these items on the NCLEX-RN examination:

1. Basic care and comfort: In this area, items focus on comfort measures and assistance with activities of daily living. Related content is on

assistive devices, complementary therapies, elimination, hygiene, mobility and immobility, non-pharmacological comfort measures, nutrition, palliative care, and rest and sleep.

2. Pharmacological and parenteral therapies: Questions are asked on blood products and administration; calculating dosages; intravenous therapy; medication administration, expected outcomes, contraindications, and side effects; and pharmacological agents, interactions, and pain management.

3. Reduction of risk potential: The content in this subcategory relates to measures for reducing the risk for developing complications or health problems. For example, items are on diagnostic tests; laboratory values; potential for complications from tests, treatments, health problems, and surgery; therapeutic procedures; and vital signs.

4. Physiological adaptation: The last subcategory on physiological adaptation includes nursing care of patients with life threatening, acute, and chronic physical health problems. Sample content areas are alterations in body systems, fluid and electrolyte abnormalities, hemodynamics, infectious diseases, management of illness and medical emergencies, and pathophysiology (NCSBN, 2003, p. 7).

Integrated Processes

There are four processes that are integrated throughout each of the categories of the test plan: (a) nursing process, (b) caring, (c) communication and documentation, and (d) teaching and learning. Thus there can be test items on teaching patients and the nurse's ethical and legal responsibilities in patient education as part of the Management of Care subcategory, teaching nursing assistants about the use of restraints in the Safety and Infection Control subcategory, health education for different age groups in the Health Promotion and Maintenance category, and discharge teaching in the Reduction of Risk Potential subcategory. The other processes are integrated similarly throughout the test plan.

Cognitive Levels

The NCLEX-RN Examination uses Bloom's taxonomy for developing items. This taxonomy was presented in chapter 1. Items are developed at the knowledge, comprehension, application, and analysis levels, with the majority of items at the application and higher cognitive levels (NCSBN, 2003; Wendt, 2003). This has implications for testing in schools of nursing. Faculty should avoid preparing only recall and comprehension items on their tests. While some of these low-level questions are essential to measure knowledge and understanding of facts and basic principles, questions also need to ask students to *use* their knowledge and think critically to arrive at an answer. Test blueprints can be developed to list not only the content and number of items in each content area but also the level of cognitive complexity at which items should be written. An example of a blueprint of this type was provided in Table 3.3 in chapter 3.

NCLEX-PN EXAMINATION TEST PLAN

The test plan for the NCLEX-PN is developed and organized similarly to the RN examination. For the 2005 test plan, practical and vocational nurses who were newly licensed were asked how frequently they performed about 150 nursing activities and their priority (NCSBN, 2004a). Those activities were then used as the framework for the development of the test plan for the PN examination.

The test plan is structured around client needs and integrated processes fundamental to the practice of practical and vocational nursing. The same four client needs categories are used for the NCLEX-PN examination with differences in some of the subcategories, related content, and percentage of items in each category and subcategory. Table 8.2 lists the percentage of items in each client

TABLE 8.2   Percentage of Items in NCLEX-PN Examination Test Plan

Client Needs	Percentage of Items from each Category or Subcategory
Safe and Effective Care Environment	
Coordinated Care	11–17
Safety and Infection Control	8–14
Health Promotion and Maintenance	7–13
Psychosocial Integrity	8–14
Physiological Integrity	
Basic Care and Comfort	11–17
Pharmacological Therapies	9–15
Reduction of Risk Potential	10–16
Physiological Adaptation	12–18

Source: National Council of State Boards of Nursing, Inc. (2004). NCLEX-PN® Examination: Test plan for the National Council Licensure Examination for Licensed Practical/Vocational Nurses. Chicago: Author, p. 3.

need category or subcategory. Similar to the NCLEX-RN Examination, the processes are integrated throughout the test. The integrated processes are: (a) the clinical problem-solving process (nursing process), (b) caring, (c) communication and documentation, and (d) teaching and learning. Items are developed at all cognitive levels with the majority written at the application or higher levels of cognitive abilities consistent with the NCLEX-RN Examination test plan (NCSBN, 2004a).

TYPES OF ITEMS ON THE NCLEX EXAMINATIONS

The NCLEX examinations contain the standard four-option multiple-choice items and alternate item formats, which were introduced in 2003. Earlier chapters described how to construct multiple-choice items and each of the alternate formats: fill-in-the-blank, hot-spot, and multiple-response. Any of these formats might include a table, a chart, or an image as part of the item. Wendt (2003) indicated that most of the items on a candidate's examination continue to be multiple-choice. However, more alternate format items might be used in the future for developing synthesis questions.

ADMINISTRATION OF NCLEX EXAMINATIONS

The NCLEX examinations are administered to candidates by computerized adaptive testing (CAT). The CAT model is such that each candidate's test is assembled interactively as the person is answering the questions. Each item on the NCLEX has a predetermined difficulty level. As each item is answered, the computer calculates a skill estimate based on whether the answer is correct or incorrect, and then selects from a large data bank the next item, calculated to measure the candidate's ability most precisely (NCSBN, 2003, 2004a). This is an efficient means of testing, avoiding questions that do not contribute to determining a candidate's level of nursing competence. The licensing examination, therefore, is tailored to the individual's knowledge and skills yet still measures competence as required by the test plan (NCSBN, 2003).

The standard for passing the NCLEX is criterion-referenced. The standard is set by the NCSBN based on an established protocol and is used as the basis for determining if the candidate has passed or failed the examination. All RN candidates must answer a minimum number of 75 items. The maximum number they can answer is 265 (NCSBN, 2003). As of October 1, 2004, the maximum time allowed to take the NCLEX-RN Examination increased from 5 to 6 hours (NCSBN, 2004b). On the NCLEX-PN Examination, practical and vocational nurse candidates must answer a minimum of 85 items. The maximum number of items they can answer is 205 during the 5-hour testing period allowed (NCSBN, 2004b).

PREPARATION OF ITEMS AT VARIED COGNITIVE LEVELS

When courses have higher-level outcomes, tests in those courses need to measure learning at the application and analysis levels rather than at recall and comprehension. This principle was discussed in earlier chapters. Items at higher levels of cognitive complexity are more difficult and time-consuming to develop, but they provide a way of evaluating ability to apply knowledge to new situations and to engage in analytical thinking. Items at these higher levels can be used to assess critical thinking (McDonald, 2002; Morrison & Free, 2001). Wendt (2003) commented that many of the more recently developed NCLEX items require candidates to problem solve in order to prioritize care and select the best response.

Students are at a disadvantage if they encounter only recall and comprehension test items as they progress through a nursing program. Low-level items measure how well students memorize specific information, not if they can use that knowledge to analyze clinical situations and arrive at the best decisions possible for those situations. Students need experience answering questions at the application and analysis levels before they take the NCLEX Examination. Morrison (2005) emphasized that content-oriented test items at the knowledge level do not prepare students to take the NCLEX-RN. More importantly, if course outcomes are at higher levels of cognitive complexity, then tests and other evaluation strategies need to assess learning at those levels. In graduate nursing programs, test items should be developed at higher cognitive levels to measure students' ability to problem solve and think critically and to prepare them for certification examinations they might take as graduates.

When developing a new test, a blueprint is important to plan the number of items at each cognitive level for the content areas to be evaluated. By using a blueprint, teachers can avoid writing too many recall and comprehensive items. For existing tests that were not developed using a blueprint, teachers can code items using Bloom's taxonomy and then decide if more higher-level items should be added.

Knowledge or Recall

In developing items at varying cognitive levels, it is important to remember the outcome of learning intended at each of these levels. Questions at the knowledge level deal with facts, principles, and other specific information that is memorized and then recalled to answer the item. An example of a multiple-choice item at the knowledge level follows.

> Your patient is taking pseudoephedrine for his stuffy nose. Which of the following side effects is common among patients using this medication?
>
> a.   Diarrhea
> b.   Dyspnea
> c.   Hallucinations
> d.   Restlessness *

Comprehension

At the comprehension level, items measure understanding of concepts and ability to explain them. These questions are written at a higher level than recall, but they do not evaluate problem solving or use of information in a new context. An example of an item at the comprehension level is:

> An adult female patient is a new admission with the diagnosis of acute renal failure. Her total urine output for the previous 24 hours was 90 mL. A urinary output of this amount is known as _____.

Application

At the application level, students apply concepts and theories as a basis for responding to the item. At this level, test questions measure *use* of knowledge in new or unique situations. One strategy for developing items at this level is to prepare stems that have information that students did not encounter in their learning about the content. The stem might present patient data, diagnoses, or treatments different from the ones discussed in class or in the readings. If examples in class related to nursing care of adults, items might test ability to use those concepts when the patient is an adolescent or has multiple co-existing problems. An example of an item at the application level is:

A mother tells you that she is worried about her 4-year-old daughter's development because her daughter seems to be "behind." You complete a developmental assessment. Which of the following behaviors suggests the need for further developmental testing?

a.   Cannot follow 5 commands in a row
b.   Has difficulty holding a crayon between thumb and forefinger *
c.   Is unable to balance on each foot for 6 seconds
d.   Keeps making mistakes when asked about the day of the week

Analysis

Questions at the analysis level are the most difficult to construct. They require analysis of a clinical or other situation to identify critical elements and relationships among them. Items should provide a new situation for students to analyze, not one encountered previously for which the student might recall the analysis. Many of these items require problem solving and making a decision about priorities or the best approach to take among the options. Or, items might ask students to identify the most immediate course of action to meet patient needs or manage the clinical situation. The difference between application and analysis items is not always readily apparent; analysis items, though, should require students to identify relevant data, critical elements, component parts, and their interrelationships.

On the NCLEX examinations, the clinical situations can involve any age group of patients in hospitals, long-term care, community health, or other types of settings. Wendt (2003) indicated that at the analysis level, NCLEX items often require candidates to distinguish between significant and non-significant information and to choose the best approaches among those cited in the alternatives.

An example of an item written at the analysis level is:

You receive a report on the following patients at the beginning of your evening shift at 3 p.m. Which patient should you assess first?

a.   An 82-year-old with pneumonia who seems confused at times *
b.   A 76-year-old patient with cancer with 300 mL remaining of an intravenous infusion
c.   A 40-year-old who had an emergency appendectomy 8 hours ago
d.   An 18-year-old with chest tubes for treatment of an pneumothorax following an accident

TESTING IN THE NURSING PROCESS FRAMEWORK

One of the processes integrated into the NCLEX test plans is the nursing process. This is also a framework taught in many nursing programs. If not presented as a series of stages, most clinical courses address, in some form, assessment, data analysis, diagnoses, interventions, and evaluation. For this reason another useful framework for developing test questions is the nursing process. Items can examine assessment of patients with varied needs and health problems, analysis of data, nursing and other diagnoses, priorities of care, nursing interventions, treatments, and evaluation of the outcomes of care.

Current practices suggest that many test questions focus on scientific rationale, principles underlying patient care, and selection of interventions. Fewer questions are developed on collecting and analyzing data, determining nursing diagnoses and patient problems, setting priorities and realistic goals of care, and evaluating the effectiveness of interventions and outcomes. Developing items on the nursing process and based on clinical scenarios provides an opportunity to examine these outcomes of learning. McDonald (2002) identified another advantage of nursing process testing as promoting the development of unique situations, which then allows for testing at a higher cognitive level. While nursing process items can be written at the recall level, they are more appropriate for testing of more complex cognitive outcomes.

Writing Items in Framework of the Nursing Process

The process of developing nursing process items begins with identifying the total number of items to be written. This includes specifying the number of items for each phase of the nursing process. On some tests, greater weight may be given to certain phases of the process, for example, assessment, if these were emphasized in the instruction. As part of this planning, the teacher also maps out the clinical situations to be tested as relevant to course content. For instance, the teacher may plan for two assessment questions on pain; three intervention questions, including two on nursing management and a third on medications; and one item on evaluating the effectiveness of pain management with children. A similar process may be used with other content areas for which this type of testing is intended. Questions may stand alone, or a series of items may be developed around one clinical scenario. In the latter format the teacher has an option of adding data to the situation and creating an unfolding case, which was discussed in chapter 7.

Test items on assessment examine knowledge of data to collect, use of varied sources of data, relevancy of selected data for a patient, verifying data, communicating information, and documenting findings. Analysis questions (referring to the nursing process, not the analysis level in Bloom's taxonomy) measure ability to interpret data, identify patient problems and needs, and determine nursing diagnoses. Questions on planning focus on identifying priorities, planning nursing measures to achieve outcomes of care, selecting effective interventions, and collaborating with others in developing interdisciplinary plans. Items on implementation relate to the principles underlying nursing and other interventions, effectiveness of interventions, priorities of care, and documentation. The last phase for which items may be written is evaluation. These items focus on patients' responses to care, the extent to which outcomes have been achieved, variables influencing care delivery, recording patient progress and outcomes, and needed revisions of the plan of care.

Examples of stems that can be used to develop items about the nursing process are provided in Table 8.3. McDonald (2002) referred to these sample stems as "item shells." Teachers can select a stem and add content from their own course, providing an easy way of writing items on the nursing process. Sample items for each phase of the nursing process follow.

Assessment

An 8-year-old boy is brought to the emergency room by his mother after falling off his bike and hitting his head. Which of the following data is most important to collect in the initial assessment?

a.   Blood pressure
b.   Level of consciousness
c.   Pupillary response
d.   Respiratory status *

Analysis

A 17-year-old adolescent girl is seen in the clinic for pelvic inflammatory disease. The nurse should anticipate which of these nursing diagnoses?

a.   Altered health maintenance
b.   Pain *
c.   Knowledge deficit
d.   Sexual dysfunction

Planning

Your patient is being discharged after a sickle cell crisis. Which of the following measures should be included in your teaching plan for this patient? Select all that apply.

- ☐ 1. Avoid warm temperatures inside and outdoors
- ☐ 2. Do not use nonsteroidal anti-inflammatory drugs (NSAIDs) for pain
- ☑ 3. Drink at least 8 glasses of water a day
- ☑ 4. Eat plenty of grains, fruits, and green leafy vegetables
- ☑ 5. Get a vaccination for pneumonia
- ☐ 6. Keep cold packs handy for joint pain

Implementation

Your patient is in active labor with contractions every 3 minutes lasting about 1 minute. She appears to have a seizure. Which of the following interventions is the top priority?

- a. Assess her breathing pattern. *
- b. Attach an external fetal monitor.
- c. Call the physician.
- d. Prepare for a cesarean delivery.

Evaluation

A male adult patient was discharged following a below-the-knee amputation. You are making the first home health visit after his discharge. Which of the following statements by the patient indicates that he needs further instruction?

- a. "I know to take my temperature if I get chills again like in the hospital."
- b. "I won't exert myself around the house until I see the doctor."
- c. "The nurse said to take more insulin when I start to eat more."*
- d. "The social worker mentioned a support group. Maybe I should call about it."

TABLE 8.3   Examples of Stems for Nursing Process Questions

Assessment

The nurse should collect which of the following data?
Which of the following information should be collected as a priority in the assessment?
Which data should be collected first?
Which questions should the nurse ask [the patient, the family, others] in the assessment?
Your patient develops [symptoms]. What data should the nurse collect now?
What additional data are needed to establish the nursing diagnosis? Patient problems?
Which resources should be used to collect the data?
Which of the following information is a priority to report to the [physician, nurse, other provider]?

Analysis

These data support the [diagnosis, problem] of _____.
Which [diagnosis, problem] is most appropriate for this patient?
The priority nursing diagnosis is _____.
The priority problem of this [patient, family, community] is _____.
A patient with [a diagnosis of, symptoms of] is at risk for developing which of the following complications?

Planning

Which outcomes are most important for a patient with a [diagnosis of]?
What are the priority outcomes for a patient receiving [treatment]?
Which nursing measures should be included in the plan of care for a patient with [diagnosis, surgery, treatment, diagnostic test]?
Which of the following nursing interventions would be most effective for a patient with [diagnosis of, problem of, symptoms of]?
The nurse is teaching a patient who is [years old]. Which teaching strategy would be most appropriate?
Which intervention is most likely to be effective in managing [symptoms of]?

Implementation

Which of the following actions should be implemented immediately?
Nursing interventions for this patient include:
Following this [procedure, surgery, treatment, test], which nursing measures should be implemented?
Which of these nursing interventions is a priority for a patient with [diagnosis]?
A patient with [a diagnosis of] complains of [symptoms]. What should the nurse do first?
Which explanation should the nurse use when teaching a patient [with a diagnosis of, prior to procedure, surgery, treatment, test]?
Which of the following instructions should be given to the [patient, family, caregiver, nurse] at discharge?
Which of the following situations should be reported immediately to a manager?

(continued)

TABLE 8.3   *(continued)*

Evaluation

Which of these responses indicates the [intervention, medication, treatment] is effective?
A patient is taking [medication] for [diagnosis, problem]. Which of these data indicate
   a side effect of the medication?
Which response by the patient indicates improvement?
Which of the following observations indicates that the [patient, caregiver] knows how
   to [perform the procedure, give the treatment, follow the protocol]?
Which statement by the [patient, caregiver] indicates the need for further teaching?

PREPARATION OF STUDENTS FOR THE NCLEX EXAMINATIONS

A number of studies have been done over the years to identify predictors of success on the NCLEX-RN. Some factors related to performance on the NCLEX-RN are: SAT scores (Crow, Handley, Morrison, & Shelton, 2004); scores on exit or pre-licensure readiness examinations (Beeson & Kissling, 2001; Morrison, Free, & Newman, 2002; Nibert, Young, & Britt, 2003); grades in nursing courses and graduation grade point average (Arathuzik & Aber, 1998; Beeman & Waterhouse, 2001; Beeson & Kissling, 2001); and grades in science prerequisite courses (Roncoli, Linsanti, & Falcone, 2000). Academic achievement, in terms of nursing course grades and overall grade point average, has been found across studies as predictive of student performance on the NCLEX-RN. In Beeman and Waterhouse's study (2001), the number of high grades earned in nursing theory courses was the best predictor of success on the NCLEX-RN, followed by grades in nursing courses. The grades correctly classified 93% of the graduates who passed the NCLEX and 92% who failed it.

Other nurse educators have examined nonacademic factors that might influence performance on the NCLEX. In qualitative interviews with graduates of a baccalaureate nursing program, Eddy and Epeneter (2002) found that those who had passed the examination on the first attempt were proactive in preparing for it, took the test when they felt ready, and used stress management strategies. Those who had failed reported they did not feel ready for the examination, were less able to cope with the stress associated with taking it, and tended to blame others for their lack of success. New graduates should be encouraged to study intensively for the examination. In a study by Beeman and Waterhouse (2003), the total number of hours studied correlated with passing the NCLEX.

A second area of the literature on the NCLEX-RN focuses on strategies for preparing students to pass the examination. One development in this area has been the use of standardized examinations designed to predict student performance on the NCLEX-RN Examination. A number of companies have published standardized tests that are intended to measure students' readiness for the NCLEX, including Assessment Technologies Institute, LLC (ATI); Educational Resources, Inc. (ERI); Mosby; the National League for Nursing; and Health Education Systems, Inc. (HESI), among others. For example, the HESI Exit Exam™ is a computerized comprehensive examination that uses a mathematical model to compare individual students with students throughout the United States, indicating their preparedness for the NCLEX and as a benchmark for remediation (Morrison, Free, & Newman, 2002). Studies have shown the HESI Exit Exam™ to be highly accurate in predicting NCLEX success and licensure failure (Lauchner, Newman, & Britt, 1999; Morrison, Adamson, Nibert, & Hsia, 2004; Nibert & Young, 2001; Nibert, Young, & Britt, 2003). By analyzing the results of standardized tests for NCLEX readiness, faculty and students can work together to design individual plans for remediation so that students will be more likely to experience first-time success on the licensure examination.

Other strategies such as self-assessment of content areas needing improvement, test-taking tips, managing test anxiety, cooperative study groups, commercial reviews, and careful planning for the day of testing have been used by nursing faculty to assist students in preparing for the NCLEX examinations (Crow, Handley, Morrison, & Shelton, 2004; Cunningham, Stacciarini, & Towle, 2004; McQueen, Shelton, & Zimmerman, 2004; Mills, Wilson, & Bar, 2001; Siktberg & Dillard, 2001; Poorman, Mastorovich, Webb, & Molcan, 2003; Stark, Feikema, & Wyngarden, 2002). Experience with test items that are similar to the NCLEX prepares students for the types of questions they will encounter on the licensing examination. In addition to this format of test items, students also need experience in taking practice tests.

SUMMARY

The chapter summarized the NCLEX test plans and their implications for nurse educators. One of the principles emphasized was the need to prepare items at different cognitive levels as indicated by the outcomes of the course. Items at the recall level measure how well students memorized facts and specific information; they do not, however, provide an indication of whether students can use that information in practice or can engage in analytical or critical thinking. To measure those higher-level outcomes, items must be written at the application or higher level or evaluated by strategies other than tests. It is worthwhile for faculty to develop a test blueprint that plans for the number of items to be developed at each cognitive level for content areas in the course. By using a blueprint, teachers can avoid writing too many recall and comprehensive items on an examination.

As students progress through a nursing program, they develop abilities to assess patients with varied needs and health problems, analyze data and derive multiple nursing diagnoses, set priorities for care, critique nursing interventions and select appropriate ones, and evaluate the effectiveness and outcomes of care. Testing within the framework of the nursing process provides an opportunity to measure these learning outcomes. Items may be written about phases of the nursing process, decisions to be made in clinical situations and consequences of each, varying judgments possible in a situation, and other questions that examine students' critical thinking as related to the situation described in the item. This format of testing also provides experience for students in answering the types of items encountered on licensure and certification examinations.

REFERENCES

Arathuzik, D., & Aber, C. (1998). Factors associated with National Council Licensure Examination–Registered Nurse success. *Journal of Professional Nursing, 14,* 119–126.

Beeman, P. B., & Waterhouse, J. K. (2001). NCLEX-RN performance: Predicting success on the computerized examination. *Journal of Professional Nursing, 17,* 158–165.

Beeman, P. B., & Waterhouse, J. K. (2003). Post-graduation factors predicting NCLEX-RN success. *Nurse Educator, 28,* 257–260.

Beeson, S. A., & Kissling, G. (2001). Predicting success for baccalaureate graduates on the NCLEX-RN. *Journal of Professional Nursing, 17,* 121–127.

Crow, C. S., Handley, M., Morrison, R. S., & Shelton, M. M. (2004). Requirements and interventions used by BSN programs to promote and predict NCLEX-RN success: A national study. *Journal of Professional Nursing, 20,* 174–186.

Cunningham, H., Stacciarini, J. M., & Towle, S. (2004). Strategies to promote success on the NCLEX-RN for students with English as a second language. *Nurse Educator, 29,* 15–19.

Eddy, L. L., & Epeneter, B. J. (2002). The NCLEX-RN experience: Qualitative interviews with graduates of a baccalaureate nursing program. *Journal of Nursing Education, 41,* 273–278.

Lauchner, K., Newman, M., & Britt, R. (1999). Predicting licensure success with a computerized comprehensive nursing exam: The HESI Exit Exam. *Computers in Nursing, 17,* 120–128.

McDonald, M. E. (2002). *Systematic assessment of learning outcomes: Developing multiple-choice exams.* Boston: Jones & Bartlett.

McQueen, L., Shelton, P., & Zimmerman, L. (2004). A collective community approach to preparing nursing students for the NCLEX RN examination. *Association of Black Nursing Faculty Journal, 15*(3), 55–58.

Mills, L. W., Wilson, C. B., & Bar, B. B. (2001). A holistic approach to promoting success on NCLEX-RN. *Journal of Holistic Nursing, 19*, 360–374.

Morrison, S. (2005). Improving NCLEX-RN pass rates through internal and external curriculum evaluation. In M. H. Oermann & K. Heinrich (Eds.), *Annual Review of Nursing Education*, Vol. 3 (pp. 77–94). New York: Springer.

Morrison, S., Adamson, C., Nibert, A., & Hsia, S. (2004). HESI Exams: An overview of reliability and validity. *CIN: Computers, Informatics, Nursing, 22*, 220–226.

Morrison, S., & Free, K. W. (2001). Writing multiple-choice test items that promote and measure critical thinking. *Journal of Nursing Education, 40*, 17–24.

Morrison, S., Free, K. W., & Newman, M. (2002). Do progression and remediation policies improve NCLEX-RN pass rates? *Nurse Educator, 27*, 94–96.

National Council of State Boards of Nursing, Inc. (2003). NCLEX-RN Examination: Test plan for the National Council Licensure Examination for Registered Nurses. Chicago: Author.

National Council of State Boards of Nursing, Inc. (2004a). NCLEX-PN® Examination: Test plan for the National Council Licensure Examination for Licensed Practical/ Vocational Nurses. Chicago: Author.

National Council of State Boards of Nursing, Inc. (2004b). Testing Services. Extended Time Length for the NCLEX-RN Examination. Retrieved October 22, 2004, from http://www.ncsbn.org/testing/candidates_90467AB73F404C0BA00C3B01C 150FB78.htm

Nibert, A., & Young, A. (2001). A third study on predicting NCLEX-RN success with the HESI Exit Exam. *Computers in Nursing, 19*, 172–178.

Nibert, A., Young, A., & Britt, R. (2003). The HESI Exit Exam: Progression benchmark and remediation guide. *Nurse Educator, 28*, 141–145.

Poorman, S. G., Mastorovich, M. L., Webb, C. A., & Molcan, K. L. (2003). *Good thinking: Test taking and study skills for nursing students* (2nd ed.). Pittsburgh, PA: STAT Nursing Consultants.

Roncoli, M., Lisanti, P., & Falcone A. (2000). Characteristics of baccalaureate graduates and NCLEX-RN performance. *Journal of the New York State Nurses Association, 31*(1), 17–19.

Siktberg, L. L., & Dillard, N. L. (2001). Assisting at-risk students in preparing for NCLEX-RN. *Nurse Educator, 26*, 150–152.

Stark, M. A., Feikema, B., & Wyngarden, K. (2002). Empowering students for NCLEX® success. *Nurse Educator, 27*, 103–105.

Wendt, A. (2003). The NCLEX-RN® Examination: Charting the course of nursing practice. *Nurse Educator, 28*, 276–280.

Chapter 9

Assembling and Administering Tests

In addition to the preparation of a test blueprint and the skillful construction of test items that correspond to it, the final appearance of the test and the way in which it is administered can affect the validity of the test results. A haphazard arrangement of test items, directions that are confusing, and typographical and other errors on the test may contribute to measurement error. By following certain design rules, teachers can avoid such errors when assembling a test. Administering a test usually is the simplest phase of the testing process. There are some common problems associated with test administration, however, that may also affect the reliability of the resulting test scores and consequently the validity of inferences made about those scores. Careful planning can help the teacher avoid or minimize such difficulties. This chapter discusses the process of assembling the test and administering it to students.

TEST DESIGN RULES

Allow Enough Time

As discussed in Chapter 3, preparing a high quality test requires time for the design phases as well as for the item writing phase. Assembling the test is not simply a clerical or technical task; the teacher should make all decisions about the arrangement of test elements and the final appearance of the test even if someone else types or prints the test. The teacher must allow enough time for this phase to avoid errors that could affect the students' test scores (Gaberson, 1996).

Arrange Test Items in a Logical Sequence

Various methods for arranging items on the test have been recommended, including by order of difficulty and according to the sequence in which the content was taught. However, if the test contains items of two or more formats, the teacher should first group items of the same format together. Since each item format requires different tasks of the student, this type of arrangement makes it easier for students to maintain the mental set required to answer each type of item, and prevents errors caused by frequent changing of tasks. Keeping items of the same format together also facilitates scoring if a scannable answer sheet is not used (Gaberson, 1996; Kubiszyn & Borich, 2003).

Within each item format group, items may be arranged to begin with the easiest items and progress in difficulty. Even well-prepared students are likely to be somewhat anxious at the beginning of a test, and encountering difficult items may increase their anxiety and interfere with their optimum performance. Beginning with easier items may build the students' confidence and allow them to answer these items quickly and reserve more time for difficult items. By answering the beginning items correctly, students may have less anxiety about the test (Kubiszyn & Borich, 2003).

Another method for arranging items is according to the order in which the content was taught, which may assist students to recall information more easily. The teacher can easily combine the difficulty and content sequence methods of ordering items within each item format section of the test.

Write Directions

The teacher cannot assume that the students know the basis on which they are to select or provide answers or how and where to record their answers to test items. The students may be well prepared, rested, and confident, but unable to perform at their best if the teacher does not tell them what to do (Gaberson, 1996).

The test should begin with a set of clear general directions. These general directions should include instructions on:

- how and where to record responses,
- what type of writing implement to use,
- whether or not students may write on the test booklet,
- the amount of time allowed,
- the number of pages and items on the exam,
- the types and point value of items,
- whether students may ask questions during the test, and

- what to do after finishing the exam (Gaberson, 1996; Hopkins, 1998; Kubiszyn & Borich, 2003).

Students may need to know some of these instructions while they are preparing for the test, for instance, if their answers to items requiring them to supply the names of medications must be spelled accurately to be scored as correct.

Each item format section should begin with specific instructions. For multiple-choice items, the student needs to know whether to select the correct or best response. Directions for completion and essay items should state whether spelling, grammar, punctuation, and organization will be considered in scoring. For computation items, directions should specify the degree of precision required, the unit of measure, whether to show the calculation work, and what method of computation to use if there is more than one. Matching exercise directions should clearly specify the basis on which the match is to be made (Kubiszyn & Borich, 2003). An example is: "For each definition in Column A, select the proper term in Column B. Use each letter in Column B only once or not at all."

Use a Cover Page

The general test directions may be printed on a cover page (Figure 9.1). A cover page also serves to keep the test items hidden from view during the distribution of the exam so that the first students to receive the test will not have more time to complete it than students who receive their copies later. If the directions on the cover page indicate the number of pages and items, the students can quickly check their test booklets for completeness and correct sequence of pages. The teacher can then replace defective test booklets before students begin answering items (Gaberson, 1996).

When a separate answer sheet is used, the cover page may be numbered to help maintain test security; students are directed to record this number on the answer sheet. With this system, the teacher can track any missing test booklets after the test is done.

Avoid Crowding

Test items are difficult to read when they are crowded together on the page; learning-disabled students and those for whom English is a second language may find crowding particularly trying. Techniques that allow students to read efficiently and to prevent errors in recording their responses include leaving sufficient white space within and between items and indenting certain elements. Kubiszyn and Borich (2003) recommended that teachers allow enough blank

Exam Number ____

PSYCHIATRIC-MENTAL HEALTH NURSING FINAL EXAM

Directions

1. This test consists of 12 pages. Please check your test booklet to make sure you have the correct number of pages in the proper sequence.

2. Parts I and II consist of 86 multiple-choice and matching items. You may write on the test booklet but **you must record your answers to these items on your answer sheet**. This part of the test will be machine-scored; read carefully and follow the instructions below:

    a. Use a #2 pencil.

    b. Notice that the items on the answer sheet are numbered **DOWN** the page in each column.

    c. Choose the **ONE BEST** response to each item. Items with multiple answer marks will be counted as incorrect. Fill in the circle completely; if you change your answer, erase your first answer thoroughly.

    d. Print your name (last name, first name) in the blocks provided, then fill in completely the corresponding circle in each column. If you wish to have your score posted, fill in an identification number of up to 9 digits (**DO NOT** use your Social Security Number) and fill in the corresponding circle in each column.

    e. Above your name, write your test booklet number.

3. Part III consists of 2 essay items. Directions for this section are found on page 12. Write your answers to these items on the lined paper provided. You may use pen or pencil. On each page of your answers, write your **TEST BOOKLET NUMBER. DO NOT** write your name on these pages.

4. If you have a question during the test, do not leave your seat—raise your hand and a proctor will come to you.

5. You have until 11:00 a.m. to complete this test.

FIGURE 9.1 Example of a cover page with general directions.

space between items so that each item is distinct from the others. If not, the students might inadvertently read a line from a preceding or following item and think it belongs to the item they are answering (p. 192). Tightly packing words on a page may minimize the amount of paper used for testing, but facilitating maximum student performance on a test is worth a small additional expense for a few more sheets of paper (Gaberson, 1996).

Optimum spacing varies for each item format. The response options for a multiple-choice item should not be printed in tandem fashion, as the following example illustrates:

1.   Which method of anesthesia involves injection of an agent into a nerve bundle that supplies the operative site?
      A. General; B. Local; C. Regional; D. Spinal; E. Topical

The options are much easier to read if listed in a single column below the stem (Haladyna, 2004), as in this example:

1.   Which method of anesthesia involves injection of an agent into a nerve bundle that supplies the operative site?

      A. General
      B. Local
      C. Regional
      D. Spinal
      E. Topical

Notice in this example that the second line of the stem is indented to the same position as the first line and that the responses are slightly indented. This spacing makes the item number and its content easier to read.

Keep Related Material Together

The stem of a multiple-choice item and all related responses should appear on the same page. Both columns of a matching exercise should also be printed side by side and on one page, including the related directions; using short lists of premises and responses makes this arrangement easier. With context-dependent items, the introductory material and all related items should be contained on the same page, if possible. This facilitates reading the material and related questions (Haladyna, 2004). Otherwise, students may be distracted as they turn pages back and forth to read and respond to the test items, and they may make careless errors unrelated to their knowledge of the content (Nitko, 2004).

Facilitate Scoring

If the test will be scored by hand, the layout of the test or the answer sheet should facilitate easy scoring. A separate answer sheet can be constructed to permit rapid scoring by comparing student responses to an answer key. If the students record their answers directly on the test booklet, the test items should be arranged with scoring in mind. For example, a series of true-false items should be organized with columns of Ts and Fs at either the right or left margin so that students need only circle their responses, as in the following example:

T   F   1.   A stethoscope is required to perform auscultation.

T   F   2.   Physical exam techniques should be performed in the order of least to most intrusive.

T   F   3.   When using percussion, it is easier to detect a change from dullness to resonance.

Circling a letter rather than writing or printing it will prevent misinterpretation of the students' handwriting. With completion items, printing blank spaces for the answers in tandem, as in the following example, makes scoring difficult:

1.   List 3 responsibilities of the circulating nurse during induction of general anesthesia.

_____, _____, _____

Instead, the blanks should be arranged in a column along one side of the page, as in this example:

1–3.   List 3 responsibilities of the   1. _____
circulating nurse during in-   2. _____
duction of general anesthe-   3. _____
sia.

Arrange the Correct Answers in a Random Pattern

Many teachers have a tendency to favor certain response positions for the correct or keyed answer to objective test items, for example, to assign the correct response to the A or D position of a multiple-choice item. Some teachers arrange test items so that the correct answers form a pattern that makes scoring easy (e.g., T-F-T-F, or A-B-C-D). Test-wise students may use such test characteristics to gain an unfair advantage (Haladyna, 2004). Response positions should be used with approximately equal frequency; there are several ways to accomplish this.

Many item analysis software programs calculate the number of times the keyed response occurs in each position, or the teacher can tally the number of Ts and Fs, or As, Bs, Cs, and Ds, on the answer key by hand. For true-false items, if either true or false statements are found to predominate, some items may be rewritten to make the distribution more equal (although it is recommended by some experts to include more false than true items).

Haladyna (2004) recommended that the position of the correct response in multiple-choice items be randomly assigned. This avoids what Attali and Bar-Hillel (2003) referred to as edge aversion. Edge aversion theory suggests that the correct answer is seldom placed in the first or last option, giving students a clue to select instead one of the middle options. By randomly assigning the correct response, the position of the correct answer is used about the same number of times and avoids the "effects of edge aversion" (Haladyna, 2004, p. 113).

Arrange Options in Logical or Numerical Order

The response alternatives for multiple-choice and matching items should be arranged according to a logical or meaningful order, such as alphabetical or chronological order, or in order of size or degree. This type of arrangement reduces reading time (Nitko, 2004); it also helps students who know the correct answer to search though the options to find it. This strategy also tends to randomly distribute the correct answer position, especially on lengthy tests.

When the options are numerical, they should always be in ascending or descending numerical order (Haladyna, 2004). This saves reading time for the test-taker. This principle can be seen in the example that follows:

Options Not Ordered	*Options in Numerical Order*
Your patient is ordered gu-aifenesin 300mg four times daily. It comes in 200mg/5mL. How many milliliters should you give per dose?	Your patient is ordered gu-aifenesin 300mg four times daily. It comes in 200mg/5mL. How many milliliters should you give per dose?
a. 5.0mL	e. 2.5mL
b. 2.5mL	f. 5.0mL
c. 10mL	g. 7.5mL*
d. 7.5mL*	h. 10mL

Number the Items Continuously Throughout the Test

Although test items should be grouped according to format, they should be numbered continuously throughout the test. That is, the teacher should not start each new item format section with item number 1 but continue numbering items in continuous sequence. This numbering system helps students to find items they may have skipped and to avoid making errors when recording their answers.

Proofread

The test items and directions should be free of spelling, punctuation, grammatical, and typing errors. Such defects are a source of measurement error and can cause confusion and distraction, particularly among students who are anxious (Haladyna, 2004). Typographical and similar errors are a problem for any student but more so for those who have learning disabilities or who use English as a second language. Often the test designer does not recognize his or her own errors; another teacher who knows the content may be asked to proofread a copy of the test before it is duplicated. The spell-check or grammar-check features of a word processing program may not recognize punctuation errors or words that are spelled correctly but used in the wrong context, nor will they detect structural errors such as giving two test items the same number or two responses the same letter (Gaberson, 1996).

Prepare an Answer Key

Whether the test will be machine-scored or hand-scored, the teacher should prepare and verify an answer key in advance to facilitate efficient scoring and to provide a final check on the accuracy of the test items. Scannable answer sheets also can be used for hand-scoring; an answer key can be produced by punching holes to indicate the correct answers. The teacher also should prepare ideal responses to essay items, identify intended responses to completion items, and make decisions regarding the point values of required answer elements if the analytical scoring method is used.

REPRODUCING THE TEST

Assure Legibility

Legibility is an important consideration when printing and duplicating the test; poor quality copies may interfere with optimum student performance. A font that includes only upper-case letters is difficult to read; upper- and lower-case lettering is recommended. The master or original copy should be letter-quality, produced with a laser or other high quality printer so that it can be clearly reproduced. For best results, the test should be photocopied on a machine that has sufficient toner to produce crisp, dark print without any stray lines or artifacts.

Print on One Side of the Page

The test should be reproduced on only one side of each sheet of paper. Printing on both sides of each page could cause students to skip items unintentionally or make errors when recording their scores on a separate answer sheet. It also creates distractions from excessive page-turning during the test. If the test is to be hand-scored and students record their answers on the test rather than on a separate answer sheet, printing only on one side makes it easier to score.

Duplicate Enough Copies

The teacher should duplicate more test copies than the number of students to allow for extra copies for proctors or to replace defective copies that may have been distributed inadvertently to students. Displaying test items on a screen from an overhead projector or computer projector, or writing them on the chalkboard or interactive whiteboard, may save money, but these procedures may cause problems for students with learning or visual disabilities. When students do not have their own copies of a test for whatever reason, they cannot control the pace at which they answer items or return to a previous item. Dictating test items is not recommended except when the objective is to test knowledge of correct spelling; in addition to creating problems for students with hearing impairments, this method wastes time that students could otherwise spend in thinking about and responding to the items. In addition, there is no record of how the items were worded, which could present a problem if a student later questions how an answer was scored.

Maintain Test Security

Teachers have a serious responsibility to maintain the security of tests by protecting them from unauthorized access. Carelessness on the part of the teacher can enable dishonest students to gain access to test materials and use them to obtain higher scores than they deserve. This contributes to measurement error, and it is unfair to honest students who are well-prepared for the test. It is up to the teacher to make arrangements to secure the test while it is being prepared, duplicated, stored, administered, and scored.

Test materials should be stored in locked areas accessible only to authorized personnel. Computer files that contain test items should be protected with passwords, encryption, or similar security devices. Only regular employees should handle test materials; student employees should not be asked to type, print, or duplicate tests. While test items are being typed, they should be protected from the view of others by turning the monitor off if an unauthorized individual enters the area. Printed drafts of tests should be destroyed by shredding pages rather than discarding them in trash or recycling receptacles.

One suggestion for preventing cheating during test administration to large groups is to prepare alternative forms of the test. This can be done by presenting the same questions but in a different order on each form. For calculation items the teacher can modify values within the same question on different forms; in that way the responses will differ (Center for Teaching Excellence, 2003). This same strategy can be used with online tests. Faculty members can prepare alternative forms of the test for students to complete online. Software is also available that allows for random sequencing of items on an online exam. The problem with this technique is that a random sequencing may not be consistent with principles for ordering items on a test. It also may result in alternative forms of a test that are not equivalent.

Similarly, the order of responses to multiple-choice and matching items might be scrambled to produce an alternative form of the test. However, the psychometric properties of alternative forms produced in these ways might be sufficiently different as to result in different scores, especially when the positions of items with unequal difficulty are switched. If there is little or no evidence for the true equivalence of these alternative forms, it is best not to use this approach. Other ways to prevent cheating are discussed in the next section of this chapter.

TEST ADMINISTRATION

Environmental Conditions: Face-to-Face and Online

The environmental conditions of test administration can be a source of measurement error if they interfere with the students' performance. If possible, the teacher should select a room that limits potential distractions during the test. For example, if windows must be open for ventilation during warm weather, the students may be distracted by lawn mowing or construction noise; requesting a room on another side of the building may prevent the problem. Placing a sign such as "Testing—Quiet Please" on the door of the classroom may reduce noise in the hallway.

For online courses, it is critical to determine prior to the test administration that students have the computer capabilities and Internet access to take the exam for the time period allotted. Students with dial-up modems may experience problems "timing out," being disconnected from the Internet by their Internet Service Providers after a set period of time or what appears to be inactivity on the part of the user. When that occurs, the students cannot transmit their completed exams, and course management systems such as BlackBoard will not permit them to access another copy.

Distributing the Test Materials

Careful organization allows the teacher to distribute test materials and give instructions to the students efficiently. With large groups of students, several proctors may be needed to assist with this process. If a separate answer sheet is used, it usually can be distributed first, followed by the test booklets. During distribution of the test booklets, the teacher should instruct students to not turn the cover page and begin the test until told to do so. At this point, the students should check their test booklets for completeness, and the proctors should replace defective booklets. The teacher then should read the general directions aloud while the students read along. Hearing the directions may help students whose anxiety may interfere with their comprehension of the written instructions. Once the teacher answers the questions about the test procedures, the students can begin the test.

Answering Questions During the Test

Some students may find it necessary to ask questions of the teacher during a test, but responding to these questions is always somewhat disturbing to other students. Distraction can be kept to a minimum by telling students to raise their hands if they have questions rather than leaving their seats to approach the teacher; a proctor then goes to each student's seat. Proctors should answer questions as quietly and briefly as possible. In answering questions, proctors certainly should address errors in the test copy and ambiguity in directions but should avoid giving clues to the correct answers. When writing items, teachers should work to eliminate cultural bias and terms that would be unfamiliar to students for whom English is not their native language. This is discussed further in chapter 14.

Preventing Cheating

Cheating is widely believed to be common on college campuses in the United States. A recent study found that a "steadily growing number of students cheat or plagiarize in college" (Hinman, 2004, p. A19). Hinman suggested that when teachers know their students, interact with them about their learning, and give meaningful assignments, they create an environment in which cheating is less likely to occur.

Cheating is defined as any activity whose purpose is to gain a higher score on a test or other academic assignment than a student is likely to earn on the basis of achievement. Cheating on a test can take the form of acquiring test materials in advance of the test or sharing these materials with others, arranging for a substitute to take a test, preparing and using unauthorized notes during the test, exchanging information with others or copying answers from another student during the test, and copying test items or retaining test booklets to share with others who may take the test later. With adequate test security and good proctoring during the test, the teacher can prevent these opportunities for cheating. Students who do act honestly resent those who cheat, especially if dishonest students are rewarded with high test scores. Honest students also resent faculty who do not recognize and deal effectively with cheating (Gaberson, 1997).

Although a number of methods for preventing cheating during a test have been proposed, one effective method is careful proctoring. In research by Kerkvliet and Sigmund (1999), having a proctor in the room was a deterrent to cheating; there was a 12% reduction in cheating when a proctor was in the room. There should be enough proctors to supervise students adequately during exams; for most groups of students, at least two proctors are suggested so that one is available to leave the room with a student in case of emergency without leaving the remaining students unsupervised (Gaberson, 1996). When proctoring a test, it is important to be serious about the task and devote full attention to it rather than bringing papers to grade and other materials to work on.

A particularly troubling situation for teachers is how to deal with a student's behavior that suggests cheating during a test. Prior to administering the test, the teacher must know the policies of the nursing program and college or university if a student cheats on an examination or another assessment. When teachers are certain that a student is cheating, they should quietly collect the test and answer sheet and ask the student to leave the room. However, if it is possible that the teacher's interpretation of the behavior is incorrect, it may be best not to confront the student at that time. In addition to preventing a potentially innocent student from completing the test, confiscating test materials and ordering a student to leave will create a distraction to other students that may affect the accuracy of all the students' test scores. A better response is to continue to observe the student, making eye contact if possible to make the student aware of the teacher's attention. If the student was attempting to cheat, this approach usually effectively stops the behavior. If the behavior continues, the teacher should attempt to verify this observation with another proctor, and if both agree, the student may be asked to leave the room (Gaberson, 1997). The appropriate penalty for cheating on a test is a score of zero for that test. The teacher should not just deduct points from the test score or lower the grade in some other way. By deducting points, it appears as though the student took the exam and achieved a low score on it when that was not the case.

If the teacher learns that a copy of a test is circulating in advance of the scheduled date of administration, the teacher should attempt to obtain verifiable evidence that some students have seen it. In this case, the teacher needs to prepare another test or develop a new way of assessing student learning. As described in this book, there are many assessment strategies applicable for measuring learning outcomes in nursing.

Online Testing. As more courses and programs are offered through distance education, teachers are faced with how to prevent cheating on an assessment when they cannot directly observe the students. There are different approaches that can be used, ranging from administering the tests in a traditional, face-to-face session to computer adaptive tests.

Examinations in an online course can be given on campus as done with face-to-face courses or in an on-campus computer testing facility. Students can be required to take tests within a designated time period, for example, one week, on campus. Some institutions with large online programs have testing facilities throughout the state where nursing students can go to take their tests in a proctored traditional way. Another option is to make arrangements for students to take the exam at a library, school, or other facility close to the student's home, or where the exam can be proctored. In these situations, whether on- or off-campus, students must provide proof of identity. One issue with this approach, though, is that it may conflict with the reasons that the student enrolled in an online course, for example, living in a rural area and scheduling conflicts, among others.

With course management systems such as BlackBoard and WebCT, teachers can administer a proctored examination online. The test can be set up to require the proctor to input his or her ID and a password known only to the proctor to start the exam (McNett, 2002). The students can only access the test with their IDs at that same time. With these course management systems, the teacher can also limit access to a test to a specific day and time, and can restrict the time allowed to complete the exam, similar to traditional test administration. By offering short tests more frequently and limiting the time for their completion, teachers provide fewer opportunities for students to look up the answers during a test. Tests that are shorter also help students who use dial-up connections, which may "time out" before the allowable testing time expires.

Another method of discouraging cheating is to post a copy of an honor code policy on a Web page that precedes the test. After reading the honor code, students can be asked to affirm that they will not use course notes, textbooks, and other resources to complete the test and will not consult with others during it.

There is also software that allows the teacher to develop a database of questions. The software program then selects items, according to principles set by the faculty member, to include in the test (McNett, 2002). This software can be used to randomly order items in a test, developing alternative forms of the exam that can be randomly assigned to the students. An important issue with this approach, as mentioned earlier, is that the psychometric properties of the alternative forms might not be the same. Without knowing if the forms are truly equal, it is best not to use this approach. Software also is available to develop computer adaptive tests like the NCLEX examinations; the student's answers determine the subsequent questions.

Collecting Test Materials

For traditional on-site tests, when students are finished with the test and are preparing to leave the room, the resulting confusion and noise can disturb students who are still working. The teacher should plan for efficient collection of test materials to minimize such distractions and to maintain test security. It is important to assure that no test materials leave the room with the students. Therefore, teachers should take care to verify that the students turn in their test booklets, answer sheets, scratch paper, and any other test materials. With a large group of students, one proctor may be assigned the task of collecting test materials from each student; this proctor should check the test booklet and answer sheet to assure that the directions for marking answers were followed, that the student's name (or number) is recorded as directed, and that the student has not omitted any items. Any such errors can then be corrected before the student leaves the room, and test security will not be compromised.

If students are still working near the end of the allotted testing time, the remaining amount of time should be announced, and they should be encouraged to finish as quickly as possible. When the time is up, all students must stop, and the teacher or proctor must collect the rest of the tests. Students who have not finished the test at that point cannot have additional time unless they have legitimate learning disabilities. In those cases, the testing time may be extended if the student's learning disability has been confirmed according to college or university policies. This decision should be made in advance of the test and the necessary arrangements made. Extended testing time is not an appropriate remedy for every learning disability, however. It should be provided only when specifically prescribed based on a psychoeducational evaluation of a student's abilities and needs.

SUMMARY

The final appearance of a test and the way in which it is administered can affect the validity of the test results. Poor arrangement of test items, confusing or missing directions, typographical errors, and careless administration may contribute to measurement error. Careful planning can help the teacher to avoid or minimize these difficulties.

Rules for good test design include allowing sufficient time, arranging test items in a logical sequence, writing general and item format directions, using a cover page, spacing test elements to avoid crowding, keeping related material together, arranging the correct answers in a random or logical pattern, numbering items consecutively throughout the test, proofreading the test, and preparing an accurate answer key. In preparing to duplicate the test, the teacher should assure legibility, print the test on one side of each page, prepare enough copies for all students and proctors, and maintain the security of test materials.

Although administering a test is usually the simplest phase of the testing process, there are some common problems that may affect the reliability of the resulting scores. Teachers should arrange for favorable environmental conditions, distribute the test materials and give directions efficiently, make appropriate plans for proctoring and answering questions during the test, and collect test materials efficiently. Strategies were described for administering tests in an online environment including approaches to prevent cheating. Teachers have an important responsibility to prevent cheating before, during, and after a test, and should respond to verified evidence of cheating with appropriate sanctions.

REFERENCES

Attali, Y., & Bar-Hillel, M. (2003). Guess where: The position of correct answers in multiple-choice test items as a psychometric variable. *Journal of Educational Measurement, 40*, 109–128.

Center for Teaching Excellence. (2003). Practical approaches to dealing with cheating on exams. University of Illinois at Urbana-Champaign. Instructional Development, Center for Teaching Excellence. Accessed February 19, 2005, from http://www.oir.uiuc.edu/Did/Resources/Illini%20Instructor/Cheating.htm

Gaberson, K. B. (1996). Test design: Putting all the pieces together. *Nurse Educator*, *21*(4), 28–33.

Gaberson, K. B. (1997). Academic dishonesty among nursing students. *Nursing Forum*, *32*(3), 14–20.

Haladyna, T. M. (2004). *Developing and validating multiple-choice test items*. Mahwah, NJ: Lawrence Erlbaum.

Hinman, L. M. (2004, September 3). How to fight college cheating. *The Washington Post*, p. A19.

Hopkins, K. D. (1998). *Educational and psychological measurement and evaluation* (8th ed.). Boston: Allyn & Bacon.

Kerkvliet, J., & Sigmund, C. L. (1999). Can we control cheating in the classroom? *The Journal of Economic Education*, *30*(4), 331–343.

Kubiszyn, T., & Borich, G. (2003). *Educational testing and measurement: Classroom application and practice* (7th ed.). New York: John Wiley.

McNett, M. (2002). Curbing academic dishonesty in online courses. *Pointers & Clickers*. Accessed February 21, 2005, from http://www.ion.illinois.edu/resources/pointersclickers/2002_05/index.asp

Nitko, A. J. (2004). *Educational assessment of students* (4th ed.). Upper Saddle River, NJ: Prentice Hall.

Chapter 10

Scoring and Analyzing Tests

After administering a test, the teacher's responsibility is to score it or arrange to have it scored. The teacher then interprets the results and uses these interpretations to make grading, selection, placement, or other decisions. To accurately interpret test scores, however, the teacher needs to analyze the performance of the test as a whole and of the individual test items, and to use these data to draw valid inferences about student performance. This information also helps faculty prepare for posttest discussions with students about the exam. This chapter discusses the processes of obtaining scores and performing test and item analysis. It also suggests ways in which teachers can use posttest discussions to contribute to student learning and seek student feedback that can lead to test item improvement.

SCORING

Many teachers say that they "grade" tests, when in fact it would be more accurate to say that they "score" tests. Scoring is the process of determining the first direct, unconverted, uninterpreted measure of performance on a test, usually called the raw score or observed score. The raw score represents the number of correct answers or number of points awarded to separate parts of an assessment (Nitko, 2004, p. 385). On the other hand, grading or marking is the process of assigning a symbol to represent the quality of the student's performance. Symbols can be letters (A, B, C, D, F, which may also include + and −); categories (pass-fail, satisfactory-unsatisfactory); integers (9 through 1); or percentages (100, 99, 98 . . .), among other options (Kubiszyn & Borich, 2003). In most cases, test scores should not be converted to grades for the purpose of later computing a final average grade. Instead the teacher should record actual test scores and then combine them into a composite score that can be converted to a final grade. Recording scores contributes to greater measurement accuracy because information is lost each time scores are converted to grades. For example, if scores from 70 to 79 are all converted to a grade of C, each score in this range receives the same grade, although scores of 71 and 78 may represent important differences in achievement. If the C grades are all converted to the same numerical grade, for example, C = 2.0, then such distinctions are lost when the teacher computes the final grade for the course. Various grading systems and their uses are discussed in Chapter 16.

Weighting Items

As a general rule, each objectively scored test item should have equal weight. It is difficult for teachers to justify that one item is worth 2 points while another is worth 1 point; such a weighting system also motivates students to argue for partial credit for some answers. Differential weighting implies that the teacher believes knowledge of one concept to be more important than knowledge of another concept. When this is true, the better approach is to write more items about the important concept; this emphasis would be reflected in the test blueprint, which specifies the number of items for each content area. Most machine-scoring systems assign 1 point to each correct answer; this seems reasonable for hand-scored tests as well. It is not necessary to adjust the numerical weight of items in order to achieve a total of 100 points. Although a test of 100 points allows the teacher to calculate a percentage score quickly, this step is not necessary to make valid interpretations of students' scores.

Correction for Guessing

The raw score sometimes is adjusted or corrected before it is interpreted. One procedure involves applying a formula intended to eliminate any advantage that a student might have gained by guessing correctly. The correction formula reduces the raw score by some fraction of the number of the student's wrong answers (Nitko, 2004, p. 312). The formula only can be used with true-false, multiple-choice, and some matching items, and is dependent upon the number of options per item. The general formula is:

$$\text{Corrected score} = R - \frac{W}{(n-1)} \qquad \text{[Equation 10.1]}$$

where R is the number of right answers, W is the number of wrong answers, and n is the number of options in each item (Nitko, 2004, p. 312). Thus, for 2-option items like true-false, the teacher merely subtracts the number of wrong answers from the number of right answers (or raw score); for 4-option items, the raw score is reduced by $1/3$ of the number of wrong answers. A correction formula obviously is difficult to use for a test that contains several different item formats.

The use of a correction formula is appropriate only when the students have been instructed to not answer any item for which they are uncertain of the answer. Even under these circumstances, students may differ in their interpretation of "certainty" and therefore may interpret the advice differently. Some students will guess regardless of the instructions given and the threat of a penalty; the risk-taking or test-wise student is likely to be rewarded with a higher score than the risk-avoiding or non-test-wise student because of guessing some answers correctly. These personality differences cannot be equalized by instructions not to guess and penalties for guessing. The use of a correction formula also is based on the assumption that the student who does not know the answer will guess blindly. However, Nitko (2004) suggested that the chance of getting a high score by random guessing was slim, though many students choose correct answers through informed guesses based on some knowledge of the content. Use of a correction formula also complicates the scoring process, allowing opportunities for scoring errors (Nitko, 2004, p. 313). Based on these limitations, the best approach is to advise all students to answer every item, even if they are uncertain about their answers, and apply no correction for guessing.

ITEM ANALYSIS

Computer software for item analysis is widely available for use with electronic answer sheet scanning equipment. Figure 10.1 is an example of a computer-generated item analysis report. For teachers who do not have access to such equipment and software, procedures for analyzing student responses to test items by hand are described in detail later in this section. Regardless of the method used for analysis, teachers should be familiar enough with the meaning of each item analysis statistic to correctly interpret the results. It is important to realize that most item analysis techniques are designed for items that are scored dichotomously, that is, either right or wrong, from tests that are intended for norm-referenced uses (Nitko, 2004).

Difficulty Index

One useful indication of test item quality is its difficulty. The most commonly employed index of difficulty is the p level; p levels range from 0 to 1.00, indicating

ITEM STATISTICS
(N = 68)

Item	Key	A	B	C	D	E	Omit	Multiple Response	Diff. Index	Discrim. Index
1	A	44	0	24	0	0	0	0	.65	.34
2	B	0	62	4	2	0	0	0	.91	.06
3	A	59	1	4	4	0	0	0	.87	.35
4	C	12	4	51	1	0	0	0	.75	.19
5	E	23	8	0	8	29	0	0	.43	.21
6	D	2	3	17	46	0	0	0	.68	.17

FIGURE 10.1   Sample computer-generated item analysis report.

Note: Diff. Index = difficulty index

Discrim. Index = discrimination index

the percentage of students who answered the item correctly. A p value of 0 indicates that no one answered the item correctly, and a value of 1.00 indicates that every student answered the item correctly (Nitko, 2004).

A simple formula for calculating the p value is:

$$p = \frac{R}{T} \qquad \text{[Equation 10.2]}$$

where R is the number of students who responded correctly and T is the total number of students who took the test (Nitko, 2004).

The difficulty index is commonly interpreted to mean that items with p values of .20 and below are difficult, and items with p values of .80 and above are easy. However, this interpretation may imply that test items are intrinsically easy or difficult and may not take into account the quality of the instruction or the abilities of the students in that group. A group of students who were taught by an expert instructor might tend to answer a test item correctly, while a group of students with similar abilities who were taught by a ineffectual instructor might tend to answer it incorrectly. Different p values might be produced by students with more or less ability. Thus, test items cannot be labeled as easy or difficult without considering how well that content was taught.

The *p* value also should be interpreted in relationship to the student's probability of guessing the correct response. For example, if all students guess the answer to a true-false item, on the basis of chance alone, the *p* value of that item should be approximately .50. On a 4-option multiple-choice item, chance alone should produce a *p* value of .25.

For most tests whose results will be interpreted in a norm-referenced way, *p* values of .30 to .70 are desirable. Very easy and very difficult items have little power to discriminate between students who know the content and students who do not, and they also decrease the reliability of the test scores. Teachers can use item difficulty information to identify content that may need to be retaught or to identify test items that are ambiguous (Nitko, 2004).

Discrimination Index

The discrimination index, *D*, is a powerful indicator of test item quality. A positively discriminating item is one that was answered correctly more often by students who scored well on the total test than by those who scored poorly on the total test. A negatively discriminating item was answered correctly more often by students who scored poorly on the test than by those who scored well. When an equal number of high and low scoring students answers the item correctly, then the item is nondiscriminating (Nitko, 2004).

A number of item discrimination indices are available; a simple method of computing *D* is:

$$D = p_h - p_l \qquad \text{[Equation 10.3]}$$

where p_h is the fraction of students in the high-scoring group who answered the item correctly and p_l is the fraction of students in the low-scoring group who answered the item correctly (Hopkins, 1998, p. 261; Nitko, 2004, p. 319). Computer item analysis programs usually calculate *D* as the correlation of the item with the total score on the test (Hopkins, 1998, p. 260).

The *D* value ranges from −1.00 to +1.00. In general, the higher the positive value, the better the test item. Hopkins (1998) indicated that *D* values of .40 and higher indicate excellent discrimination (i.e., very good items), values between 0.30 and 0.39 indicate good discrimination (i.e., reasonably good items), values between .10 and .29 suggest fair discrimination (i.e., that the item needs to be improved), and values below 0.10 indicate poor discrimination (i.e., items that should be revised or not used again) (p. 260). One possible interpretation of a negative *D* value is that the item was misinterpreted by high scorers (Hopkins, 1998), who thought that the item meant something different from what the teacher intended. Negative D values signal items that should be reviewed carefully; they may need to be revised or eliminated (Nitko, 2004, p. 320).

When interpreting a D value, it is important to keep in mind that an item's ability to discriminate is highly related to its difficulty index. An item that is answered correctly by all students has a difficulty index of 1.00; the discrimination index for this item is 0.00, because there is no difference in performance on that item between students whose overall test scores were high and those whose scores were low. Similarly, if all students answered the item incorrectly, the difficulty index is 0.00, and the discrimination index is also 0.00 because there is no discrimination power.

Distractor Analysis

As previously indicated, item analysis statistics can serve as indicators of test item quality. No teacher, however, should make decisions about retaining a test item in its present form, revising it, or eliminating it from future use on the basis of the item statistics alone. The teacher should carefully examine each questionable test item for evidence of poorly functioning distractors, ambiguous alternatives, and miskeying.

Every distractor should be selected by at least one lower-group student, and more lower-group students should select it than higher-group students. A distractor that is not selected by any student in the lower group may contain a technical flaw or may be so implausible as to be obvious even to students who lack knowledge of the correct answer. A distractor is ambiguous if upper-group students tend to choose it with about the same frequency as the keyed, or correct, response. This result usually indicates that there is no one clearly correct or best answer. Poorly functioning and ambiguous distractors may be revised to make them more plausible or to eliminate the ambiguity. If a large number of higher-scoring students select a particular incorrect response, the teacher should check to see if the answer key is correct. In each case, the content of the item, not the statistics alone, should guide the teacher's decision-making (Nitko, 2004).

Performing an Item Analysis by Hand

The following process for performing item analysis by hand is adapted from Hopkins (1998) and Nitko (2004):

Step 1. After the test is scored, arrange the test scores in rank order, highest to lowest.

Step 2. Divide the scores into a high-scoring half and a low-scoring half. For this step, some sources recommend dividing scores into equal thirds (Hopkins,

1998; Nitko, 2004) or identifying scores in the upper and lower 25% of the distribution and not using the remaining scores for analysis. The use of two groups is recommended for the purpose of this discussion because it is more useful with scores from small groups of students and because the resulting calculations are easy to perform.

Step 3. For each item, tally the number of students in each group who chose each alternative. Record these counts on a copy of the test item next to each response option. The keyed response for the following sample item is d; the group of 20 students is divided into 2 groups of 10 students each.

1. What is the most likely explanation for breast asymmetry in an adolescent girl?

		Higher	*Lower*
A.	Blocked mammary duct in the larger breast	0	3
B.	Endocrine disorder	2	3
C.	Mastitis in the larger breast	0	0
*D.	Normal variation in growth	8	4

Step 4. Calculate the difficulty index for each item. The following formula is a variation of the one presented earlier, to account for the division of scores into two groups:

$$p = \frac{R_h + R_l}{T} \qquad \text{[Equation 10.4]}$$

where R_h is the number of students in the high-scoring half who answered correctly, R_l is the number of students in the low-scoring half who answered correctly, and T is the total number of students. For the purpose of calculating the difficulty index, consider omitted responses and multiple responses as incorrect. For the example in Step 4, the p value is .60, indicating a moderately difficult item.

Step 5. Calculate the discrimination index for each item. Using the data from Step 4, divide R_h by the total number of students in that group to obtain p_h. Repeat the process to calculate p_l from R_l. Subtract p_l from p_h to obtain D, as in Equation 9.3. For the example in Step 4, the discrimination index is .40, indicating that the item discriminates well between high-scoring and low-scoring students.

Step 6. Check each item for implausible distractors, ambiguity, and miskeying. It is obvious that in the sample item, no students chose "Mastitis in the larger breast" as the correct answer. This distractor does not contribute to the discrimination power of the item, and the teacher should consider replacing it with an alternative that might be more plausible.

TEST CHARACTERISTICS

In addition to item analysis results, information about how the test performed as a whole also helps teachers to interpret test results. Measures of central tendency and variability, reliability estimates, and the shape of the score distribution can assist the teacher to make judgments about the quality of the test; difficulty and discrimination indices are related to these test characteristics. Test statistics are discussed in detail in chapter 15.

In addition, teachers should examine test items in the aggregate for evidence of bias. For example, although there may be no obvious gender bias in any single test item, such a bias may be apparent when all items are reviewed as a group. Similar cases of ethnic, racial, religious, and cultural bias may be found when items are grouped and examined together. The effect of bias on testing and evaluation is discussed in detail in chapter 14.

CONDUCTING POSTTEST DISCUSSIONS

Giving students feedback about test results can be an opportunity to reinforce learning, to correct misinformation, and to solicit their input for improvement of test items. But a feedback session also can be an invitation to engage in battle, with students attacking to gain extra points and the teacher defending the honor of the test and, it often seems, the very right to give tests. Discussions with students about the test should be rational rather than the teacher asserting power and authority (Kubiszyn & Borich, 2003). Posttest discussions can be beneficial to both teachers and students if they are planned in advance and not emotionally charged. The teacher should prepare for a posttest discussion by completing a test and item analysis and reviewing the items that were most difficult for the majority of students. Discussion should focus on items missed and possible reasons why. Student comments about how the test is designed, its directions, and individual test items provide an opportunity for the teacher to improve the test (Kubiszyn & Borich).

To use time efficiently, the teacher should give the correct answers quickly. If the test is hand-scored, correct answers may be indicated by the teacher on the students' answer sheets or test booklets. If machine-scoring is used, the answer key may be reproduced on a transparency and displayed. Teachers should continue to protect the security of the test during the posttest discussion by accounting for all test booklets and answer sheets and by eliminating other opportunities for cheating. Some teachers do not allow students to use pens or pencils during the feedback session to prevent answer-changing and subsequent complaints that scoring errors were made. Another approach is to distribute pens with red or green ink and permit only those pens to be used to mark answers. Teachers also should decide in advance whether to permit students to take notes during the session.

Some teachers allow students to record their answers on the test booklets, where the students also record their names. At the completion of the exam, students submit the answer sheets and their test booklets to the teacher. Students then are able to return to the room to check their answers using their test booklets. The teacher might project the answers onto a screen using overhead, opaque, or computer projection. At the conclusion of this session, the test booklets are then collected by the teacher or proctor. It is important not to review and discuss individual items because the test has not yet been scored and analyzed. However, students can be asked to write down problematic questions with a rationale that the teacher can use in conjunction with the item analysis (Kubiszyn & Borich, 2003). One disadvantage to this method of giving posttest feedback is that because the test has not yet been scored and analyzed, the teacher would not have an opportunity to thoroughly prepare for the session; feedback consists only of the correct answers, and no discussion takes place.

Whatever the structure of the posttest discussion, the teacher should control the session so that it produces maximum benefit for all students. While discussing an item that was answered incorrectly by a majority of students, the teacher should maintain a calm, matter-of-fact, nondefensive attitude. Students who answered the item incorrectly may be asked to provide their rationale for choosing an incorrect response; students who supplied or chose the right answer may be asked to explain why it is correct. The teacher should avoid arguing with students about individual items and engaging in emotionally charged discussion; instead, the teacher should either invite written comments as described above or schedule individual appointments to discuss the items in question. Students who need additional help are encouraged to make appointments with the teacher for individual review sessions.

Eliminating Items or Adding Points

Teachers often debate the merits of adjusting test scores by eliminating items or adding points to compensate for real or perceived deficiencies in test construction or performance. For example, during a posttest discussion, students may argue that if they all answered an item incorrectly, the item should be omitted or all students should be awarded an extra point to compensate for the "bad item." It is interesting to note that students seldom propose subtracting a point from their scores if they all answer an item correctly. In any case, how should the teacher respond to such requests? In this discussion, a distinction is made between test items that are technically flawed and those that do not function as intended.

If test items are properly constructed, critiqued, and proofread, it is unlikely that serious flaws will appear on the test. However, errors that do appear may have varying effects on students' scores. For example, if the correct answer to a multiple-choice item is inadvertently omitted from the test, no student will be able to answer the item correctly. In this case, the item simply should not be scored. That is, if the error is discovered during or after test administration and before the test is scored, the item is omitted from the answer key; a test that was intended to be worth 73 points then is worth 72 points. If the error is discovered after the tests are scored, they can be re-scored. Students often worry about the effect of this change on their scores and may argue that they should be awarded an extra point in this case. The possible effects of both adjustments on a hypothetical score are as follows:

	Total possible points	Raw score	Percent correct
Original test	73	62	84.9
Flawed item not scored	72	62	86.1
Point added to raw score	73	63	86.3

It is obvious that omitting the flawed item and adding a point to the raw score produce nearly identical results. Although students might view adding a point to their scores as more satisfying, it makes little sense to award a point for an item that was not answered correctly. The "extra" point in fact does not represent knowledge of any content area or achievement of an objective, and therefore it does not contribute to a valid interpretation of the test scores. Teachers should inform students matter-of-factly that an item was eliminated from the test and reassure them that their relative standing with regard to performance on the test has not changed.

If the technical flaw consists of a misspelled word in a true–false item that does not change the meaning of the statement, no adjustment should be made.

The teacher should avoid lengthy debate about item semantics if it is clear that such errors are unlikely to have affected the students' scores. Feedback from students can be used to revise items for later use and sometimes make changes in the instruction.

Teachers should resist the temptation to eliminate items from the test solely on the basis of low difficulty and discrimination indices. Omission of items may affect the validity of the scores from the test, particularly if several items related to one content area or objective are eliminated, resulting in inadequate sampling of that content (Flynn & Reese, 1988).

Because identified flaws in test construction do contribute to measurement error, the teacher should consider taking them into account when using the test scores to make grading decisions and set cut-off scores. That is, the teacher should not fix cutoff scores for assigning grades until after all tests have been given and analyzed. The proposed grading scale then can be adjusted if necessary to compensate for deficiencies in test construction. It should be made clear to students that any changes in the grading scale because of flaws in test construction would not adversely affect their grades.

DEVELOPING A TEST ITEM BANK

Because considerable effort goes into developing, administering, and analyzing test items, teachers should develop a system for maintaining and expanding a pool or bank of items from which to select items for future tests. Teachers can maintain databases of test items on their computers with backups on computer media such as computer discs or other storage devices. When storing test item databases on computers, the computer must be password protected and test security maintained. When developing test banks, the teacher can record the following data with each test item: (a) the correct response for objective-type items and a brief scoring key for completion or essay items; (b) the course, unit, content area, or objective for which it was designed; and (c) the item analysis results for a specified period of time. Figure 10.2 is one such example.

Commercially produced software programs can be used in a similar way to develop a database of test items. Each test item is a record in the database. The test items can then be sorted according to the fields in which the data are entered; for example, the teacher could retrieve all items that are classified as Objective 3, with a moderate difficulty index.

Many publishers also offer test-item banks that relate to the content contained in their textbooks. However, faculty members need to be cautious about using these items for their own examinations. The purpose of the test, relevant characteristics of the students to be tested, and the balance and emphasis of

Content Area: Physical Assessment
Unit 5
Objective 3

1.   What is the most likely explanation for breast asymmetry in an adolescent girl?

    A.   Blocked mammary duct in the larger breast
    B.   Endocrine disorder
    C.   Mastitis in the larger breast
  *D.   Normal variation in growth

Test date	Difficulty index	Discrimination index
10/22	.72	.25
2/20	.56	.33
10/23	.60	.40

FIGURE 10.2   Sample information to include with items in test bank.

content as reflected on the teacher's test blueprint are the most important criteria for selecting test items. Although some teachers would consider these item banks to be a shortcut to the development and selection of test items, they should be evaluated carefully before they are used. There is no guarantee that the quality of test items in a published item bank is superior to that of test items that a skilled teacher can construct. Many of the items may be of questionable quality. Masters and colleagues (2001) examined a random sample of 2,913 multiple-choice items from 17 test banks accompanying selected nursing textbooks. Items were evaluated to determine if they met accepted guidelines for writing multiple-choice items and were coded as to their cognitive level based on Bloom's taxonomy. The researchers found 2,233 violations of item-writing guidelines; while most were minor problems, some were more serious flaws. Nearly half of the items were at the recall level.

In addition, published test-item banks seldom contain item analysis information such as difficulty and discrimination indices. However, this information can be calculated for each item that a teacher uses from a published item bank, and a teacher-made item file can be developed and maintained.

SUMMARY

After administering a test, the teacher must score it and interpret the results. In order to accurately interpret test scores, the teacher needs to analyze the performance of the test as a whole and the individual test items. Information about how the test performed helps teachers to give feedback to students about test results and to improve test items for future use.

Scoring is the process of determining the first direct, uninterpreted measure of performance on a test, usually called the raw score. The raw score usually represents the number of right answers. Test scores should not be converted to grades for the purpose of later computing a final average grade. Instead, the teacher should record actual test scores and then combine them into a composite score that can be converted to a final grade.

As a general rule, each objectively-scored test item should have equal weight. If knowledge of one concept is more important than knowledge of another concept, the teacher should sample the more important domain more heavily by writing more items in that area. Most machine-scoring systems assign 1 point to each correct answer; this seems reasonable for hand-scored tests as well.

A raw score sometimes is adjusted or corrected before it is interpreted. One procedure involves applying a formula intended to eliminate any advantage that a student might have gained by guessing correctly. Correcting for guessing is appropriate only when students have been instructed to not answer any item for which they are uncertain of the answer; students may interpret and follow this advice differently. Therefore, the best approach is to advise all students to answer every item, and no correction for guessing should be applied.

Item analysis can be performed by hand or by the use of a computer program. Teachers should be familiar enough with the meaning of each item analysis statistic to correctly interpret the results. The difficulty index, ranging from 0 to 1.00, indicates the percentage of students who answered the item correctly. Items with p values of .20 and below are considered to be difficult, and those with p values of .80 and above are considered to be easy. However, interpretation of the difficulty index should take into account the quality of the instruction and the abilities of the students in the group. The discrimination index, ranging from −1.00 to +1.00, is an indication of the extent to which the item was answered correctly more often by high-scoring students than by low-scoring students. In general, the higher the positive value, the better the test item; discrimination indices of .40 and higher indicate very good items. An item's ability to discriminate is highly related to its difficulty index. An item that is answered correctly by all students has a difficulty index of 1.00; the discrimination index for this item is 0.00, because there is no difference in performance on that item between high scorers and low scorers.

Flaws in test construction may have varying effects on students' scores and therefore should be handled differently. If the correct answer to a multiple-choice item is inadvertently omitted from the test, no student will be able to answer the item correctly. In this case, the item simply should not be scored. If a flaw consists of a misspelled word that does not change the meaning of the item, no adjustment should be made.

Teachers should develop a system for maintaining a pool or bank of items from which to select items for future tests. Item banks can be developed by the faculty and stored electronically. Use of published test-item banks should be based on the teacher's evaluation of the quality of the items as well as on the purpose for testing, relevant characteristics of the students, and the desired emphasis and balance of content as reflected in the teacher's test blueprint.

REFERENCES

Flynn, M. K., & Reese, J. L. (1988). Development and evaluation of classroom tests: A practical application. *Journal of Nursing Education, 27,* 61–65.

Hopkins, K. D. (1998). *Educational and psychological measurement and evaluation* (8th ed.). Boston: Allyn & Bacon.

Kubiszyn, T., & Borich, G. (2003). *Educational testing and measurement: Classroom application and practice* (7th ed.). New York: John Wiley.

Masters, J. C., Hulsmeyer, B. S., Pike, M. E., Leichty, K., Miller, M. T., & Verst, A. L. (2001). Assessment of multiple-choice questions in selected test banks accompanying text books used in nursing education. *Journal of Nursing Education, 40,* 25–32.

Nitko, A. J. (2004). *Educational assessment of students* (4th ed.). Upper Saddle River, NJ: Prentice Hall.

Chapter 11

Evaluation of Written Assignments

In most nursing courses, students complete some type of written assignment. With these assignments students can develop their critical thinking skills, gain experience with different types of writing, and achieve other outcomes specific to a course. Written assignments with feedback from the teacher help students develop their writing ability, an important outcome in any nursing program from the beginning level through graduate study. This chapter focuses on developing and evaluating written assignments for nursing courses.

PURPOSES OF WRITTEN ASSIGNMENTS

Written assignments are a major instructional and evaluation method in nursing in both the classroom and clinical practice components of a course. They can be used to achieve many learning outcomes but need to be carefully selected and designed considering the instructional goals. With written assignments students can: (a) critique the literature, integrate the literature and other sources of information, and report on their findings; (b) analyze concepts and theories and apply them to clinical situations; (c) improve their problem-solving and critical-thinking skills; (d) gain experience in formulating their ideas and communicating them in a clear and coherent way to others; and (e) develop writing skills. Many of the written assignments in clinical courses assist students in mapping out their plan of care and identifying areas in which they need further instruction. Some assignments such as keeping journals also encourage students to examine their own feelings, beliefs, and values and to reflect on their learning in a course.

Not all written assignments achieve each of these purposes, and the teacher plans the assignment based on the intended goals of learning. Assignments should meet *specific* objectives of a course and should not be included only for the purpose of having a written assignment as a course requirement. Instead, they should be carefully selected to help students improve their writing and achieve course outcomes.

Because writing is a developmental process that improves with practice, writing assignments should build on one another throughout a course and nursing program. A sequence of papers across courses encourages the improvement of writing more effectively than having students complete a different type of paper in each course. This planning also eliminates excessive repetition of assignments in the program. Along the same line, faculty should decide on the number of written assignments needed by students to achieve the outcomes of a course or clinical practice experience. In some clinical nursing courses, students complete the same assignments repeatedly throughout a course, leading to their frustration with the "paperwork" in the course. How many times do students need to submit a written assessment of a patient? Written assignments are time consuming for students to prepare and teachers to read and respond to. Thus, they should be carefully selected to meet course goals and should benefit the students in terms of their learning.

Drafts and Rewrites

Written assignments enable the teacher to evaluate students' ability to present, organize, and express ideas effectively in writing. Through papers and other written assignments, students develop an understanding of the content they are writing about, and they learn how to communicate their ideas in writing. To improve their writing abilities, though, students need to complete drafts of writing on which they get feedback from the teacher.

Drafts and rewrites of papers are essential if the goal is to develop skill in writing (Oermann, 1999a, 1999b, 2002, 2004). Teachers should critique papers for quality of the content; organization; process of developing ideas and arguments; and writing style such as clarity of expression, sentence structure, punctuation, grammar, spelling, length of the paper, and accuracy and format of the references (Oermann, 2002). This critique should be accompanied by feedback on how to improve writing. Students need specific suggestions about revisions, not general statements such as "*writing is unclear.*" Instead, the teacher should identify the problem with the writing and give suggestions as to how to improve it, for example, "*Introductory sentence does not relate to the content in the paragraph. Replace it with a sentence that incorporates the three nursing measures you discuss in the paragraph.*" Drafts combined with feedback from the teacher are intended to improve students' writing skills. Since they are used for this purpose, they should not be graded.

Providing feedback on writing is time consuming for teachers. Another strategy that can be used is for students to critique each other's writing in small groups or pairs. Peers can provide valuable feedback on content, organization, how the ideas are developed, and if the writing is clear. While they may not identify errors in grammar and sentence structure, they often can find problems with errors in content and clarity of writing. Peers can evaluate writing in small group activities in the classroom and in post-clinical conference if the writing assignment deals with clinical practice. Small group critique provides a basis for subsequent revisions.

TYPES OF WRITTEN ASSIGNMENTS

There are many types of writing assignments appropriate for evaluation in nursing. Some of these assignments provide information on how well students have learned the content but not necessarily on writing skill. For example, structured assignments that involve short sentences and phrases, such as nursing care plans and teaching plans, do not foster development of writing skills nor do they provide data for evaluating writing. Other assignments such as papers on analyses of theories and critiques of the literature provide data for judging acquisition of knowledge as well as writing ability. Therefore, not all written assignments provide data for evaluating writing skill, and again the teacher needs to be clear about the outcomes to be judged with the assignment.

Many written assignments can be used in nursing courses. These include:

- Term paper
- Research paper and development of research protocol
- Evidence-based practice paper in which students analyze and integrate the literature and then report on evidence for practice
- Paper analyzing concepts and theories and their application to clinical practice
- Paper comparing different interventions with their underlying rationale and research base
- Paper on how the class content compares with what the students read in their textbook and in other sources, and how it applies to patient care
- Short paper designed for critical thinking in which students analyze different options, weigh alternatives, consider alternative points of view, analyze issues, and develop arguments for a position

- Case study analysis with written rationale
- Journals in which students share their feelings and thoughts with the teacher about their experiences in the classroom.

For clinical courses, written assignments that accompany the clinical practicum are valuable for encouraging critical thinking and development of problem-solving and decision-making skills. They also provide a strategy for students to analyze ethical issues in the clinical setting and reflect on their personal experiences with patients and staff.

Written assignments for clinical learning include:

- Concept map, a graphic arrangement of key concepts related to a patient's care, that includes a written description of the meaning of the interrelationships
- Concept analysis paper in which students describe a concept, its characteristics, and how it relates to care of a simulated or an actual patient situation
- Analysis of a clinical experience, the care given by the student, and alternative approaches that could have been used
- Paper that examines how readings apply to care of patient
- Teaching plan
- Nursing care plan
- Analysis of interactions with individuals and groups in the clinical setting
- Report of observations made in clinical settings
- Journal and other writings about personal reflections of patient care experiences and meaning to students, and
- Portfolio.

In-class and Small-Group Writing Activities

Not all written assignments need to be prepared by students individually as out-of-class work that is evaluated by the teacher. In-class writing assignments provide practice in expressing ideas and an opportunity for faculty and peers to give feedback on writing. For example, students can write down their thoughts about the content presented in class. They can list 1 to 2 questions about the content and pass them to other students to answer in writing. The teacher can ask a question about how the content just discussed could be applied in a different context, and ask students to write a response to the question. Several students can volunteer or be called on to read their responses aloud, and the teacher can collect all written responses for later analysis. This activity assists students in organizing their thoughts before making an oral contribution to a class discussion. Another option is for students to write a few paragraphs about how the content compares with their readings: What new learning did they gain from the class not in their readings?

For another in-class writing activity, the teacher can give students short case studies related to the content presented in class. In small groups or individually, students analyze these cases, identify diagnoses, and develop plans of care, and then report in a few paragraphs the results of their analysis and rationale for their plan. They also can describe in writing how the case is similar to or differs from what they learned in class or from their readings.

These short written activities are valuable at the end of a class to summarize the new content and actively involve students in learning. With any of these in-class activities, students can "pass their writing" to peers whose task is to critique both content and writing, adding their own thoughts about the topic and assessing the writing. The teacher can also review the written work to provide feedback.

Students can work in pairs or small groups for writing assignments. For example, a small group of students can write an editorial or a letter to the editor; develop a protocol for patient care based on the content presented in the lecture and readings for class; and review, critique, and summarize literature that relates to patient care. Students also can prepare a manuscript or work through the steps in writing for publication beginning with an outline, preparing a draft, and revising the draft for a final product. These assignments among others encourage acquisition of content and development of skill in writing; they also provide experience in group writing, learning about its benefits and pitfalls.

Writing Activities for Post-clinical Conferences

In post-clinical conferences, students can work in pairs or in small groups to critically analyze a clinical situation, decide on alternate interventions that might be used, and then write a short paper about their discussion. They can write about their own clinical activities and document the care they provided during that clinical experience. "Pass the writing" assignments work well in clinical conferences because they encourage peers to critically analyze the content, adding their own perspectives, and to identify how writing can be improved. These assignments also actively involve students in learning, which is important following a tiring clinical practice day. Group writing exercises are effective in post-clinical conferences as long as the groups are small and the exercises are carefully focused.

EVALUATING WRITTEN ASSIGNMENTS

Papers and other types of written assignments should be evaluated using predetermined criteria that address quality of content; organization of ideas; the process of arriving at decisions and, depending on the assignment, at developing an argument; and writing style. General criteria for this purpose, which can be adapted for most written assignments, are found in Table 11.1. Scoring rubrics work well for evaluating papers. An example of a rubric for scoring papers and other written assignments, which is based on these general criteria, is in Table 11.2.

Consistent with other evaluation methods, written assignments may be assessed either formatively (not graded) or summatively (graded). With formative evaluation the intent is to give feedback on the content and writing so that students can further develop their writing ability. Feedback is of value only if given promptly and with enough detail for students to understand how they can improve their writing. With some assignments, such as reflective journals, only formative evaluation may be appropriate.

Suggestions for Evaluating and Grading Written Assignments

The suggestions that follow for evaluating papers and other written assignments do not apply to every written assignment used in a course, as these are general recommendations to guide teachers in this process.

1. *Relate the assignments to the learning outcomes of the course.* Papers and other written assignments should be planned to meet particular learning objectives. All too often students complete papers that may have a questionable relationship to course goals.

2. *Consider the number of written assignments to be completed by students, including drafts of papers.* How many teaching plans, concept papers, research proposals, one-page papers, and so forth are needed to meet the goals of the course? Students should not complete repetitive assignments unless they are essential to meet course goals or personal learning needs.

TABLE 11.1   Criteria for Evaluating Papers and Other Written Assignments

Content

Content is relevant.
Content is accurate.
Significant concepts and theories are presented.
Concepts and theories are used appropriately for analysis.
Content is comprehensive.
Content reflects current research.
Hypotheses, conclusions, and decisions are supported.

Organization

Content is organized logically.
Ideas are presented in logical sequence.
Paragraph structure is appropriate.
Headings are used appropriately to indicate new content areas.

Process

Process used to arrive at solutions, approaches, decisions, and so forth is adequate.
Consequences of decisions are considered and weighed.
Sound rationale is provided based on theory and research as appropriate.
For papers analyzing issues, rationale supports position taken.
Multiple perspectives and new approaches are considered.

Writing Style

Ideas are described clearly.
Sentence structure is clear.
There are no grammatical errors.
There are no spelling errors.
Appropriate punctuation is used.
Writing does not reveal bias related to gender, sexual orientation, racial or ethnic identity,
    or disabilities.
Length of paper is consistent with requirements.
References are cited appropriately throughout paper.
References are cited accurately according to required format.

Source: Gaberson, K., & Oermann, M. H. (1999). *Clinical teaching strategies in nursing education.*
New York: Springer, p. 200. Copyright 1999 by Springer. Adapted with permission.

TABLE 11.2   Sample Scoring Rubric for Term Papers and Other Written Assignments

---

Content

Content relevant to purpose of paper, comprehensive and in depth	Content relevant to purpose of paper	Some content not relevant to purpose of paper, lacks depth
10 9 8	7 6 5 4	3 2 1
Content accurate	Most of content accurate	Major errors in content
10 9 8	7 6 5 4	3 2 1
Sound background developed from concepts, theories, and literature	Background relevant to topic but limited development	Background not developed, limited support for ideas
20–15	14–7	6–1
Current research synthesized and integrated effectively in paper	Relevant research summarized in paper	Limited research in paper, not used to support ideas
10 9 8	7 6 5 4	3 2 1

Organization

Purpose of paper/thesis well developed and clearly stated	Purpose/thesis apparent but not developed sufficiently	Purpose/thesis poorly developed, not clear
5	4 3 2	1
I deas well organized and logically presented, organization supports arguments and development of ideas	Clear organization of main points and ideas	Poorly organized, ideas not developed adequately in paper
10 9 8	7 6 5 4	3 2 1
Thorough discussion of ideas, includes multiple perspectives and new approaches	Adequate discussion of ideas, some alternate perspectives considered	Discussion not thorough, lacks detail, no alternate perspectives considered
10 9 8	7 6 5 4	3 2 1

TABLE 11.2 *(continued)*

Effective conclusion and integration of ideas in summary	Adequate conclusion, summary of main ideas	Poor conclusion, no integration of ideas
5	4 3 2	1

Writing Style and Format

Sentence structure clear, smooth transitions, correct grammar and punctuation, no spelling errors	Adequate sentence structure and transitions; few grammar, punctuation, and spelling errors	Poor sentence structure and transitions; errors in grammar, punctuation, and spelling
10 9 8	7 6 5 4	3 2 1
Professional appearance of paper, all parts included, length consistent with requirements	Paper legible, some parts missing or too short/too long considering requirements	Unprofessional appearance, missing sections, paper too short/too long considering requirements
5	4 3 2	1
References used appropriately in paper, references current, no errors in references, correct use of APA style for references	References used appropriately in paper but limited, most references current, some citations or references with errors and/or some errors in APA style for references	Few references and limited breadth, old references (not classic), errors in references, errors in APA style for references
5	4 3 2	1

Total Points _____ (sum points for total score)

3. *Avoid assignments that require only summarizing the literature and substance of class discussions unless this is the intended purpose of the assignment.* Otherwise students merely report on their readings often without thinking about the content and how it relates to varied clinical situations. If a review of the literature is the outcome intended, have students read these articles critically and synthesize them as part of the written assignment, not merely report on each article.

4. *Include clear directions about the purpose and format of the written assignment.* The goals of the written assignment—why students are writing the paper

and how it relates to the course outcomes—should be identified clearly, and generally the more detailed the directions, the better for both students and the teacher grading the papers. If there is a particular format to be followed, the teacher should review this with students and provide a written copy for their use in preparing the paper. Students need the criteria for grading and scoring rubric before they begin the assignment so it is clear how it will be evaluated.

5. *Specify the number of drafts to be submitted, each with required due dates, and provide prompt feedback on the quality of the content and writing, including specific suggestions about revisions.* These drafts are a significant component of written assignments because the intent is to improve thinking and writing through them. Drafts in most instances are used as a means of providing feedback to students and should not be graded.

6. *Develop specific criteria for evaluation and review those with the students prior to their beginning the assignment.* Include criteria related to quality of the content; organization of content; process of developing ideas and arguments; and writing style such as clarity of expression, sentence structure, punctuation, grammar, spelling, length of the paper, and accuracy and format of the references. Table 11.3 is a checklist that teachers can use in assessing writing structure and style. Other criteria would be specific to the outcomes to be met through the assignment. If a scoring rubric is used, it should be shared and discussed with the students before they begin the paper.

7. *For papers dealing with analysis of issues, focus the evaluation and criteria on the rationale developed for the position taken rather than the actual position.* This type of assignment is particularly appropriate as a group activity with critique of each other's work.

8. *Read all papers and written assignments anonymously.* The rationale for this is the same as with essay testing—the teacher needs to remove potential bias from the assessment process. Reading papers anonymously helps avoid the chance of a carryover effect in which the teacher develops an impression of the quality of a student's work, for example from prior papers, tests, and/or clinical practice, and is then influenced by that impression when grading other assignments. By grading papers anonymously, the teacher also avoids a halo effect.

9. *Skim a random sample of papers to gain an overview of how the students approached the topic of the paper, developed their ideas, and addressed other aspects of the paper that would be graded.* In some instances the evaluation criteria and scoring rubric might be modified, for example, if no students included a particular content area that was reflected in the grading criteria.

TABLE 11.3   Checking Writing Structure and Style

✓ Content organized clearly
✓ Each paragraph focuses on one topic and presents details about it
✓ Clear sequence of ideas developed within paragraphs
✓ Clear transitions between paragraphs
✓ First sentence of paragraph introduces subject and provides transition from preceding paragraph
✓ Paragraphs appropriate length
✓ Sentences clearly written and convey intended meaning
✓ Sentences appropriate length
✓ Clear transitions between sentences
✓ Words express intended meaning and used correctly
✓ Clear antecedents for pronouns
✓ No misplaced modifiers
✓ Excessive and unnecessary words omitted
✓ Stereotypes, impersonal writing, jargon, and abbreviated terms avoided
✓ Active voice used
✓ Grammar: Correct?
✓ Punctuation: Correct?
✓ Capitalization: Correct?
✓ Spelling: Correct?
✓ Writing keeps reader's interest
✓ References used appropriately in paper
✓ References current
✓ No errors in references
✓ Correct use of APA or other style for references

Adapted from Oermann, M. H. (2002). *Writing for publication in nursing*. Philadelphia: Lippincott Williams & Wilkins, p. 200. Copyright 2002 by Lippincott Williams & Wilkins. Adapted with permission.

10. *Read papers in random order.* Papers read first in the group may be scored higher than those read at the end. To avoid any bias in the order of the paper, it is best to read papers in a random order instead of always organizing papers in the same order (e.g., alphabetical) before reading them. The teacher also should take frequent breaks from grading papers to keep focused on the criteria for evaluation and avoid fatigue that could influence scoring papers near the end.

11. *Read each paper twice before scoring.* In the first reading, note omissions of and errors in content, problems with organization and development of ideas, issues with the process used for developing the paper, and writing style concerns. Record comments and suggestions on post-it notes or in

pencil in case they need to be modified once the paper is read in its entirety. If papers are submitted online, the teacher can insert comments and suggestions in the paper using the "track changes" or "comments" tools, or by using a different colored highlighting, making it easy to identify them.

12. *If unsure about the evaluation of the paper, have a colleague also read and evaluate it.* The second reader should review the paper anonymously, without knowledge of the grade given by the original teacher, and without information about the reason for the additional review. Scores can be averaged, or the teacher might decide to read the paper again depending on the situation. A second reader also might be used if the grade on the paper will determine whether the student passes the course and progresses in the program. In decisions such as these, it is helpful to obtain a "second opinion" about the quality of the paper.

13. *Consider incorporating student self-critique, peer critique, and group writing exercises within the sequence of writing assignments.*

14. *Prepare students for written assignments by incorporating learning activities in the course, completed in- and out-of-class.* These activities provide practice in organizing and expressing ideas in writing.

SUMMARY

Through papers and other written assignments, students develop an understanding of the content they are writing about and improve their ability to communicate their ideas in writing. With written assignments, students can analyze and integrate the literature and report on their findings, analyze theories and how they apply to nursing practice, improve their critical thinking skills, and learn how to write more effectively. To improve their writing abilities, though, students need to complete drafts and rewrites on which they get prompt feedback from the teacher on both content and writing.

There are many types of papers and written assignments that students can complete individually or in small groups in a nursing course. Written assignments should be evaluated using predetermined criteria that address quality of content, organization of ideas, the process of arriving at decisions and developing arguments, and writing style. General criteria for evaluating papers, an example of a scoring rubric, and suggestions for assessing and grading written assignments were provided in the chapter.

REFERENCES

Gaberson, K., & Oermann, M. H. (1999). *Clinical teaching strategies in nursing education*. New York: Springer.

Oermann, M. H. (1999a). Extensive writing projects: Tips for completing them on time. *Nurse Author & Editor, 9*(1), 8–10.

Oermann, M. H. (1999b). Writing for publication as an advanced practice nurse. *Nursing Connections, 12*(3), 5–13.

Oermann, M. H. (2002). *Writing for publication in nursing.* Philadelphia: Lippincott, Williams, & Wilkins.

Oermann, M. H. (2004). Writing for publication in nursing: What every nurse educator needs to know. In L. Caputi & L. Engelmann (Eds.), *A guide for teaching nursing in higher education* (Vol. 3, pp. 126–177). Glen Ellyn, IL: College of DuPage.

Chapter 12

Clinical Evaluation

Nursing as a practice discipline requires development of higher-level cognitive skills, values, and psychomotor and technological skills for care of patients across settings. Acquisition of knowledge alone is not sufficient; professional education includes a practice dimension where students develop competencies for care of patients and learn to think and act like professionals. Through clinical evaluation the teacher arrives at judgments about the students' competencies, that is, their performance, in practice. This chapter describes the process of clinical evaluation in nursing; in the next chapter specific clinical evaluation methods are presented.

OUTCOMES OF CLINICAL PRACTICE

There are many outcomes that students can achieve through their clinical practice experiences. In clinical courses students acquire knowledge and learn about concepts and theories to guide their patient care. They have an opportunity to transfer learning from readings, face-to-face lectures and discussions, online classes, and other experiences to care of patients.

Clinical experiences also provide an opportunity for students to use research findings and evidence for making decisions about interventions and other aspects of patient care. In the practice setting, with guidance from the teacher, students learn the process of evidence-based nursing and how to use that framework for their clinical decision making. Equally important is for students to be committed to providing evidence-based care as graduates (Pierce, 2005); the teacher can promote and reinforce this value through clinical learning activities.

In practice students deal with ambiguous patient situations and unique cases that do not fit the textbook description and require students to think critically about what to do. For this reason, clinical practice, whether in the patient care setting or simulation laboratory, is important for developing higher-level cognitive skills and for learning to make clinical decisions based on available information. Schön (1990) emphasized the need for such learning in preparing for professional practice. Clinical experiences present problems and situations that may not lend themselves to resolution through the rational application of scientific theory learned in class and through one's readings. Schön referred to these problems as ones in the swampy lowlands, problems that may be difficult to identify, may present themselves as unique cases, and may be known by the professional but have no clear solutions. Cohen (2005) suggested that through reflective thinking, students learn to cope with practice situations characterized by uncertainty and uniqueness and where the theory they have learned is of limited usefulness. When faced with these clinical situations, students have an opportunity to develop their critical thinking and decision-making skills, important outcomes of clinical practice (Gaberson & Oermann, 1999).

Through practice experiences with patients and in learning and simulation laboratories, students develop their psychomotor skills, learn how to use technology, and gain necessary skills for implementing nursing and other interventions. This practice is essential for initial learning, to refine competencies, and to maintain them over a period of time.

Having technical skills, though, is only one aspect of professional practice. In caring for patients and working with nurses and other health providers, students gain an understanding of how professionals approach their patients' problems, how they interact with each other, and behaviors important in carrying out their roles in the practice setting. By observing others in the clinical setting, students learn important role behaviors of nurses as professionals. Practice as a professional is contingent not only on having knowledge to guide decisions but also on having a value system that recognizes the worth, dignity, and rights of patients and others in the health system. As part of this value system, students need to develop cultural competence and gain the knowledge and attitudes essential to provide multicultural health care—outcomes that can be met in clinical practice. Covington (2004) recommended that students begin their clinical experiences in settings with culturally diverse populations to allow them to understand the cultural meaning of health and illness, and then learn to provide culturally competent care in later courses in the curriculum.

Most clinical experiences involve an interpersonal dimension, enabling students to develop their communication skills and learn how to collaborate with others. Some clinical courses focus on management and leadership outcomes, providing learning opportunities for students in managing groups of patients, providing leadership to staff, and delegating, among other competencies.

In clinical practice students learn to accept responsibility for their actions and decisions about patients. They also should be willing to accept errors in judgment and learn from them. These are important outcomes of clinical practice in any nursing and health professions program.

Another outcome of clinical practice is learning to learn. Professionals in any field are perpetual learners throughout the duration of their careers. Continually expanding knowledge, developments in health care, and new technology alone create the need for lifelong learners in nursing. In clinical practice, students are faced with situations of which they are unsure; they are challenged to raise questions about patient care and seek further learning. There are three related skills to be developed, all of which are critical to maintaining competence in practice as a professional: the ability to evaluate one's own knowledge and skills for clinical practice, a willingness to engage in this self-assessment, and an awareness of resources available for the development of new knowledge and competencies (Oermann, 1998b, 2002). In the clinical component of nursing courses as students are faced with gaps in their learning, they should be guided in this self-assessment process, directed to resources for learning, and supported by the teacher. All too often students are hesitant to express their learning needs to their teachers for fear of the effect it will have on their grade or on the teacher's impression of the student's competence in clinical practice.

These outcomes of clinical practice are listed in Table 12.1. They provide a framework for faculty to use in planning their clinical courses and how to evaluate student performance in them. Not all outcomes are applicable to every nursing course; for instance, some courses may not have technological or delega-

TABLE 12.1   Outcomes of Clinical Practice in Nursing Programs

- Acquire concepts, theories, and other knowledge for clinical practice.
- Use research and other evidence for clinical decision making and evidence-based nursing practice.
- Use critical thinking in clinical practice.
- Develop psychomotor and technological skills and competence in other types of interventions.
- Develop professional values and knowledge essential to providing health care to a diverse and multicultural client population.
- Communicate effectively with patients and others in the health system.
- Demonstrate leadership skills and behaviors of a professional.
- Accept responsibility for actions and decisions.
- Accept need for continued learning and self development.

tion skills to be acquired, but overall most courses will move students toward achievement of these outcomes as they progress through the nursing program.

CONCEPT OF CLINICAL EVALUATION

Clinical evaluation is a process by which judgments are made about learners' competencies in practice. This practice may involve care of patients, families, and communities; other types of experiences in the clinical setting; simulated experiences; and performance of varied skills. Most frequently, clinical evaluation involves observing performance and arriving at judgments about the student's competence. Judgments influence the data collected, i.e., the specific types of observations made to evaluate the student's performance, and the inferences and conclusions drawn from the data about the quality of that performance. Teachers may collect different data to evaluate the same outcomes, and when presented with a series of observations about a student's performance in clinical practice, there may be minimal consistency in their judgments about how well that student performed. Clinical evaluation is not an objective process; it is subjective involving judgments of the teacher and others involved in the process.

As discussed in Chapter 1, the teacher's values influence evaluation. This is most apparent in clinical evaluation, where our values influence the observations we make of students and the judgments we make about the quality of their performance. Thus, it is important for teachers to be aware of which of their own values might bias their judgments of students. This is not to suggest that clinical evaluation can be value-free; the teacher's observations of performance and conclusions will always be influenced by the teacher's values. The key is to develop an awareness of these values to avoid their influencing clinical evaluation to a point of unfairness to the student. For example, if the teacher prefers students who initiate discussions and participate actively in conferences, this value should not influence judgments about students' competencies in other areas. The teacher needs to be aware of this preference to avoid an unfair evaluation of other dimensions of the students' clinical performance. Or, if the teacher is used to the fast pace of most acute care settings, when working with beginning students or someone who "moves slowly," the teacher should be cautious not to let this prior experience influence expectations of performance. Faculty should examine their own values, attitudes, and beliefs so that they are aware of them as they teach and evaluate students in practice settings.

Clinical Evaluation vs. Grading

Clinical evaluation is not the same as grading. In evaluation the teacher makes observations of performance and collects other types of data, then compares this information to a set of standards to arrive at a judgment. From this assessment, a quantitative symbol or grade may be applied to reflect the evaluation data and judgments made about performance. The clinical grade, such as pass-fail or A through F, is the symbol to represent the evaluation. Clinical performance may be evaluated and not graded, such as with formative evaluation or feedback to the learner, or it may be graded. Grades, however, should not be assigned without sufficient data about clinical performance.

Norm- and Criterion-Referenced Clinical Evaluation

Clinical evaluation may be norm- or criterion-referenced as described in Chapter 1. In norm-referenced evaluation, the student's clinical performance is compared with that of other students, indicating that the performance is better than, worse than, or equivalent to that of others in the comparison group or that the student has more or less knowledge, skill, or ability than the other students. Rating students' clinical competencies in relation to others in the clinical group, for example indicating that the student was "average," is a norm-referenced interpretation.

In contrast, criterion-referenced clinical evaluation involves comparing the student's clinical performance to predetermined criteria, not to the performance of other students in the group. In this type of clinical evaluation, the criteria are known in advance and used as the basis for evaluation. Indicating that the student has met the clinical outcomes or achieved the clinical competencies, regardless of how other students performed, represents a criterion-referenced interpretation.

Formative and Summative Clinical Evaluation

Clinical evaluation may be formative or summative. Formative evaluation in clinical practice provides feedback to learners about their progress in meeting the outcomes of the clinical course or in developing the clinical competencies. The purposes of formative evaluation are to enable students to develop further their clinical knowledge, skills, and values; indicate areas in which learning and practice are needed; and provide a basis for suggesting additional instruction to improve performance. With this type of evaluation, after identifying the learning needs, instruction is provided to move students forward in their learning. Formative evaluation, therefore, is diagnostic; it should not be graded (Nitko, 2004). For example, the clinical teacher or preceptor might observe a student perform wound care and give feedback on changes to make with the technique. The goal of this evaluation is to improve subsequent performance, not to grade how well the student carried out the procedure.

Summative clinical evaluation, however, is designed for determining clinical grades because it summarizes competencies the student has developed in clinical practice. Summative evaluation is done at the end of a period of time, e.g., at midterm or at the end of the clinical practicum, to assess the extent to which learners have achieved the clinical outcomes or competencies. Summative evaluation is not diagnostic; it summarizes the performance of students at a particular point in time. For much of clinical practice in a nursing program, summative evaluation comes too late for students to have an opportunity to improve performance. At the end of a course involving care of mothers and children, for instance, there may be many behaviors the student would not have an opportunity to practice in subsequent courses.

Any protocol for clinical evaluation should include extensive formative evaluation and periodic summative evaluation. Formative evaluation is essential to provide feedback to improve performance while practice experiences are still available. A third type of clinical evaluation, confirmative, determines if learners have maintained their clinical competencies over time.

FAIRNESS IN CLINICAL EVALUATION

Considering that clinical evaluation is not objective, the goal is to establish a *fair* evaluation system. Fairness requires that:

1. the teacher identify own values, attitudes, beliefs, and biases that may influence the evaluation process,
2. clinical evaluation be based on predetermined outcomes or competencies, and
3. the teacher develop a supportive clinical learning environment.

Identify One's Own Values

Teachers need to be aware of their personal values, attitudes, beliefs, and biases that may influence the evaluation process. These can affect both the data collected about students and the inferences made. In addition, students have their own set of values and attitudes that influence their self-evaluations of performance and their responses to the teacher's evaluations and feedback. Students' acceptance of the teacher's guidance in clinical practice and information provided to them for improving performance is affected by their past experiences in clinical courses with other faculty. Students may have had problems in prior clinical courses, receiving only negative feedback and limited support from the teacher, staff, and others. In situations in which student responses inhibit learning, the teacher may need to intervene to guide students in more self-awareness of their own values and the effect they are having on their learning.

Base Clinical Evaluation on Predetermined Outcomes or Competencies

Clinical evaluation should be based on preset outcomes, clinical objectives, or competencies that are then used to guide the evaluation process. Without these, neither the teacher nor the student has any basis for evaluating clinical practice. What are the outcomes of the clinical course (or in some nursing education programs, the clinical objectives) to be met? What clinical competencies should the student develop? These outcomes or competencies provide a framework for faculty to use in observing performance and for arriving at judgments about achievement in clinical practice. For example, if the competencies relate to developing communication skills, then the learning activities, whether in the patient care setting or laboratory, should assist the students in learning how to communicate. The teacher's observations and subsequent evaluation should focus on communication behaviors, not on other competencies unrelated to the learning activities.

Develop a Supportive Learning Environment

It is up to the teacher to develop a supportive learning environment where students view the teacher as someone who will facilitate their learning and development of clinical competencies. Students need to be comfortable asking faculty and staff questions and seeking their guidance rather than avoiding them in the clinical setting. A supportive environment is critical for effective evaluation because students need to recognize that the teacher's feedback is intended to help them improve performance. Developing a "climate" for learning is also important because clinical practice is inherently stressful for students. This learning environment includes the physical, human, interpersonal, and organizational properties of the clinical setting and the trust and respect between teacher and students (Chan, 2003).

STUDENT STRESS IN CLINICAL PRACTICE

There have been a number of studies in nursing education on student stress in the clinical setting. Some of the stresses students have identified are:

- the fear of making a mistake that would harm the patient
- having insufficient knowledge and skills for patient care
- changing patient conditions and uncertainty about how to respond
- being unfamiliar with the staff, policies, and other aspects of the clinical setting
- caring for difficult patients
- having the teacher observe and evaluate clinical performance, and
- interacting with the patient, the family, nursing staff, and other health providers (Oermann, 1998a; Oermann, 2004).

The stresses that students experience in clinical practice, however, may not be the same in each course. For example, Oermann and Lukomski (2001) found that students were more stressed in their pediatric nursing course than in other courses in the curriculum; they were concerned most about giving medications to children. Other courses such as foundations of nursing were not as stressful for students. For faculty, though, beginning clinical courses may be more demanding and stressful to teach than upper-level courses (Oermann, 1998c).

Learning in the clinical setting is a *public experience*. Students cannot hide their lack of understanding or skills as they might in class or in an online discussion board. In clinical practice the possibility exists for many people to observe the student's performance—the teacher, patient, peers, nursing staff, and other health providers. Being observed and evaluated by others is stressful for students in any health field.

The potential stress that students might experience in the clinical setting reinforces the need for faculty to be aware of the learning environment they set when working with students in a clinical course. The student is a learner, not a nurse, although some faculty and staff expect students to perform at an expert level without giving them sufficient time to practice and refine their performance (Gaberson & Oermann, 1999). Simulated experiences may be effective in reducing some of the anxieties of students in the clinical setting by allowing them to practice their skills, both cognitive and psychomotor, prior to care of patients. Now that more schools are using simulators, the effect of these experiences on student performance and stress in clinical practice needs to be examined.

FEEDBACK IN CLINICAL EVALUATION

For clinical evaluation to be effective, the teacher should provide continuous feedback to students about their performance and how they can improve it. This feedback may be verbal, by describing observations of performance and explaining what to do differently, or visual, by demonstrating correct performance. Feedback should be accompanied by further instruction either from the teacher or by directing the student to other resources for learning. The ultimate goal is for students to progress to a point at which they can judge their own performance, identify resources for their learning, and use those resources to further develop competencies.

Students must have an underlying knowledge base and beginning skills to judge their own performance. Nitko (2004) suggested that feedback on performance also identifies the possible causes or reasons why the student has not mastered the learning outcomes. Sometimes the reason is that the student does not have the prerequisite knowledge and skills for developing the new competencies. As such it is critical for faculty and preceptors to begin their clinical instruction by assessing if students have learned the necessary concepts and skills and if not, to start there.

Principles of Providing Feedback as Part of Clinical Evaluation

There are five principles for providing feedback to students as part of the clinical evaluation process. First, the feedback should be precise and specific. General information about performance, such as "You need to work on your assessment" or "You need more practice in the simulation laboratory," does not indicate what behaviors need improvement or how to develop them. Instead of using general statements, the teacher should indicate what specific areas of knowledge are lacking, where there are problems in decision making and critical thinking, and what particular competencies need more development (Gaberson & Oermann, 1999). Rather than saying to a student, "You need to work on your assessment," the student would be better served if the teacher identified the specific areas of data collection omitted and the physical examination techniques that need improvement. Specific feedback is more valuable to learners than a general description of their behavior.

2 Second, for procedures, use of technologies, and any psychomotor skill, the teacher should provide both verbal and visual feedback to students. This means that the teacher should explain first, either orally or in writing, where the errors were made in performance and then demonstrate the correct procedure or skill. This should be followed by student practice of the skill with the teacher guiding performance. By allowing immediate practice, with the teacher available to correct problems, students can more easily *use* the feedback to further develop their skills.

3 Third, feedback about performance should be given to students at the time of learning or immediately following it. The longer the period of time between

performance and feedback from the teacher, the less effective is the feedback (Gaberson & Oermann, 1999). As time passes, neither student nor teacher may remember specific areas of clinical practice to be improved. This principle holds true whether the performance relates to decision making and critical thinking, a procedure or technical skill, or an attitude or value expressed by the student, among other areas. With the hectic pace of many clinical settings and the number of students in a clinical group, the teacher needs to develop a strategy for giving focused and immediate feedback to students during the clinical day and following up with further discussion as needed. Recording short anecdotal notes on paper, in Personal Digital Assistants (PDAs), or on flow sheets for later discussion with individual students helps the teacher remember important points about performance.

④ Fourth, students need different amounts of feedback and positive reinforcement. In beginning practice and with clinical situations that are new to learners, most students will need frequent and extensive feedback. As students progress through the program and become more competent, they usually can evaluate their own performance. Some students need more feedback and direction from the teacher than others do. Similar to many aspects of education, one approach does not fit all students.

⑤ One final principle is that feedback should be diagnostic. This means that after identifying areas in which further learning is needed, the teacher's responsibility is to guide students so that they can improve their performance. The process is cyclical—the teacher observes and evaluates performance, gives students feedback about that performance, and then guides their learning and practice so that they can become more competent.

CLINICAL OUTCOMES AND COMPETENCIES

There are different ways of specifying the outcomes to be achieved in clinical practice, which in turn provide the basis for clinical evaluation. These may be stated in the form of outcomes to be met or as competencies to be demonstrated in clinical practice. Some schools of nursing specify the outcomes in the form of clinical objectives. Regardless of how these are stated, they represent *what* is evaluated in clinical practice.

The outcomes of clinical practice in Table 12.1 can be used for developing specific outcomes or competencies for a clinical course. Not all clinical courses will have outcomes in each of these areas, and in some courses there may be other types of competencies unique to practice in that clinical specialty. Some faculty identify common outcomes or competencies that are used for each clinical course in the program and then level those to illustrate their progressive development through the nursing program (Ignatavicus & Caputi, 2004). For example, with this model, each course would have an outcome on communication. In a beginning clinical course, the outcome might be, "Identifies verbal and nonverbal techniques for communicating with patients." In a later course in the curriculum, the communication outcome might focus on the family and working with caregivers, e.g., "Develops interpersonal relationships with families and caregivers." Then in the community health course the outcome might be, "Collaborates with other health care providers in care of patients in the community and the community as client."

As another approach, some faculty state the outcomes broadly and then indicate specific behaviors students should demonstrate in order to meet those outcomes in a particular course. For example, the outcome on communication might be stated as "Communicates effectively with patients and others in the health system." Examples of behaviors that indicate achievement of this outcome in a course on care of children include, "Uses appropriate verbal and nonverbal communication based on the child's age, developmental status, and health condition" and "Interacts effectively with parents, caregivers, and others." Generally, the outcomes or competencies are then used for developing the clinical evaluation tool or form, which is discussed in the next chapter.

Regardless of how the outcomes are stated for a clinical course, they need to be specific enough to guide the evaluation of students in clinical practice. An outcome such as "Use the nursing process in care of children" is too broad to guide evaluation. More specific outcomes such as "Carries out a systematic assessment of children reflecting their developmental stage," "Evaluates the impact of health problems on the child and family," and "Identifies resources for managing the child's care at home" are clearer to students as to what is expected of them in clinical practice.

Competencies are the abilities to be demonstrated by the learner in clinical practice. For nurses in practice, these competencies reflect the proficiencies needed to perform a particular task or carry out their defined role in the health care setting. Competencies for nurses are assessed as part of the initial employment and orientation to the health care setting and on an ongoing basis. For each of the competencies identified for clinical practice, there may be performance criteria or critical behaviors established for determining achievement of the competency (Lockhart, 2004). Table 12.2 illustrates a competency with related performance criteria. These criteria are important in clinical evaluation because they illustrate the behaviors or actions as evidence of competency in that area.

Caution must be exercised in developing clinical outcomes and competencies to avoid having too many for evaluation, considering the number of learners for whom the teacher is responsible, types of clinical experiences available, and

TABLE 12.2   Sample Competency and Performance Criteria

Competency: IV Injection of Medication

Performance Criteria:

☐ Checks physician's order.
☐ Checks medication administration record.
☐ Adheres to rights of medication administration.
☐ Assembles appropriate equipment.
☐ Checks compatibility with existing IV if present.
☐ Explains procedure to patient.
☐ Positions patient appropriately.
☐ Checks patency of administration port or line.
☐ Administers medication at proper rate.
☐ Monitors patient response.
☐ Flushes tubing as necessary.
☐ Documents IV medication correctly.

time allotted for clinical learning activities. In preparing outcomes or competencies for a clinical course, teachers should keep in mind that they need to collect sufficient data for the group of students for each outcome or competency specified for that course. Too many outcomes makes it nearly impossible to collect enough data on the performance of all of the students in the clinical group. Regardless of how the evaluation system is developed, the clinical outcomes or competencies need to be realistic and useful for guiding the evaluation.

SUMMARY

Through clinical evaluation the teacher arrives at judgments about students' performance in clinical practice. The teacher's observations of performance should focus on the outcomes to be met or competencies to be developed in the clinical course. These provide the framework for learning in clinical practice and the basis for evaluating performance.

While a framework such as this is essential in clinical evaluation, teachers also need to examine their own beliefs about the evaluation process and purposes it serves in nursing. Clarifying one's own values, beliefs, attitudes, and biases that may affect evaluation is an important first step. Recognizing the inherent stress of clinical practice for many students and developing a supportive learning environment are also important. Other concepts of evaluation, presented in chapter 1, apply to clinical evaluation. Specific methods for clinical evaluation are described in the next chapter.

REFERENCES

Chan, D. S. K. (2003). Validation of the Clinical Learning Environment Inventory. *Western Journal of Nursing Research, 25*, 519–532.

Cohen, J. A. (2005). The mirror as metaphor for the reflective practitioner. In M. H. Oermann & K. Heinrich (Eds.), *Annual review of nursing education* (Vol. 3, pp. 313–330). New York: Springer.

Covington, L. W. (2004). Cultural diversity: Teaching students to provide culturally-competent nursing care. In L. Caputi & L. Engelmann, *Teaching nursing: The art and science* (Vol. 1, pp. 519–554). Glen Ellyn, IL: College of DuPage Press.

Gaberson, K. B., & Oermann, M. H. (1999). *Clinical teaching strategies in nursing education.* New York: Springer.

Ignatavicus, D., & Caputi, L. (2004). Evaluating students in the clinical setting. In L. Caputi & L. Engelmann, *Teaching nursing: The art and science* (Vol. 1, pp. 178–195). Glen Ellyn, IL: College of DuPage Press.

Lockhart, J. S. (2004). *Unit-based staff development for clinical nurses.* Pittsburgh, PA: Oncology Nursing Society.

Nitko, A. J. (2004). *Educational assessment of students* (4th ed.). Upper Saddle River, NJ: Prentice Hall.

Oermann, M. H. (1998a). Differences in clinical experiences of ADN and BSN students. *Journal of Nursing Education, 37*(5), 197–201.

Oermann, M. H. (1998b). Professional reflection: Have you looked in the mirror lately? *Orthopaedic Nursing, 17*(4), 22–26.

Oermann, M. H. (1998c). Role strain of clinical nursing faculty. *Journal of Professional Nursing, 14*, 329–334.

Oermann, M. H. (2002). Developing a professional portfolio. *Orthopaedic Nursing, 21*(2), 73–78.

Oermann, M. H. (2004). Reflections on undergraduate nursing education: A look to the future. *Journal of Nursing Education Scholarship, 1*(1), 1–15. Available at http://www.bepress.com/ijnes/vol1/iss1/art5

Oermann, M. H., & Lukomski, A. P. (2001). Experiences of students in pediatric nursing clinical courses. *Journal of the Society of Pediatric Nurses, 9*(2), 65–72.

Pierce, S. T. (2005). Integrating evidence-based practice into nursing curricula. In M. H. Oermann & K. Heinrich (Eds.), *Annual review of nursing education* (Vol. 3, pp. 233–248). New York: Springer.

Schön, D. A. (1990). *Educating the reflective practitioner.* San Francisco: Jossey-Bass.

Chapter 13

Clinical Evaluation Methods

After establishing a framework for evaluating students in clinical practice and exploring one's own values, attitudes, and biases that may influence evaluation, the teacher identifies a variety of methods for collecting data on student performance. Evaluation methods are strategies for assessing learning outcomes in clinical practice. That practice may be with patients in hospitals and other health care facilities, with families and communities, in simulation and learning laboratories, and involving other activities using multimedia. Some evaluation methods are most appropriate for use by faculty or preceptors who are onsite with students and can observe their performance; other evaluation methods assess students' knowledge, cognitive skills, and other competencies but do not involve direct observation of their performance.

There are many evaluation methods for use in nursing education. Some methods, such as journals, are most appropriate for formative evaluation while others are useful for either formative or summative evaluation. In this chapter varied strategies are presented for evaluating clinical performance.

SELECTING CLINICAL EVALUATION METHODS

There are several factors to consider when selecting clinical evaluation methods to use in a course. First, the evaluation methods should provide information on student performance of the clinical competencies associated with the course. With the evaluation methods, the teacher collects data on performance to judge if students are developing the clinical competencies or have achieved them by the end of the course. For many outcomes of a course, there are different strategies that can be used, thereby providing flexibility in choosing methods for evaluation.

Most evaluation methods provide data on multiple clinical outcomes. For example, a short written assignment in which students compare two different data sets might relate to outcomes on assessment, critical thinking, and writing. In planning the evaluation for a clinical course, the teacher reviews the outcomes or competencies to be developed and decides which evaluation methods will be used for assessing them, recognizing that most methods provide information on more than one outcome or competency.

Second, there are many different clinical evaluation strategies that might be used to assess performance. Varying the methods maintains student interest and takes into account individual needs, abilities, and characteristics of learners. Some students may be more proficient in methods that depend on writing, while others prefer strategies such as conferences and other discussions. Planning for multiple evaluation methods in clinical courses as long as congruent with the outcomes to be evaluated reflects these differences among students. It also avoids relying on one method, such as a rating scale, for determining the entire clinical grade.

Third, the teacher should always select evaluation methods that are realistic considering the number of students to be evaluated, available practice or simulation activities, and constraints such as the teacher's or preceptor's time. Planning for an evaluation method that depends on patients with specific health problems or particular clinical situations may not be realistic considering the types of experiences with actual or simulated patients available to students. Some methods are not appropriate because of the number of students that would need to use them within the timeframe of the course. Others may be too costly or require resources not available in the nursing education program or health care setting.

Fourth, evaluation methods can be used for formative or summative evaluation. In the process of deciding how to evaluate students' clinical performance, the teacher should identify if the methods will be used to provide feedback to learners (formative) or for grading (summative). Students should know this ahead of time. Some of the strategies designed for clinical evaluation provide feedback to students on areas for improvement and should not be graded. Other methods such as rating scales and written assignments can be used for summative purposes and therefore can be computed as part of the course or clinical grade.

Fifth, before finalizing the protocol for evaluating clinical performance in a course, the teacher should review the purpose and number required of each assignment completed by students in clinical practice. What are the purposes of these assignments, and how many are needed to demonstrate competency? For example, in some clinical courses, students complete an excessive number of written assignments. How many assignments, regardless of whether they are for formative or summative purposes, are needed to meet the outcomes of the course? Students benefit from continuous feedback from the teacher, not from repetitive assignments that contribute little to their development of clinical knowledge and skills. Instead of daily or weekly care plans or other assignments, which may not even be consistent with current practice, once students develop the competencies, they can progress to other more relevant learning activities.

Sixth, in deciding how to evaluate clinical performance, the teacher should consider the time needed to complete the evaluation, provide feedback, and grade the assignment. Instead of requiring a series of written assignments in a clinical course, the same outcomes might be met through discussions with students, cases analyzed by students in clinical conferences, group writing activities, and other methods requiring less teacher time and accomplishing the same purposes. Considering the demands on nursing faculty, it is important to consider one's own time when planning how to evaluate students' performance in clinical practice (Oermann, 2004).

The rest of the chapter presents clinical evaluation methods for use in nursing education programs. Some of these methods such as written assignments were examined in earlier chapters.

OBSERVATION

The predominant strategy for evaluating clinical performance is observing students in clinical practice, simulation and learning laboratories, and other settings. Although observation is widely used, there are threats to its validity and reliability. First, observations of students may be influenced by the teacher's values, attitudes, and biases, as discussed in the last chapter. There also may be over-reliance on first impressions, which might change as the teacher or preceptor observes the student over a period of time and in different situations. In any performance assessment there needs to be a series of observations made before drawing conclusions about performance.

Second, in observing performance, there are many aspects of that performance on which the teacher may focus attention. For example, while observing a student administer an IV medication, the teacher may focus mainly on the technique used for its administration, ask limited questions about the purpose of the medication, and make no observations of how the student interacts with the patient. Another teacher observing this same student may focus on those other aspects. The same practice situation, therefore, may yield different observations.

Third, the teacher may arrive at incorrect judgments about the observation, such as inferring that a student is inattentive during conference when in fact the student is thinking about the comments made by others in the group. It is important to discuss observations with students, obtain their perceptions of their behavior, and be willing to modify one's own inferences when new data are presented.

Fourth, every observation in the clinical setting reflects only a sampling of the learner's performance during a clinical activity. An observation of the same student at another time may reveal a different level of performance. The same holds true for observations of the teacher; on some clinical days and for some classes the teacher's behaviors do not represent a typical level of performance. An observation of the same teacher during another clinical activity and class may reveal a different quality of teaching.

Finally, similar to other clinical evaluation methods, the outcomes or competencies guide the teacher on *what* to observe. They help the teacher focus the observations of performance. However, all observed behaviors should be shared with the students.

Anecdotal Notes

It is difficult if not impossible to remember the observations made of each student for each clinical activity. For this reason teachers need a strategy to help them remember their observations and the context in which the performance occurred. There are several ways of recording observations of students in clinical settings, simulation and learning laboratories, and other settings: anecdotal notes, checklists, and rating scales. These are summarized in Table 13.1.

Anecdotal notes are narrative descriptions of observations made of students. Some teachers include only a description of the observations, and then after a series of observations, review the pattern of the performance and draw conclusions about it. Other teachers record their observations and include a judgment about

TABLE 13.1 Methods for Recording Observations

Anecdotal Notes	Used for recording descriptions of observations made of students in clinical setting, simulation laboratory, and experiences in which teachers, preceptors, and others observe performance. May also include interpretations or conclusions about the performance
Checklists	Used primarily for recording observations of specific competencies, procedures, and skills performed by students; includes list of behaviors to demonstrate competency and steps for carrying out the procedure or skill. May also include errors in performance to check
Rating Scales	Used for recording judgments about students' performance in clinical practice. Includes a set of defined clinical outcomes, behaviors, or competencies and scale for rating the degree of competence (graduated scale or pass-fail)

how well the student performed (Case & Oermann, 2004). Anecdotal notes should be recorded as close to the time of the observation as possible; otherwise it is difficult to remember what was observed and the context, e.g., patient and clinical situation, of that observation. In the clinical setting, notes can be handwritten on flow sheets, on other forms, or as narratives. They also can be recorded in Personal Digital Assistants (PDAs). Software is available for teachers to keep a running anecdotal record for each student, or they can use the available software on their PDA. The anecdotal notes can then be exported to the computer for formatting and printing.

The goal of the anecdotal note is to provide a description of the student's performance as observed by the teacher or preceptor. Liberto, Roncher, and Shellenbarger (1999) identified five key areas to include in an anecdotal note:

- Date of the observation
- Student name
- Faculty signature
- Setting of the observation, and
- Record of student actions, with an objective and a detailed description of the observed performance (p. 16).

Anecdotal notes should be shared with students as frequently as possible; otherwise they are not effective for feedback. Considering the issues associated with observations of clinical performance, the teacher should discuss observations with the students and be willing to incorporate their own judgments about the performance. Anecdotal notes are also useful in conferences with students, for example, at midterm and end-of-term, as a way of reviewing a pattern of performance over time. When there are sufficient observations about performance, the notes can serve as documentation for ratings on the clinical evaluation tool.

Checklists

A checklist is a list of specific behaviors or activities to be observed with a place for marking whether or not they were present during the performance (Nitko, 2004). A checklist often lists the steps to be followed in performing a procedure or demonstrating a skill. Some checklists also include errors in performance that are commonly made. Checklists not only facilitate the teacher's observation of procedures and behaviors performed by students, but they also provide a way for students to assess their own performance. With checklists, students can review and evaluate their performance prior to assessment by the teacher.

For common procedures and skills, teachers can often find checklists already prepared that can be used for evaluation, and some nursing textbooks have accompanying skills checklists. When these resources are not available, there are four steps to follow in developing a checklist for rating performance:

1. Review the procedure or competency to understand critical elements in performance and rationale.

2. List each step or behavior to be demonstrated in the correct order.

3. Add to the list specific errors students often make (to alert the evaluator to observe for these).

4. Develop the list into a form to check off the steps or behaviors as they are performed in the proper sequence. (Nitko, 2004)

In designing checklists, it is important not to include every possible step, which makes the checklist too cumbersome to use, but to focus instead on critical items and where they fit into the sequence. The goal is for students to learn how to perform a procedure safely and to understand the order of steps in the procedure. When there are different ways of performing a skill, the students should be allowed that flexibility when evaluated. Table 13.2 provides an example of a checklist developed from the sample competency and performance criteria in Table 12.2.

Rating Scales

Rating scales, also referred to as clinical evaluation tools or instruments, provide a means of recording judgments about the observed performance of students in clinical practice. A rating scale has two parts: (a) a list of outcomes, competencies, or behaviors the student is to demonstrate in clinical practice and (b) a scale for rating their performance of them.

Rating scales are most useful for summative evaluation of performance; after observing students over a period of time, the teacher draws conclusions about performance, rating it according to the scale provided with the instrument. They also may be used to evaluate specific activities that the students complete in clinical practice, for example, rating a student's presentation of a case in clinical conference or the quality of teaching provided to a patient. Other uses of rating scales are to: (a) help students focus their attention on critical behaviors to be performed in clinical practice; (b) give specific feedback to students about the performance; and (c) demonstrate growth in clinical competencies over a designated time period if the same rating scale is used.

TABLE 13.2   Sample Checklist

Student Name _____

Instructions to teacher/examiner: Observe the student performing the following procedure and check the steps completed properly by the student. Check only those steps that the student performed properly. After competing the checklist, discuss performance with the student, reviewing aspects of the procedure to be improved.

IV Injection of Medication

Checklist:

☐ Checks physician's order.
☐ Checks medication administration record.
☐ Adheres to rights of medication administration.
☐ Assembles appropriate equipment.
☐ Checks compatibility with existing IV if present.
☐ Explains procedure to patient.
☐ Positions patient appropriately.
☐ Checks patency of administration port or line.
☐ Administers medication at proper rate.
☐ Monitors patient response.
☐ Flushes tubing as necessary.
☐ Documents IV medication correctly.

Types of Rating Scales

Many types of rating scales are used for evaluating clinical performance. The scales may be multidimensional with descriptors such as:

- Letters: A, B, C, D, E or A, B, C, D, F

- Numbers: 1, 2, 3, 4, 5

- Qualitative labels: Excellent, very good, good, fair, and poor; Exceptional, above-average, average, and below-average, and

- Frequency labels: Always, usually, frequently, sometimes, and never.

Other scales have been developed such as Bondy's Criterion Matrix that uses a 5-point scale to rate the quality of a student's performance based on appropriate performance, qualitative aspects of the performance, and the degree of assistance needed by the student (Bondy, Jenkins, Seymour, Lancaster, & Ishee, 1997).

A short description included with the letters, numbers, and labels for each of the outcomes, competencies, or behaviors rated improves objectivity and consistency (Nitko, 2004). For example, if teachers were using a scale of exceptional, above-average, average, and below-average, or based on the numbers 4, 3, 2, and 1, short descriptions of each level in the scale could be written to clarify the performance expected at each level. For the clinical outcome "Collects relevant data from patient," the descriptors might be:

> *Exceptional (or 4):* Differentiates relevant from irrelevant data, analyzes multiple sources of data, establishes comprehensive data base, identifies data needed for evaluating all possible nursing diagnoses and patient problems
>
> *Above-Average (or 3):* Collects significant data from patients, uses multiple sources of data as part of assessment, identifies possible nursing diagnoses and patient problems based on the data
>
> *Average (or 2):* Collects significant data from patients, uses data to develop main nursing diagnoses and patient problems
>
> *Below-Average (or 1):* Does not collect significant data and misses important cues in data; unable to explain relevance of data for nursing diagnoses and patient problems

Rating scales for clinical evaluation may be two-dimensional such as pass-fail and satisfactory-unsatisfactory. In a survey of 79 nursing programs, randomly selected, Alfaro-LeFevre (2004) found that 75% (n = 59) of the programs used pass-fail rating scales for their clinical evaluation, consistent with earlier studies. Both types of scales are appropriate for clinical evaluation.

Issues with Rating Scales

One problem in using rating scales is apparent by a review of the sample scale descriptors. What are the differences between above-average and average? Between a "2" and "1"? Is there consensus among faculty using the rating scale as to what constitutes different levels of performance for each outcome, competency, or behavior evaluated? This problem exists even when descriptions are provided for each level of the rating scale. Teachers may differ in their judgments of whether the student collected *relevant* data, if *multiple* sources of data were used, if the data base was *comprehensive* or not, if *all possible* nursing diagnoses were considered, and so forth. Scales based on frequency labels are often difficult to implement because of limited experiences for students to practice and demonstrate a level of skill rated as "always, usually, frequently, sometimes, and never." How should faculty rate students' performance in situations in which they practiced the skill perhaps once or twice? Even with two-dimensional scales such as pass-fail, there is room for variability among faculty.

Nitko (2004) identified six common errors that occur with rating scales applicable to rating clinical performance:

1. *Leniency error* results when the teacher tends to rate all students toward the high end of the scale.

2. *Severity error* is the opposite of leniency, tending to rate all students toward the low end of the scale.

3. *Central tendency error* is hesitancy to mark either end of the rating scale and instead use only the midpoint of the scale. Rating students only at the extremes or only at the midpoint of the scale limits the validity of the ratings for all students and introduces the teacher's own biases into the evaluation (Nitko, 2004).

4. *The halo effect* is a judgment based on a general impression of the student. With this error the teacher lets an overall impression of the student influence the ratings of specific aspects of the student's performance. This impression is considered a "halo" around the student that affects the teacher's ability to objectively evaluate and rate specific competencies or behaviors on the tool. This halo may be positive, giving the student a higher rating than is deserved, or negative, letting a general negative impression of the student result in lower ratings of specific aspects of the performance.

5. *Personal bias* occurs when the teacher's biases influence ratings such as favoring nursing students who do not work while attending school over those who are employed while attending school.

6. *Logical error* results when similar ratings are given for items on the scale that are logically related to one another. This is a problem with rating scales in nursing that are too long and often too detailed. For example, there may be multiple behaviors on communication skills to be rated. The teacher observes some of these behaviors but not all of them. In completing the clinical evaluation form, the teacher gives the same rating to all behaviors on communication on the tool. When this occurs, often some of the behaviors on the rating scale can be combined.

Table 13.3 provides guidelines for using rating scales for clinical evaluation in nursing.

TABLE 13.3   Guidelines for Using Rating Scales for Clinical Evaluation

---

1. Be alert to the possible influence of your own values, attitudes, beliefs, and biases in observing performance and drawing conclusions about it.

2. Use the clinical outcomes, competencies, or behaviors to focus your observations. Give students feedback on other observations made about their performance.

3. Collect sufficient data on students' performance before drawing conclusions about it.

4. Observe the student more than one time before rating performance. Rating scales when used for clinical evaluation should represent a *pattern* of the students' performance over a period of time.

5. If possible observe students' performance in different clinical situations either in the patient care or simulated setting. When not possible, develop additional strategies for evaluation so that performance is evaluated with different methods and at different times.

6. Do not rely on first impressions; they may not be accurate.

7. Always discuss observations with students, obtain their perceptions of performance, and be willing to modify own judgments and ratings when new data are presented.

8. Review the available clinical learning activities and opportunities in the simulation and learning laboratories. Are they providing sufficient data for completing the rating scale? If not, new learning activities may need to be developed, or the behaviors on the tool may need to be modified to be more realistic considering the clinical teaching circumstances.

9. Avoid using rating scales as the only source of data about a student's performance—use multiple evaluation methods for clinical practice.

10. Rate each outcome, competency, or behavior individually based on the observations made of performance and conclusions drawn. If you have insufficient information about achievement of a particular competency, do not rate it—leave it blank.

11. Do not rate all students high, low, or in the middle; similarly, do not let your general impression of the student or personal biases influence the ratings.

12. If the rating form is ineffective for judging student performance, then revise and re-evaluate it. Consider these questions: Does use of the form yield data that can be used to make valid decisions about students' competence? Does it yield reliable, stable data? Is it easy to use? Is it realistic for the types of learning activities students complete and available in clinical settings?

Although there are issues with rating scales, they remain an important clinical evaluation method because they allow teachers, preceptors, and others to rate performance over time and to note patterns of performance. Many different types of rating scales are used for evaluating clinical performance in nursing programs. Sample forms are included in Appendix A.

SIMULATIONS

Simulation is an event or a situation made to resemble clinical practice (Rauen, 2004). With simulations students can develop their psychomotor and technological skills and practice those skills to maintain their competence. Simulations, however, particularly those involving patient simulators, enable students to gain critical-thinking and problem-solving skills. With patient simulators and more complex simulations presented through multimedia, students can assess a patient or clinical situation, analyze data, make decisions about priority problems and actions to take, implement those interventions, and evaluate outcomes. Students can also practice interacting with patients, staff, and others in a safe environment and making decisions as a health team (Oermann, in press). In a study done with beginning nursing students, Ham and O'Rourke (2004) found that the simulated activity eased the transition of the students into their first clinical setting.

Simulations are increasingly important as a clinical teaching strategy, given the limited time for clinical practice in many programs and the complexity of skills to be developed by students. In a simulation laboratory, students can practice those skills without the constraints of a real-life situation. With human patient simulators (HPSs), students can respond to changing situations offered by the simulator without harming a patient (Rauen, 2004). Learners can practice skills, conduct assessments, analyze physiological and other types of data, give medications, and observe the outcomes of interventions and treatments they select.

Using Simulations for Clinical Evaluation

Simulations are not only effective for instruction in nursing, but they also are useful for clinical evaluation. Students can demonstrate procedures and technologies, conduct assessments, analyze clinical scenarios and make decisions about problems and actions to take, carry out care, and evaluate the effects of their decisions. Each of these outcomes can be evaluated for feedback to students or for summative grading.

There are different types of simulations that can be used for clinical evaluation. Case scenarios that students analyze can be presented in paper-and-pencil format or though multimedia, such as with interactive video and CD-ROMs. Many computer simulations are available for use in evaluation. Simulations can be developed with models and manikins for evaluating skills and procedures, and for evaluation with standardized patients. With HPSs, teachers can identify outcomes and clinical competencies to be evaluated, present various clinical events and situations on the simulator for students to analyze and take action, and evaluate student decision making and performance in these scenarios.

Many nursing education programs have set up simulation laboratories with HPSs, clinically-equipped examination rooms, manikins and models for skill practice and assessment, areas for simulated patients, and a wide range of multimedia that facilitate performance evaluations. The rooms can be equipped with two-way mirrors, video cameras, microphones, and other media for observing and rating performance by faculty and others. Videoconferencing technology is being used to conduct clinical evaluations of students in settings at a distance from the nursing education program, effectively replacing onsite performance evaluations by faculty. For example, in one program, an examination room in an Emergency Department was set up for patient assessments by graduate students. Using videoconferencing, students' performance is videotaped and transmitted to faculty at a different site for evaluation (Sackett & Dickerson, 2003).

Incorporating Simulations into Clinical Evaluation Protocol

The same principles for evaluating student performance in the clinical setting apply to using simulations. The first task is to identify which clinical outcomes will be evaluated with a simulation. This decision should be made during the course planning phase as part of the protocol developed for clinical evaluation in the course. It is important to remember when deciding on evaluation methods that evaluation can be done for feedback to students and thus remain ungraded, or be used for grading purposes. Simulations can be used in both instances.

Once the outcomes or clinical competencies to be evaluated with simulations are identified, the teacher can plan the specifics of the evaluation. Some questions to guide teachers in using simulations for clinical evaluation are:

- What are the specific clinical outcomes or competencies to be evaluated using simulations? These should be designated in the plan or protocol for clinical evaluation in a course.

- What types of simulations are needed to evaluate the designated outcomes, e.g., simulations to demonstrate psychomotor and technological skills; ability to identify problems, treatments, and interventions; and pharmacological management?

- Do the simulations need to be developed by faculty, or are they already available in the nursing education program?

- If the simulations need to be developed, who will be responsible for their development? Who will manage their implementation? Because simulations are time consuming to develop and use, decisions need to be made about faculty workload.

- Are the simulations for formative evaluation only? If so, how many practice sessions should be planned? What is the extent of faculty and expert guidance needed? Who will provide that supervision and guidance?

- Are the simulations for summative evaluation (i.e., for grading purposes)? If used for summative clinical evaluation, then faculty need to determine the process for rating performance and how those ratings will be incorporated into the clinical grade, whether pass-fail or a multidimensional system for grading.

- Who will develop or obtain checklists or other methods for rating performance in the simulations?

- When will the simulations be implemented in the course?

- How will the effectiveness of the simulations be evaluated, and who will be responsible?

These are only a few of the questions for faculty planning to use simulations for clinical evaluation in their course.

Standardized Patients

One type of simulation for clinical evaluation uses standardized patients. Standardized patients are individuals who have been trained to accurately portray the role of a patient with a specific diagnosis or condition. With simulations using standardized patients, students can be evaluated on a history and physical examination, related skills and procedures, and communication techniques, among other outcomes. Standardized patients are effective for evaluation because the actors are trained to recreate the same patient condition and clinical situation each time they are with a student, providing for consistency in the performance evaluation. When standardized patients are used for formative evaluation, they provide feedback to the students, an important aid to their learning.

In a study using standardized patients for teaching and evaluating health assessment skills in an advanced practice nursing program, Gibbons and colleagues (2002) found that student learning increased with this method. Improvement was indicated by the end-of-course evaluations and in ratings of the final videotaped physical examinations. Students and faculty were satisfied with this method of teaching and evaluation.

Objective Structured Clinical Examination

An Objective Structured Clinical Examination (OSCE) provides a means of evaluating performance in a simulation laboratory rather than in the clinical setting. In an OSCE students rotate through a series of stations; at each station they complete an activity or perform a task, which is then evaluated. Some stations assess the student's ability to take a patient's history, perform a physical examination, and implement other interventions while being observed by the teacher or an examiner. The student's performance then can be rated using a rating scale or checklist. At other stations, students might be tested on their knowledge and cognitive skills—they might be asked to analyze data, select interventions and treatments, and manage the patient's condition. Most often OSCEs are used for summative clinical evaluation; however, Alinier (2003) described how they can be used formatively to enhance skill acquisition among nursing students.

Newble and Reed (2004) identified three types of stations that can be used in an OSCE. At *clinical stations* the focus is on clinical competence, e.g., taking a history and performing a physical examination, collecting appropriate data, and communicating effectively. Typically at clinical stations there is interaction between the student and a simulated patient (Newble & Reed). At these stations the teacher or examiner can evaluate students' understanding of varied patient conditions and management of them and can rate their performance.

At *practical stations* students perform psychomotor skills, procedures, and technologies, and demonstrate other technical competencies. Performance at these stations is evaluated by the teacher or examiner usually with checklists.

At the third type of station, a *static station,* there is no interaction with a simulated or standardized patient (Newble & Reed, 2004). This station facilitates the evaluation of cognitive skills such as interpreting lab results and other data, developing management plans, and making other types of decisions about patient care. At these stations the teacher or examiner is not present to observe students.

GAMES

Games are teaching methods that involve competition, rules (structure), and collaboration among team members. There are individual games such as cross-word puzzles or games played against other students either individually or in teams; many games require props or other equipment. Games actively involve learners, promote teamwork, reduce stress, and enable students to relax while learning (Henderson, 2005). Games, however, are not intended for grading; they should be used only for instructional purposes and formative evaluation.

Henderson (2005) described the development of a game lab for nursing students, entitled "Is That Your Final Nursing Answer?" Students rotate in small groups to "play" Nursing Feud, Nursing Jeopardy, So You Want to be a Millionaire Nurse?, and Wheel of Nursing Fortune, all of which review content from a clinical nursing course. A fifth area in the learning laboratory set up for "play" is titled "What's Wrong with this Nursing Picture?" (Henderson). In this game, students find violations of nursing principles and common nursing errors made in clinical practice. Answers to game questions by the student teams are accompanied by a rationale. This is one example of how games can be used for instruction, review, and feedback in nursing education.

MEDIA CLIPS

Media clips, short segments of a videotape, a CD, a DVD, an interactive video, and other forms of multimedia, may be viewed by students as a basis for discussions in post-clinical conferences, on discussion boards, and for other online activities; for small group activities; and for critique and write-up as an assignment. Media clips often are more effective than written descriptions of a scenario because they allow the student to visualize the patient and clinical situation. The segment viewed by the students should be short so they can focus on critical aspects related to the outcomes to be evaluated. Media clips are appropriate for assessing if students can apply concepts and theories to the patient or clinical situation depicted in the media clip, observe and collect data, identify possible problems, identify priority actions and interventions, and evaluate outcomes.

Students can answer questions about the media clips as part of a graded learning activity. Otherwise media clips are valuable for formative evaluation, particularly in a group format in which students discuss their ideas and receive feedback from the teacher and peers.

WRITTEN ASSIGNMENTS

Written assignments accompanying the clinical experience are effective strategies for evaluating students' problem solving, critical thinking, and higher-level learning; understanding of content relevant to clinical practice; and ability to express ideas in writing. Evaluation of written assignments was described in Chapter 11. There are many types of written assignments appropriate for clinical evaluation. The teacher should first specify the outcomes to be evaluated with written assignments and then decide which assignments would best assess if those outcomes were met. The final decision is how many assignments will be required in a clinical course.

Written assignments are valuable for evaluating outcomes in face-to-face, Web-based, and other distance education courses in nursing. However, they are misused when students complete the same assignments repetitively throughout a course once the outcomes have been met. At that point students should progress to other more challenging learning activities. Some of the written assignments might be done in post-clinical conferences as small group activities or as part of the discussion board interaction—teachers can still assess student progress toward meeting the outcomes but with fewer demands on their time for reviewing the assignments and providing prompt feedback on them.

Journals

Journals provide an opportunity for students to describe events and experiences in their clinical practice and to reflect on them. With journals students can "think aloud" and share their feelings with teachers. Journals are not intended to develop students' writing skills; instead they provide a means of expressing feelings and reflections on clinical practice and engaging in a dialogue with the teacher about them. When used in clinical courses throughout a nursing program, journals demonstrate a pattern of accomplishments and integration of knowledge and skills over time (Ruthman et al., 2004).

Cohen and Welch (2002) described Web journaling as a means of encouraging reflection on clinical learning. Students share their reflections with the teacher through private emails or with peers on discussion boards. Through Web journaling students examine their behaviors, beliefs, and values and how they influence their interactions with patients. By sharing journal reflections with the teacher and their peers, students expand their awareness of their personal experiences in clinical practice that extend beyond merely describing a clinical situation (Cohen & Welch).

Journals are not the same as diaries and logs. In a diary, students document their experiences in clinical practice with personal reflections; these reflections are meant to remain "personal" and thus are not shared with the teacher or others. A log is typically a structured record of activities completed in the clinical course without reflections about the experience. Students may complete any or all of these activities in a nursing program.

When journals are used in a clinical course, students need to be clear about the objectives—what are the purposes of the journal? For example, a journal intended for reflection in practice would require different entries than one for documenting events and activities in the clinical setting as a means of communicating them to faculty. Students also need written guidelines for journal entries, including how many and what types of entries to make. Depending on the outcomes, journals may be done throughout a clinical course or at periodic intervals. Regardless of the frequency, students need immediate and meaningful feedback about their reflections and entries.

One of the issues in using journals is whether they should be graded or used solely for reflection and self growth. For those educators who support grading journals, a number of strategies have been used such as:

- indicating a grade based on the number of journals submitted rather than on the comments and reflections in them,

- grading papers written from the journals,

- incorporating journals as part of portfolios, which are then graded,

- having students evaluate their own journals based on preset criteria developed by the students themselves, and

- requiring a journal as one component among others for passing a clinical course.

There are some teachers who grade the entries of a journal similar to other written assignments. However, when the purpose of the journal is to reflect on experiences in clinical practice and on the students' own behaviors, beliefs, and values, journals should not be graded. By grading journals the teacher inhibits the student's reflection and dialogue about feelings and perceptions of clinical experiences.

Nursing Care Plans

Nursing care plans enable the student to learn the components of the nursing process and how to use the literature and other resources for writing the plan. However, a linear kind of care planning does not help students learn how problems interrelate nor does it encourage the thinking that nurses do in clinical practice (Mueller, Johnston, & Bligh, 2001). If care plans are used for clinical evaluation, teachers should be cautious about the number of plans required in a course and the outcomes of such an assignment. Short assignments in which students analyze data, examine competing diagnoses, evaluate different interventions and their evidence for practice, suggest alternative approaches, and evaluate outcomes of care may be more effective than a care plan that students often paraphrase from their textbooks.

Concept Maps

Concept maps are tools for visually displaying relationships among concepts. An example is provided in Figure 13.1. Other names for concept maps are clinical correlation maps, clinical maps, and mind-mapped care plans. Concept maps are an effective way of helping students organize data they collect as they plan for their clinical experience; the map can be presented in pre-clinical conference, revised during the clinical learning activity, and then discussed in post-clinical conference (All, Huycke, & Fisher, 2003). With a concept map students can "see" graphically how assessment data, diagnoses, interventions, and other aspects of care relate to one another.

Mueller et al. (2001) combined concept maps and care plans into a strategy they called mind-mapped nursing care plans. Students first develop a generic concept map about something that requires planning such as a trip they might take. They then learn how to develop concept maps for general nursing concepts such as immobility. In small groups, students develop the concept map, illustrate how the concept (e.g., immobility) affects various body systems, and identify their assessment, actions, and outcomes for each branch on the map. Students also prepare a concept map from a case study and then proceed to using concept maps in clinical practice.

In most cases, concept maps are best used for formative evaluation. However, with criteria established for evaluation, they can also be graded. Couey (2004) suggested that one way to grade concept maps is to ask students to explain the relationships and cross-links among concepts. This could be done in short papers that accompany the concept map, which are then graded by the teacher similar to other written assignments. Other areas to evaluate in a concept map for patient care, depending on the goal of the assignment, are: if the assessment data are comprehensive, if the data are linked with the correct diagnoses and problems, if nursing interventions and treatments are specific and relevant, and if the relationships among the concepts are indicated and are accurate.

Case Method, Unfolding Cases, and Case Study

Case method, unfolding cases, and case study were described in chapter 7 because these are strategies for evaluating problem solving, decision making, and higher-level learning. Cases that require application of knowledge from readings and the classroom or an online component of the course can be developed for analysis by students. The scenarios can focus on patients, families, communities, the health care system, and other clinical situations that students might encounter in their clinical practice.

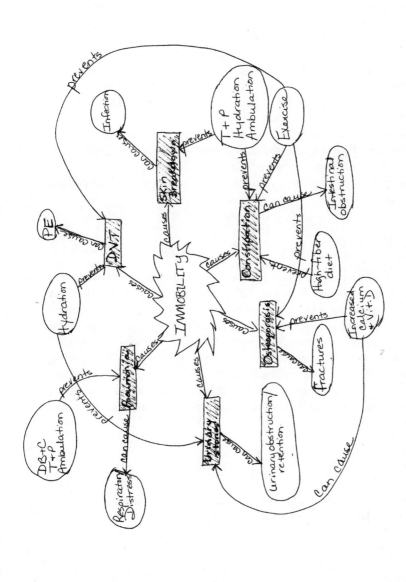

FIGURE 13.1 Example of concept map.

Source: Ignatavicius, D. D. (2004). From traditional care plans to innovative concept maps. In M. H. Oermann & K. Heinrich (Eds.), *Annual review of nursing education* (Vol. 2, pp. 205–216). New York: Springer, p. 210. © Springer Publishing Company. Reprinted with permission.

While these assignments may be completed as individual activities, they are also appropriate for group work. Cases may be presented for group discussion and peer review in clinical conferences and discussion boards. In online courses, the case scenario can be presented with open-ended questions, and based on student responses, other questions can be introduced for discussion. Using this approach, cases are effective for encouraging critical thinking. By discussing cases as a clinical group, students are exposed to other possible approaches and perspectives that they may not have identified themselves. With this method, the teacher can provide feedback on the content and thought process used by students to arrive at their answers.

One advantage of short cases, unfolding cases, and case studies is that they can be graded. By using the principles described for scoring essay tests, the teacher can establish criteria for grading and score responses to the questions with the case. Otherwise cases are useful for formative evaluation and student self-assessment.

Process Recording

Process recordings provide a way of evaluating students' ability to analyze interactions they have had with patients or in simulated clinical activities. Process recordings are useful for providing feedback to students about their interactional skills, but the analysis of the communication also may be graded. With process recordings, students can reflect on their interactions and what they might have done differently. For distance education courses, they provide one source of information about student learning in clinical practice and development of communication skills. When portfolios are used for clinical evaluation, process recordings might be included for outcomes related to communication and interpersonal relationships.

Papers

Short papers for assessing critical thinking and other cognitive skills were described in chapter 7. In short papers about clinical practice, students can:

- Given a data set, identify patient problems and what additional data need to be collected

- Compare data and problems of patients for whom they have provided nursing care, identifying similarities and differences

- Given a hypothetical patient or community problem, identify possible interventions with a rationale
- Select a patient, family, or community diagnosis, and describe relevant interventions with evidence for their use
- Identify one intervention they used with a patient, family, or community; identify one alternative approach that could be used; and provide a rationale
- Identify a decision made in clinical practice involving patients or staff; describe why they made that decision; and propose one other approach that could be used
- Identify a problem or an issue they had in clinical practice, critique the approaches they used for resolving it, and identify alternate approaches.

Short written assignments in clinical courses may be more beneficial than longer assignments because with long papers students often summarize from the textbook and other literature without engaging in any of their own thinking about the content (Oermann, 2004). Short papers can be used for formative evaluation or graded.

Term papers also may be written about clinical practice. With term papers, students can critique and synthesize relevant literature and write a paper about how that literature relates to patient care. Or they might prepare a paper on the use of selected concepts and theories in clinical practice. If the term paper includes the submission of drafts combined with prompt feedback on writing from the teacher, it can be used as a strategy for improving writing skills. While drafts of papers would be evaluated but not graded, the final product would be graded by the teacher.

There are many other written assignments that can be used for clinical evaluation in a nursing course. Similar to any assignment in a course, requirements for papers should be carefully thought out: What outcomes will be met with the assignment, how will they contribute to clinical evaluation in the course, and how many of those assignments does a student need to complete for competency? In planning the clinical evaluation protocol, the teacher should exercise caution in the type and number of written assignments so that they promote learning without unnecessary repetition. Guidelines for evaluating written assignments were presented in chapter 11 and therefore are not repeated here.

PORTFOLIO

A portfolio is a collection of projects and materials developed by the student that document achievement of the objectives of the clinical course. With a portfolio, students can demonstrate what they have learned in clinical practice and the competencies they have developed. Portfolios are valuable for clinical evaluation because students provide evidence in their portfolios to confirm their clinical competencies and document new learning and skills acquired in a course. The portfolio can include evidence of student learning for a series of clinical experiences or over the duration of a clinical course. Portfolios also can be developed for program evaluation purposes to document achievement of curriculum or program outcomes.

Portfolios can be evaluated and graded by faculty based on predetermined criteria. They can also be used for students' self-assessment of their progress in meeting personal and professional goals. Students can continue using their portfolios after graduation—for career development, job applications, as part of their annual performance appraisals, applications for educational programs, and documentation of continuing competence (Oermann, 2002).

Nitko (2004) identified two types of portfolios: best-work, and growth and learning-progress. Best-work portfolios provide evidence that the student has demonstrated certain competencies and achievements in clinical practice; these are appropriate for summative clinical evaluation. Growth and learning-progress portfolios are designed for monitoring students' progress and for self-reflection on learning outcomes at several points in time. These contain products and work of the students in process, at the intermediate stages, for the teacher to review and provide feedback (Nitko).

For clinical evaluation, these purposes can be combined. The portfolio can be developed initially for growth and learning, with products and entries reviewed periodically by the teacher for formative evaluation, and then as a best-work portfolio with completed products providing evidence of clinical competencies. The best-work portfolio can then be graded. Because portfolios are time consuming to develop, they should be used for determining if students met the objectives and passed the clinical course, and should be graded rather than prepared only for self-reflection.

The contents of the portfolio depend on the clinical objectives and competencies to be achieved in the course. Many types of materials and documentation can be included in a portfolio. For example, students can include short papers they completed in the course, a term paper, reports of group work, reports and analyses of observations made in the clinical setting, self-reflections on clinical experiences, and other products they developed in their clinical practice. The key is for students to choose materials that demonstrate their learning and development of their clinical competencies. By assessing the portfolio, the teacher should be able to determine if the students met the outcomes of the course.

There are several steps to follow in using portfolios for clinical evaluation in nursing. Nitko (2004) emphasized that the first step guides faculty in deciding whether a portfolio is an appropriate evaluation method for the course.

Step 1: Identify the purposes of the portfolio.

- Will the portfolio serve as a means of assessing students' development of clinical competencies, focusing predominantly on the growth of the students? Will the portfolio provide evidence of the students' best work in clinical practice, including products reflecting their learning over a period of time? Or, will the portfolio meet both demands, enabling the teacher to give continual feedback to students on the process of learning and projects on which they are working as well as providing evidence of their accomplishments and achievements in clinical practice?

- Will the portfolio be used for formative or summative evaluation? Or, both?

- Will the portfolio provide evaluation data for use in a clinical course? Or, will it be used for curriculum and program evaluation?

- Will the portfolio serve as a means of assessing prior learning and therefore have an impact on the types of learning activities or courses that students complete, for instance, for assessing the prior learning of registered nurses entering a higher degree program or for licensed practical nurses entering an associate degree program?

- What is the role of the students, if any, in defining the focus and content of the portfolio?

Step 2: Identify the type of entries and content to be included in the portfolio.

- What types of entries are required in the portfolio, for example, products developed by students, descriptions of projects with which the students are involved, descriptions of clinical learning activities and reactions to them, observations made in clinical practice and analysis of them, and papers completed by the students, among others?

- In addition to required entries, what other types of content and entries might be included in the portfolio?

- Who determines the content of the portfolio and the types of entries? Teacher only? Student only? Or, both?

- Will the entries be the same for all students or individualized by the student?

- What is the minimum number of entries to be considered satisfactory?

- How should the entries in the portfolio be organized, or will the students choose how to organize them?

- Are there required times for entries to be made in the portfolio, and when should the portfolio be submitted to the teacher for review and feedback?

- Will teacher and student meet in a conference to discuss the portfolio?

Step 3: Decide on the evaluation of the portfolio entries including criteria for evaluation of individual entries and the portfolio overall.

- How will the portfolio be integrated within the clinical evaluation grade and course grade, if at all?

- What criteria will be used to evaluate, and perhaps score, each type of entry and the portfolio as a whole?

- Will only the teacher evaluate the portfolio and its entries? Will only the students evaluate their own progress and work? Or, will the evaluation be a collaborative effort?

- Should a rubric be developed for scoring the portfolio and individual entries? Is there one available in the nursing program that could be used?

These steps and questions to be answered provide guidelines for teachers in developing a portfolio system for clinical evaluation in a course or for other purposes in the nursing program.

Electronic Portfolios

Portfolios can be developed electronically, which facilitates updating and revision of entries, compared with portfolios that include hard copies of materials. In addition to easy updating, prior versions of the portfolio can be archived. Students can develop an electronic portfolio in a nursing course and then reformat it for program evaluation purposes, use it in a capstone nursing course, or for a job application. The electronic portfolio can be saved on a local computer, course Web site, or CD, and can be easily sent to others for feedback or scoring. Day (2004) identified these reasons for using electronic portfolios in a course:

- They are easy to store and reproduce.

- They can be shared with others at limited or no cost (e.g., on the Web, by email, or as a CD).

- They can be updated easily.

- They can be modified for class and program assessment, graduation requirements, or a job search.

- They can include a variety of multimedia.

- They are interactive, allowing students to link documents and to other resources.

- They can be designed for review by the student for self-assessment, the teacher and student, other students in the clinical course or nursing program, or prospective employers, depending on the purpose of the portfolio.

CONFERENCES

The ability to present ideas orally is an important outcome of clinical practice. Sharing information about a patient, leading others in discussions about clinical practice, presenting ideas in a group format, and giving lectures and other types of presentations are skills that students need to develop in a nursing program. Working with nursing staff and other disciplines requires the ability to communicate effectively. Conferences provide a method for developing oral communication skills and for evaluating competency in this area. Discussions also lead to problem solving and critical thinking if questions are open-ended and geared to those outcomes, as discussed in chapter 7.

Many types of conferences are appropriate for clinical evaluation, depending on the outcomes to be met. Pre-clinical conferences take place prior to beginning a clinical learning activity and allow students to clarify their understanding of patient problems, interventions, and other aspects of clinical practice. In these conferences, the teacher can assess students' knowledge and provide feedback to them. Post-clinical conferences, held at the end of a clinical learning activity or a predetermined time during the clinical practicum, provide an opportunity for the teacher to evaluate students' ability to use concepts and theories in patient care, plan care, assess the effectiveness of interventions, problem solve and think critically, collaborate with peers, and achieve other outcomes, depending on the focus of the discussion. In clinical conferences students also can examine ethical dilemmas; cultural aspects of care; and issues facing patients, families, communities, providers, and the health care system. In discussions such as these, students can examine different perspectives and approaches that could be taken. One other conference in which students might participate is an interdisciplinary conference, providing an opportunity to work with other health providers in planning and evaluating care of patients, families, and communities.

While many clinical conferences will be face-to-face with the teacher or preceptor onsite with the students, conferences also can be conducted online. In a study by Cooper, Taft, and Thelen (2004), students identified flexibility and an opportunity for equal participation as two benefits of holding clinical conferences online versus face-to-face.

Criteria for evaluating conferences include the ability of students to:

- Present ideas clearly and in a logical sequence to the group

- Participate actively in the group discussion

- Offer ideas relevant to the topic

- Demonstrate knowledge of the content discussed in the conference

- Offer different perspectives to the topic, engaging the group in critical thinking

- Assume a leadership role, if relevant, in promoting group discussion and arriving at group decisions.

Most conferences are evaluated for formative purposes, with the teacher giving feedback to students as a group or to the individual who led the group discussion. When conferences are evaluated as a portion of the clinical or course grade, the teacher should have specific criteria to guide the evaluation and should use a scoring rubric. Figure 13.2 provides a sample form that can be used to evaluate how well a student leads a clinical conference or to assess student participation in a conference.

GROUP PROJECTS

Most of the clinical evaluation methods presented in this chapter focus on individual student performance, but group projects also can be assessed as part of the clinical evaluation in a course. Some group work is short term—only for the time it takes to develop a product such as a teaching plan or group presentation. Other groups may be formed for the purpose of cooperative learning with students working in small groups or teams in clinical practice over a longer period of time. With any of these group formats, both the products developed by the group and the ability of the students to work cooperatively can be assessed.

There are different approaches for grading group projects. The same grade can be given to every student in the group, i.e., a group grade, although this

Student's name _____

Conference topic _____

Date _____

Rate the behaviors listed below by circling the appropriate number. Some behaviors will not be applicable depending on student role in conference; mark those as not applicable (na).

Behaviors	Rating					
	Poor				Excellent	
States goals of conference	1	2	3	4	5	na
Leads group in discussion	1	2	3	4	5	na
Asks thought-provoking questions	1	2	3	4	5	na
Uses strategies that encourage all students to participate	1	2	3	4	5	na
Participates actively in discussion	1	2	3	4	5	na
Includes important content	1	2	3	4	5	na
Bases interventions on evidence for practice	1	2	3	4	5	na
Offers new perspectives to group	1	2	3	4	5	na
Considers different points of view	1	2	3	4	5	na
Assists group members in recognizing biases and values that may influence decision making	1	2	3	4	5	na
Is enthusiastic about conference topic	1	2	3	4	5	na
Is well prepared for conference discussion	1	2	3	4	5	na
If leading group, monitors time	1	2	3	4	5	na
Develops quality materials to support discussion	1	2	3	4	5	na
Summarizes at end of conference major points discussed	1	2	3	4	5	na

FIGURE 13.2 Evaluation of participation in clinical conference.

does not take into consideration individual student effort and contribution to the group product. Another approach is for the students to indicate in the finished product the parts they contributed to, providing a way of assigning individual student grades, with or without a group grade. Students also can provide an assessment of how much they contributed to the group project, which can then be integrated into their grade. Alternatively, students can prepare both a group and an individual product. Nitko (2004) emphasized that rubrics should be used for evaluating group projects and should be geared specifically to the project. An example of a scoring rubric for assessing a paper was provided in Table 11.2. This rubric could be used for grading a paper prepared by either a group or an individual student.

To assess students' participation and collaboration in the group, the rubric also needs to reflect the goals of group work. With small groups, the teacher can observe and rate individual student cooperation and contributions to the group. However, this is often difficult because the teacher is not a member of the group, and the group dynamics change when the teacher is present. As another approach, students can evaluate the participation and cooperation of their peers. These peer evaluations can be used for the students' own development, and shared among peers but not with the teacher, or can be incorporated by the teacher in the grade for the group project. Students also can be asked to assess their own participation in the group. In a study by Elliott and Higgins (2005), students reported that self and peer assessment was an effective strategy to ensure fairness and equity in grading of group projects in nursing. An easy-to-use form for peer evaluation of group participation is found in Figure 13.3.

SELF-EVALUATION

Self-evaluation is the ability of students to assess their own clinical competencies and identify where further learning is needed. Self-evaluation begins with the first clinical course and develops throughout the nursing program, continuing into professional practice. Through self-evaluation, students judge their clinical performance and identify both strengths and areas for improvement. Using students' self-evaluations, teachers can develop plans to assist students in gaining the knowledge and skills they need to meet the outcomes of the course. It is important for teachers to establish a positive climate for learning in the course, or students will not be likely to share their self-assessment with them.

In addition to developing a supportive learning environment, the teacher should hold planned conferences with each student to review performance. In these conferences, the teacher can

- give specific feedback on performance,
- obtain the student's own perceptions of competencies,
- identify strengths and areas for learning from the teacher's and student's perspectives,

Participation Rubric

Directions: Complete for each group member.

NAME _____

Score	Excellent = 5	Good = 4	Average = 3	Poor = 2
	Did a full share of the work—or more	Did an equal share of the work	Did almost as much work as others	Did less work than others
	Took the initiative in helping the group get organized	Worked agreeably with group members concerning times and places to meet	Could be coaxed into meeting with other group members	Did not meet members at agreed times and places
	Provided many ideas for group project	Participated in discussions about group project	Listened to others; on some occasions, made suggestions	Seemed bored with conversations about the group project
	Assisted other group members	Offered encouragement to other group members	Seemed preoccupied with own part of project	Took little pride in group project
	Work was ready on time or sometimes ahead of time	Work was ready very close to the agreed upon time	Work was usually late but was completed in time to be graded	Some work never got completed and other members completed the assignment
	Clearly communicated desires, ideas, personal needs and feelings	Usually shared feelings and thoughts with other group members	Rarely expressed feelings, preferences	Never spoke up to express excitement and/or frustration

(continued)

FIGURE 13.3 Rubric for peer evaluation of participation in group project.

FIGURE 13.3   *(continued)*

Score	Excellent = 5	Good = 4	Average = 3	Poor = 2
	Expressed frequent appreciation for other group members	Often encouraged and appreciated other group members	Encouraged and appreciated other group members. Seemed to take the work of others for granted	Group members often wondered, "What is going on here?"
	Gave feedback to others that dignified	Gave feedback in ways that did not offend	Sometimes hurt feelings of others with feedback	Was openly rude when giving feedback
	Accepted feedback from others willingly	Reluctantly accepted feedback	Argued own point of view over feedback	Refused to listen to feedback

Adapted with permission from Participation Rubric for Unit Development by Dr. Barbara Frandsen © Barbara Frandsen, St. Edward's University, Austin, Texas, 2005. Available at http://www.stedwards.edu/cte/resources/grub.htm1.

- plan with the student learning activities for improving performance, which is critical if the student is not passing the clinical course, and

- enhance communication between teacher and student.

Some students have difficulty assessing their own performance. For this reason, Ridley and Eversole (2004) suggested providing students with a list of terms that might prompt their self-evaluation. They ask students to circle the words that best describe their strengths and check terms that suggest areas for improvement. The students include examples of their clinical performance to validate their self-assessment. Self-evaluation is appropriate only for formative evaluation and should never be graded.

CLINICAL EVALUATION IN DISTANCE EDUCATION

Nursing education programs use different strategies for offering the clinical component of distance education courses. Often preceptors in the local area guide student learning in the clinical setting and evaluate performance. If cohorts of students are available in an area, adjunct or part-time faculty might be hired to teach a small group of students in the clinical setting. In other programs, students independently complete clinical learning activities to gain the clinical knowledge and competencies of a course. Hugie (2003) reported that her school of nursing offered concentrated clinical learning activities, for example, a one-week clinical practicum in an inpatient psychiatric facility, for students in rural areas of the state where there were no opportunities for clinical learning. Students and a faculty member traveled to the setting for the concentrated clinical experience. Regardless of how the clinical component is structured, the course syllabus, competencies to be developed, rating forms, guidelines for clinical practice, and other materials associated with the clinical course can be placed online. This provides easy access for students, their preceptors, other individuals with whom they are working, and agency personnel. Course management systems such as BlackBoard and WebCT facilitate communication among students, preceptors, course faculty, and others involved in the students' clinical activities.

The clinical evaluation methods presented in this chapter can be used for distance education. The critical decision for faculty is to identify which clinical competencies and skills, if any, need to be observed and the performance rated because that decision suggests different evaluation methods than if the focus of the evaluation is on the cognitive outcomes of the clinical course. In programs in which preceptors or adjunct faculty are available on-site, any of the clinical evaluation methods presented in this chapter can be used as long as congruent with the outcomes and competencies. There should be consistency, though, in how the evaluation is done across preceptors and clinical settings.

Even in clinical courses involving preceptors, faculty members may decide to evaluate clinical skills themselves by reviewing videotapes of performance or observing students through videoconferencing and other technology with faculty at the receiving end. Videotaping performance is valuable not only as a strategy for summative evaluation, to assess competencies at the end of a clinical course or another designated point in time, but also for review by students for self-assessment and by faculty to give feedback. Research has suggested that viewing their own performance on videotapes enables students to identify those skills needing improvement (Birnbach et al., 2002).

Some schools incorporate intensive skill acquisitions workshops in centralized settings for formative evaluation followed by end-of-course ratings by preceptors and others guiding the clinical practicum. In other programs, students travel to regional settings for evaluation of clinical skills (Fullerton & Ingle, 2003).

Another approach is to set up simulated clinical experiences for the evaluation of performance. Patient simulators and other virtual reality devices are effective for this purpose. With these simulators, students can be evaluated on their decision making and clinical judgment, assessment skills, interventions and treatments, and a range of clinical skills. Kaufmann and Liu (2001) described the use of virtual reality simulators for teaching and evaluating trauma care. The simulators have built-in scenarios and multiple patients, enabling the evaluator to vary the clinical situation and increase the level of required technical expertise.

Another clinical evaluation method for distance education is the use of standardized patients. Stroud, Smith, Edlund, and Erkel (1999) described their development of the Clinical Competency Evaluation (CCE), a standardized patient encounter for evaluating students' clinical skills in a controlled environment. Performance with standardized patients can be videotaped for faculty evaluation, and students can submit their patient histories and other written documentation that would commonly be done in practice in that situation. Students also can complete case analyses related to the standardized patient encounter for evaluating their knowledge base and rationale for their decisions.

Students can perform clinical skills and procedures on manikins and models, with performance videotaped and transmitted to faculty for evaluation. Some students may need to create videotapes themselves with personal or rented equipment as a means of demonstrating their development of clinical skills over time and documenting performance at the completion of the course. In those circumstances a portfolio would be a useful evaluation method because it would allow the students to provide materials that indicate their achievement of the course outcomes and clinical competencies.

Any rating scales, checklists, and other tools for evaluating clinical performance need to be carefully selected and validated prior to their use. If preceptors and other examiners will be involved in the performance evaluation, they should be well oriented to these tools and how to use them.

Computer simulations, analyses of cases, case presentations, written assignments, and other strategies presented in this chapter can be used to evaluate students' decision making and other cognitive skills in distance education courses. Similar to clinical evaluation in general, a combination of approaches is more effective than one strategy alone. Table 13.4 summarizes clinical evaluation methods useful for distance education courses.

SUMMARY

This chapter built on concepts of clinical evaluation examined in chapter 12. Many clinical evaluation methods are available for assessing student competencies in clinical practice. The teacher should choose evaluation methods that provide information on how well students are meeting or have met the clinical objectives or are performing the clinical competencies. The teacher also decides

TABLE 13.4   Clinical Evaluation Methods for Distance Education Courses

Evaluation of Psychomotor, Technological, and Other Clinical Skills

- Observation of performance (by faculty onsite or at distance, preceptors, examiners, others)

    With patients, patient simulators and other virtual reality devices, models, manikins, standardized patients

    Objective Structured Clinical Examinations and other types of clinical simulations (in laboratories onsite, regional assessment centers, other settings)

- Rating of performance

    Using rating scales, checklists, performance algorithms

    By faculty, preceptors, examiners, others onsite

    By videotaping, videoconferencing, other transmission to faculty at a distance

- Anecdotal notes of clinical performance by preceptor, examiner, others in local area

Evaluation of Cognitive Outcomes and Skills

- Computer simulations: Questions, short assignments, other written activities about content in computer simulations and application to practice

- Analyses of clinical situations in own practice, interactive videos, CDs, DVDs, and other media

    Reported in a paper, in discussion board, as part of other online activities

- Case method and analyses of cases

    Reported in a paper, in discussion board, as part of other online activities

- Written assignments

    Write-ups of cases, analyses of patient care, and other clinical experiences

    Electronic journals

    Analyses of interactions in clinical setting and simulated experiences

    Short assignments for critical thinking

    Nursing care and management plans

    Sample documentation

    Term papers

    Development of teaching materials, and others

- Case presentations (with or without videotaping or videoconferencing to faculty at a distance)

- Online conferences, discussions

- Portfolio (with materials documenting clinical competencies developed in practicum)

- Test items on clinical knowledge and higher-level cognitive skills

(continued)

TABLE 13.4 *(continued)*

Evaluation of Affective Outcomes

- Online conferences and discussions about values, attitudes, and biases that might influence patient care and decisions; about cultural dimensions of care

- Analyses and discussions of cases presented online, of clinical scenarios shown in video clips and other multimedia

- Written assignments (e.g., reflective papers, journals, others)

- Debates about ethical decisions

- Value clarification strategies

- Questionnaires for self-reflection

---

if the evaluation strategy is intended for formative or summative evaluation. Some of the strategies designed for clinical evaluation are strictly to provide feedback to students on areas for improvement and are not graded. Other methods, such as rating forms and certain written assignments, may be used for summative purposes.

The predominant method for clinical evaluation is in observing the performance of students in clinical practice. Although observation is widely used, there are threats to its validity and reliability. Observations of students may be influenced by the teacher's or preceptor's values, attitudes, and biases, as discussed in the previous chapter. In observing clinical performance, there are many aspects of that performance on which the teacher may focus attention. Every observation reflects only a sampling of the learner's performance during a clinical experience. Issues such as these point to the need for a series of observations before drawing conclusions about performance. There are several ways of recording observations of students—anecdotal notes, checklists, and rating scales. These were described in the chapter.

A simulation creates a situation that represents reality. A major advantage of simulation is that it provides a clinical learning activity for students without the constraints of a real-life situation. With patient simulators, students can respond to changing situations offered by the simulator and can practice skills, conduct assessments, analyze physiological and other types of data, give medications, and observe the outcomes of interventions and treatments they select. One type of simulation for clinical evaluation uses standardized patients, that is, individuals who have been trained to accurately portray the role of a patient with a specific diagnosis or condition. Another form of simulation for clinical evaluation is an Objective Structured Clinical Examination, in which students rotate through a series of stations completing activities or performing skills that are then evaluated.

There are many types of written assignments useful for clinical evaluation depending on the outcomes to be assessed: journal, nursing care plan, concept map, case analysis, process recording, and a paper on some aspect of clinical practice. Written assignments can be developed as a learning activity and reviewed by the teacher and/or peers for formative evaluation, or they can be graded.

A portfolio is a collection of materials that the student has developed in clinical practice over a period of time. With a portfolio, students provide evidence to confirm their clinical competencies and document the learning that occurred in the clinical setting. Other clinical evaluation methods are conference, group project, and self-evaluation. The evaluation methods presented in this chapter provide the teacher with a wealth of methods from which to choose in evaluating students' clinical performance.

REFERENCES

Alfaro-LeFevre, R. (2004). Should clinical courses get a letter grade? *The Critical Thinking Indicator*, *1*(1), 1–5. Available at http://www.alfaroteachsmart.com/clinicalgrade newsletter.pdf

Alinier, G. (2003). Nursing students' and lecturers' perspectives of objective structured clinical examination incorporating simulation. *Nurse Education Today*, *23*(6), 419–426.

All, A. C., Huycke, L. I., & Fisher, M. J. (2003). Instructional tools for nursing education: Concept maps. *Nursing Education Perspectives*, *24*(6), 311–317.

Birnbach, D. J., Santos, A. C., Bourlier, R. A., Meadoes, W. E., Datta, S., Stein, D. J., et al. (2002). The effectiveness of video technology as an adjunct to teach and evaluate epidural anesthesia performance skills. *Anesthesiology*, *96*(1), 5–9.

Bondy, K. N., Jenkins, K., Seymour, L., Lancaster, R., & Ishee, J. (1997). The development and testing of a competency-focused psychiatric nursing clinical evaluation instrument. *Archives of Psychiatric Nursing*, *11*(2), 66–73.

Case, B., & Oermann, M. H. (2004). Clinical teaching and evaluation. In L. Caputi & L. Engelmann (Eds.), *Teaching nursing: The art and science* (pp. 126–177). Glen Ellyn, IL: College of DuPage Press.

Cohen, J. A., & Welch, L. M. (2002). Web journaling: Using informational technology to teach reflective practice. *Nursing Leadership Forum*, *6*(4), 108–112.

Cooper, C., Taft, L. B., & Thelen, M. (2004). Examining the role of technology in learning: An evaluation of online clinical conferencing. *Journal of Professional Nursing*, *20*(3), 160–166.

Couey, D. (2004). Using concept maps to foster critical thinking. In L. Caputi & L. Engelmann, *Teaching nursing: The art and science* (pp. 634–651). Glen Ellyn, IL: College of DuPage Press.

Day, M. (2004, May 18). *Faculty exemplar: Electronic portfolios.* Paper presented at Faculty Summer Institute, University of Illinois at Urbana-Champaign. Retrieved January 25, 2005, from http://www.engl.niu.edu/mday/fsi04.html

Elliott, N., & Higgins, A. (2005). Self and peer assessment—does it make a difference to student group work? *Nurse Education in Practice, 5,* 40–48.

Fullerton, J. T., & Ingle, H. T. (2003). Evaluation strategies for midwifery education linked to digital media and distance delivery technology. *Journal of Midwifery & Women's Health, 48,* 426–436.

Gibbons, S. W., Adamo, G., Padden, D., Ricciardi, R., Graziano, M., Levine, E., & Hawkins, R. (2002). Clinical evaluation in advanced practice nursing education: Using standardized patients in health assessment. *Journal of Nursing Education, 41,* 215–221.

Ham, K., & O'Rourke, E. (2004). Clinical preparation for beginning nursing students: An experiential learning activity. *Nurse Educator, 29,* 139–141.

Henderson, D. (2005). Games: Making learning fun. In M. H. Oermann & K. Heinrich (Eds.), *Annual review of nursing education* (Vol. 3, pp. 165–183). New York: Springer.

Hugie, P. E. (2003). Distance technology in nursing education on a taxpayer's budget: Lessons learned from 22 years of experience. In M. H. Oermann & K. Heinrich (Eds.), *Annual review of nursing education* (Vol. 1, pp. 297–307). New York: Springer.

Kaufmann, C., & Liu, A. (2001). Trauma training: Virtual reality applications. *Studies in Health Technology and Informatics, 81,* 236–241.

Liberto, T., Roncher, M., & Shellenbarger, T. (1999). Anecdotal notes: Effective clinical evaluation and record keeping. *Nurse Educator, 24*(6), 15–18.

Mueller, A., Johnston, M., & Bligh, D. (2001). Mind-mapped care plans: A remarkable alternative to traditional nursing care plans. *Nurse Educator, 26,* 75–80.

Newble, D., & Reed, M. (2004). *Developing and running an Objective Structured Clinical Examination (OSCE).* Retrieved January 25, 2005, from http://www.shef.ac.uk/~dme/oscehandbook.doc

Nitko, A. J. (2004). *Educational assessment of students* (4th ed.). Upper Saddle River, NJ: Prentice Hall.

Oermann, M. H. (2002). Developing a professional portfolio. *Orthopaedic Nursing, 21*(2), 73–78.

Oermann, M. H. (2004). Reflections on undergraduate nursing education: A look to the future. *Journal of Nursing Education Scholarship, 1*(1), 1–15. Available at http://www.bepress.com/ijnes/vol1/iss1/art5

Oermann, M. H. (in press). Program innovations and technology in nursing education: Are we moving too quickly? In J. Novotny & R. Davis, *Distance education in nursing* (2nd ed.). New York: Springer.

Rauen, C. A. (2004). Simulation as a teaching strategy for nursing education and orientation in cardiac surgery. *Critical Care Nurse, 24*(3), 46–51.

Ridley, R. T., & Eversole, M. (2004). Mirrors of change: Student self-reflection. *Nurse Educator, 29,* 181–182.

Ruthman, J., Jackson, J., Cluskey, M., Flannigan, P., Folse, V. N., & Bunten, J. (2004). Using clinical journaling to capture critical thinking across the curriculum. *Nursing Education Perspectives, 25*(3), 120–123.

Sackett, K., & Dickerson, S. S. (2003). Videoconferencing innovations in nursing education. In M. H. Oermann & K. Heinrich (Eds.), *Annual review of nursing education*
(Vol. 1, pp. 281–295). New York: Springer.
Stroud, S., Smith, C., Edlund, B., & Erkel, E. (1999). Evaluating clinical decision-
making skills of nurse practitioner students. *Clinical Excellence for Nurse Practitioners*,
3, 230–237.

Chapter 14

Social, Ethical, and Legal Issues

Educational testing and evaluation have grown in use and importance for students in general and nursing students in particular over the last decade. One only has to read the newspapers and watch television to appreciate the prevalence of testing and evaluation in contemporary American society. With policies such as No Child Left Behind, high school mandatory graduation tests in some states, and the emphasis on standardized achievement tests in many schools, testing and evaluation have taken a prominent role in the educational system. From the moment of birth, when we are weighed, measured, and rated according to the Apgar scale, throughout all of our educational and work experiences, and even in our personal and social lives, we are used to being tested and evaluated. In addition, nursing and other professional disciplines have come under increasing public pressure to be accountable for the quality of educational programs and the competency of their practitioners; thus testing and evaluation often are used to provide evidence of quality and competence.

With the increasing use of evaluation and testing come intensified interest and concern about fairness, appropriateness, and impact. This chapter discusses selected social, ethical, and legal issues related to testing and evaluation practices in nursing education.

SOCIAL ISSUES

Testing has tremendous social impact because test scores can have positive and negative consequences for individuals. Tests can provide information to assist in decision making; some of these decisions have more importance to society and to individuals than other decisions. The licensure of drivers is a good example. Written and performance tests provide information for deciding who may drive a vehicle. Society has a vested interest in the outcome because a bad

251

decision can affect the safety of a great many people. Licensure to drive a vehicle also may be an important issue to an individual; some jobs require the employee to drive a car or truck, so a person who lacks a valid operator's license will not have access to these employment opportunities.

Tests also are used to sort individuals into occupational roles. This sorting has important implications because a person's occupation to some extent determines their status and economic and political power. Because modern society depends heavily on scientific knowledge and technical competence, occupational role selection to a significant degree is based on what individuals know and can do. Therefore, by controlling who enters certain educational programs, institutions have a role in determining the possible career path of an individual.

The way in which schools should select candidates for occupational roles is a matter of controversy, however. Some individuals and groups hold the view that schools should provide equal opportunity and access to educational programs. Others believe that equal opportunity is not sufficient to allow some categories of people to overcome discrimination and oppression that has handicapped their ability and opportunity.

Decisions about which individuals should be admitted to a nursing education program are important because of nursing's commitment to the good of society and to the health and welfare of current and future patients (American Nurses Association, 2003). Nursing faculty must select individuals for admission to nursing programs who are likely to practice nursing competently and safely; tests frequently are used to assist educators in selecting candidates for admission. Improper use of testing or the misinterpretation of test scores can result in two types of poor admission decisions. If an individual is selected who is later found to be incompetent to practice nursing safely, the public may suffer harm; if an individual who would be competent to practice nursing is not admitted, that individual is denied access to an occupational role. The use of testing in employment situations and for the purpose of professional certification can produce similar results. Employers have a stake in making these decisions because they are responsible for ensuring the competence of their employees. Tests for employment, to ensure competencies at the end of orientation, and to certify continuing knowledge and skills are important not only to the employee but also to the employer. Through assessments such as these, the employer certifies that the individual is competent for the role. Selection decisions therefore have social implications for individuals, institutions, and society as a whole.

Although educational and occupational uses of testing are growing in use and importance, the public often expresses concerns about testing. Some of these concerns are rational and relevant; others are unjustified.

Test Bias

One common concern is that tests are biased or unfair to certain groups of test-takers. A major purpose of testing is to discriminate among people, that is, to identify important differences among them with regard to their knowledge, skills, or attitudes. To the extent that differences in scores represent real differences in achievement of objectives, this discrimination is not necessarily unfair (Nitko, 2004). Bias can occur though when scores from an assessment are misinterpreted, or conclusions are drawn about performance that go well beyond the assessment (Nitko, 2004, p. 93). For example, if a test is found to discriminate between men and women on variables that are not relevant to educational or occupational success, it would be unfair to use that test to select applicants for admission to a program or for a job. Thus, the question of test bias really is one of measurement validity, the degree to which inferences about test results are justifiable in relation to the purpose and intended use of the test.

Test bias also has been defined as the differential validity of a test score for a group of test-takers. With test bias, a given score does not have the same meaning for all students who took that test. "Bias favors one group of test takers over another" (Haladyna, 2004, p. 231). The teacher may interpret a low test score to mean inadequate knowledge of the content, but there may be a relevant subgroup of individuals, for example, students with learning disabilities, for whom that score interpretation is not accurate. The test score may be low for a student with a learning disability because he or she did not have enough time to complete the exam, not because of a lack of knowledge about the content.

Individual test items can also discriminate against subgroups of test-takers, such as students from ethnic minority groups; this is termed differential item functioning (Nitko, 2004, p. 93; Wessling, 2003). Test items are considered to function differentially when students of different subgroups but of equal ability, as evidenced by equal total test scores, perform differently on the item. Item bias exists in two forms, cultural bias and linguistic/structural bias (Boscher, 2003).

A culturally biased item contains references to a particular culture and is more likely to be answered incorrectly by students from a minority group. An example of a culturally biased test item follows:

1. While discussing her health patterns with the nurse, Ms. A. says that she enjoys all of the following leisure activities. Which one is an aerobic activity?

    A. Attending ballet performances
    B. Cultivating house plants
    C. Line dancing
    D. Singing in the church choir

The correct answer is "line dancing," but students for whom English is a second language (ESL) and other minority students may be unfamiliar with this term and therefore may not select this response. In this case, an incorrect response may mean that the student is unfamiliar with this type of dancing, not that the student is unable to differentiate between aerobic and nonaerobic activities.

Careful peer review of test items for discernible bias allows the teacher to reword items to remove references to American or English literature, music, art, history, customs, or regional terminology that are not essential to the nursing content being tested. The inclusion of jokes, puns, and other forms of humor may also contribute to cultural bias, as these forms of expression may not be interpreted correctly by ESL students. It is appropriate, however, to include cultural references that are essential to safe nursing practice. Students and graduate nurses must be culturally competent if they are to meet the needs of patients from a variety of cultures.

A test item with linguistic/structural bias is poorly written. It may be lengthy, unclear, or awkwardly worded, interfering with the student's understanding of the teacher's intent (Boscher, 2003). Structurally biased items create problems for all students, but they are more likely to discriminate against ESL students or those with learning disabilities. Additionally, students from minority cultures may be less likely than dominant-culture students to ask the test proctor to clarify a poorly written item, usually because it is inappropriate to question a teacher in certain cultures. Following the general rules for writing test items in this book will help the teacher to avoid structural bias.

An evaluation practice that helps to protect students from potential bias is anonymous or blinded scoring and grading. The importance of grading essay items and written assignments anonymously was discussed earlier in the book. Anonymous grading also can be used for an entire course. The process is similar to that of peer review of manuscripts and grant proposals: the teacher is unaware of the student's identity until the end of the course. Students choose a number or are randomly assigned an "Anonymous Grading System" number (Caceci, nd) at the beginning of a course. That number is recorded on every test, quiz, written assignment, and other evaluations during the semester, and scores are recorded according to these code numbers. The teacher does not know the identity of the students until the end of the course. This method of grading prevents the influence of a teacher's previous impressions of a student on the scoring of a test or written assignment.

Grade and Test Score Inflation

Another common criticism of testing concerns the general trend toward inflation of test scores and grades at all educational levels. Scanlan and Care (2004) found that grade inflation occurred throughout their university but more so in their nursing program. Grade inflation distorts the meaning of test scores, making it difficult for teachers to use them wisely in decision making. If an A is intended to represent exceptional or superior performance, then all students cannot earn As because if everyone is exceptional then no one is. With grade inflation all grades are compressed near the top, which makes it difficult to discriminate among students (Mansfield, 2001). When there is no distribution of scores or grades, there is little value in testing.

One factor contributing to grade inflation is the increasing pressure of accountability for educational outcomes. When the effectiveness of a teacher's instruction is judged on the basis of students' test performance, the teacher may "teach to the test." Teaching to the test may involve using actual test items as practice exercises, distributing copies of a previously used test for review and then using the same test, or focusing exclusively on test content in teaching. It is important, however, to distinguish between teaching to the test and purposeful teaching of content to be sampled by the test and the practice of relevant test-taking skills. However, nursing faculty members who understand the NCLEX® test plan and ensure that their nursing curricula include content and learning activities that will enable students to be successful on the NCLEX are not teaching to the test.

The Effect of Tests and Grades on Self-Esteem

Some critics of tests claim that testing results in emotional or psychological harm to students. The concern is that tests threaten students and make them anxious, fearful, and discouraged, resulting in harm to their self-esteem. There is no empirical evidence to support these claims. Feelings of anxiety about an upcoming test are both normal and helpful to the extent that they motivate students to prepare thoroughly in order to demonstrate their best performance. Since testing is a common life event, learning how to cope with these challenges is a necessary part of student development.

Nitko (2004) identified three types of test-anxious students: (a) students who have poor study skills and become anxious prior to a test because they do not understand the content that will be tested; (b) students who believe that they have good study skills but in essence do not; and (c) students who have good study skills and understand the content but fear they will do poorly no matter how much they prepare for the exam. If the teacher can identify why students are anxious about testing, they can be directed to specific resources such as those on study skills, test-taking strategies, and techniques to reduce their stress.

Most nursing students will benefit from developing good test-taking skills, particularly learners who are anxious. For example, students should be told to follow the directions carefully, read the item stems and questions without rushing to avoid misreading critical information; to read each option for multiple-choice items before choosing one; to manage time during the test, answer easy items first, and check their answers (Kubiszyn & Borich, 2003). Arranging the test with the easy items first often helps relieve anxiety as students begin the test. Since highly anxious students are easily distracted (Nitko, 2004), the teacher should ensure quiet during the testing session.

Goonan (2003) provided general guidelines for the teacher to intervene with students who have test anxiety:

1. Identify the problem to be certain it is test anxiety and not a learning disability or a problem such as a depression.

2. Encourage more than the usual test preparation.

3. Encourage the student to develop study skills (e.g., outlining material) and good study habits (e.g., how to organize the material to learn it and how to manage time).

4. Guide the student to outside resources as needed.

5. Suggest desensitization strategies such as taking timed practice tests and relaxation techniques.

While it is probably true that a certain level of self-esteem is necessary before a student will attempt the challenges associated with nursing education, high self-esteem is not essential to perform well on a test. In fact, if students are able to perform at their best, their self-esteem is enhanced. An important part of a teacher's role is to prepare students to do well on tests by helping them improve their study and test-taking skills and to learn to manage their anxiety.

Testing as a Means of Social Control

All societies sanction some form of social control of behavior; some teachers use the threat of tests and the implied threat of low test grades to control student behavior. In an attempt to motivate students to prepare for and attend class, a teacher may decide to give unannounced tests; the student who is absent that day will earn a score of zero, and the student who does not do the assigned readings will likely earn a low score. This practice is unfair to students because they need sufficient time to prepare for a test in order to demonstrate their maximum performance as discussed in Chapter 3. Using tests in a punitive, threatening, or vindictive way is unethical (Nitko, 2004).

ETHICAL ISSUES

Ethical standards make it possible for nurses and patients to achieve understanding of and respect for each other (Husted & Husted, 2001). These standards should also govern the relationships of teachers and students. Contemporary bioethical standards include those of autonomy, freedom, veracity, privacy, beneficence, and fidelity. Several of these standards are discussed here as they apply to common issues in testing and evaluation.

The standards of privacy, autonomy, and veracity relate to the ownership and security of tests and test results. Some of the questions that have been raised are: Who owns the test? Who owns the test results? Who has or should have access to the test results? Should test takers have access to standardized test items and their own responses?

Since educational institutions and employers started using standardized tests to make decisions about admission and employment, the public has been concerned about the potential discriminatory use of test results. The result of this public concern was the passage of federal and state "Truth in Testing" laws, requiring greater access to tests and test results. Some of these laws require publishers of standardized tests to supply copies of the test, the answer key, and the test-taker's own responses upon request, allowing the student to verify the accuracy of the test score.

Test-takers have the right to expect that certain information about them will be held in confidence. Teachers, therefore, have an obligation to maintain a privacy standard regarding students' test scores. Such practices as public posting of test scores and grades should be examined in light of this privacy standard. Teachers should not post assessment results if individual students' identities can be linked with their results; for this reason, many educational programs do not allow scores to be posted with student names or identification numbers. During posttest discussions, teachers should not ask students to raise their hands to indicate if they answered an item correctly or incorrectly; this practice can be considered invasion of students' privacy (Nitko, 2004).

An additional privacy concern relates to the practice of keeping student records that include test scores and other assessment results. Questions often arise about who should have access to these files and the information they contain. Access to a student's test scores and other assessment results is limited by laws such as the Family Educational Rights and Privacy Act of 1974 (FERPA). This federal law gives students certain rights with respect to their education records. For example, they can review their education records maintained by the school and request that the school correct records they believe to be inaccurate or misleading. Schools must have written permission from the student to release information from the student's record except in selected situations such as accreditation or for program evaluation purposes (U.S. Department of Education, n.d.). The FERPA limits access to a student's records to those who have legitimate rights to the information in order to meet the educational needs of the student. This law also specifies that a student's assessment results may not be transferred to another institution without written authorization from the student. In addition to these limits on access to student records, teachers should assure that the information in the records is accurate and should correct errors when they are discovered. Files should be purged of anecdotal material when this information is no longer needed (Nitko, 2004, p. 87).

Another way to violate students' privacy is to share confidential information about their assessment results with other teachers. To a certain extent, a teacher should communicate information about a student's strengths and weaknesses to other teachers to help them meet that student's learning needs. In most cases, however, this information can be communicated through student records to which other teachers have legitimate access. Informal conversations about students, especially if those conversations center on the teacher's impressions and judgments rather than on verifiable data such as test scores, can be construed as gossip.

Test results sometimes are used for research and program evaluation purposes. As long as students' identities are not revealed, their scores usually can be used for these purposes (Nitko, 2004, p. 87). One way to assure that this use of test results is ethical is to announce to the students when they enter an educational program that test results occasionally will be used to assess program effectiveness. Students may be asked for their informed consent for their scores to be used, or their consent may be implied by their voluntary participation in optional program evaluation activities. For example, if a questionnaire about student satisfaction with the program is distributed or mailed to students, those who wish to participate simply complete the questionnaire and return it; no written consent form is required.

Standards for Ethical Testing Practice

Several codes of ethical conduct in using tests and other assessments have been published by professional associations. These include the *Code of Fair Testing Practices in Education* (Joint Committee on Testing Practices, 2004) and the *Code of Professional Responsibilities in Educational Measurement* (National Council on Measurement in Education [NCME], 1995). These two codes are found in Appendix B. Another document to guide student assessment is 9 *Principles of Good Practice for Assessing Student Learning* from the American Association for Higher Education (2003) (Appendix C). The *Standards for Educational and*

Psychological Testing (American Education Research Association, American Psychological Association, & NCME, 1999) describe standards for test construction, administration, scoring, and reporting; supporting documentation for tests; fairness in testing; and a range of testing applications. The *Standards* also address testing individuals with disabilities and different linguistic backgrounds.

Common elements of these codes and standards are:

- Teachers are responsible for the quality of the tests they develop and for selecting tests that are appropriate for the intended use.

- Test administration procedures must be fair to all students and protect their safety, health, and welfare.

- Teachers are responsible for the accurate scoring of tests and reporting test results to students in a timely manner.

- Students should receive prompt and meaningful feedback.

- Test results should be interpreted and used in valid ways.

- Teachers also must communicate test results accurately and anticipate the consequences of using results to minimize negative results to students (Nitko, 2004, pp. 79–85).

LEGAL ASPECTS OF EVALUATION

It is beyond the scope of this book to interpret laws that affect the use of tests and other assessments, and the authors are not qualified to give legal advice to teachers concerning their evaluation practices. However, it is appropriate to discuss a few legal issues to provide guidance to teachers in using tests.

A number of issues have been raised in the courts by students claiming violations of their rights by testing programs. These issues include race or gender discrimination, violation of due process, unfairness of particular tests, various psychometric aspects such as measurement validity and reliability, and accommodations for students with disabilities (Nitko, 2004, pp. 91–92).

Evaluation of Students with Disabilities

The Americans with Disabilities Act (ADA) of 1990 has influenced testing and evaluation practices in nursing education and employment settings. This law prohibits discrimination against qualified individuals with disabilities. A qualified individual with a disability is defined as a person with a physical or mental impairment that substantially limits major life activities. Qualified individuals with disabilities meet the requirements for admission to and participation in a nursing program. Nursing education programs have a legal and an ethical obligation to accept and educate qualified individuals with disabilities (Carroll, 2004). It is up to the nursing education program to provide reasonable accommodations, additional services and aids as needed, and removal of barriers (Carroll). This does not mean that institutions lower their standards to comply with the ADA (Steckler, 1999).

The ADA requires teachers to make reasonable accommodations for disabled students in order to assess them properly. Such accommodations may include oral testing, computer testing, modified answer format, extended time for exams, test readers or sign language interpreters, a private testing area, or the use of large type for printed tests (Nitko, 2004, p. 82). NCLEX policies permit test-takers with documented learning disabilities to have extended testing time as well as other reasonable accommodations. Persons of a cultural or racial minority or those who speak English as a second language, however, are not considered to be qualified persons with disabilities (Klisch, 1994).

A number of concerns have been raised regarding the provision of reasonable testing accommodations for students with disabilities. One issue is the validity of the test result interpretations if the test was administered under standard conditions for one group of students and under accommodating conditions for other students. The privacy rights of students with disabilities is another issue: Should the use of accommodating conditions be noted along with the student's test score? Such a notation would identify the student as disabled to anyone who had access to the record. There are no easy answers to such questions. In general, faculty members should be guided by accommodation policies developed by their institution and have any additional policies reviewed by legal counsel to ensure compliance with the ADA.

SUMMARY

Educational testing and evaluation are growing in use and importance for society in general and for nursing in particular. Nursing has come under increasing public pressure to be accountable for the quality of educational programs and the competency of its practitioners, and testing and evaluation often are used to provide evidence of quality and competence. With the increasing use of evaluation and testing come intensified interest and concern about fairness, appropriateness, and impact.

The social impact of testing can have positive and negative consequences for individuals. Tests can provide information to assist in decision making, such as selecting individuals for admission to education programs or for employment. The way in which selection decisions are made can be a matter of controversy, however, regarding equality of opportunity and access to educational programs and jobs.

The public often expresses concerns about testing. Common criticisms of tests include: tests are biased or unfair to some groups of test-takers; test scores have little meaning because of the grade inflation; testing causes emotional or psychological harm to students; and tests are sometimes used in a punitive, threatening, or vindictive way. By understanding and applying codes for the responsible and ethical use of tests, teachers can assure the proper use of assessment procedures and the valid interpretation of test results. Teachers must be responsible for the quality of the tests they develop and for selecting tests that are appropriate for the intended use.

The Americans with Disabilities Act of 1990 has implications for the proper assessment of students with physical and mental disabilities. This law requires educational programs to make reasonable testing accommodations for qualified individuals with learning as well as physical disabilities.

REFERENCES

American Association for Higher Education. (2003). 9 principles of good practice for assessing student learning. Accessed February 6, 2005, from http://www.aahe.org/assessment/principl.htm

American Education Research Association, American Psychological Association, and National Council on Measurement in Education. (1999). Standards for educational and psychological testing. Washington, DC: American Psychological Association.

American Nurses Association. (2003). Nursing's social policy statement (2nd ed.). Washington, DC: Author.

Boscher, S. (2003). Barriers to creating a more culturally diverse nursing profession: Linguistic bias in multiple-choice nursing exams. Nursing Education Perspectives, 24, 25–34.

Caceci, T. (n.d.). Anonymous grading redux: Student reaction to a blinded grading system. Journal of Veterinary Medical Education, 20(3). Accessed February 27, 2005, from http://www.utpjournals.com/jour.ihtml?lp=jvme/jvme203/AnonymousGrading Redux.html

Carroll, S. M. (2004). Inclusion of people with physical disabilities in nursing education. Journal of Nursing Education, 43, 207–212.

Goonan, B. (2003). Overcoming test anxiety: Giving students the ability to show what they know. In J. E. Wall & G. R. Walz (Eds.), Measuring up: Assessment issues for teachers, counselors, and administrators (pp. 257–272). Greensboro, NC: ERIC Counseling and Student Services Clearinghouse. (ERIC Document Reproduction Service No. ED 480053)

Haladyna, T. M. (2004). *Developing and validating multiple-choice test items* (3rd ed.). Mahwah, NJ: Lawrence Erlbaum.

Husted, G. L., & Husted, J. H. (2001). *Ethical decision making in nursing* (3rd ed.). New York: Springer.

Joint Committee on Testing Practices. (2004). *Code of fair testing practices in education.* Washington, DC: American Psychological Association.

Klisch, M. L. (1994). Guidelines for reducing bias in nursing examinations. *Nurse Educator, 19*(2), 35–39.

Kubiszyn, T., & Borich, G. (2003). *Educational testing and measurement: Classroom application and practice* (7th ed.). New York: John Wiley.

Mansfield, H. C. (2001, April 6). Grade inflation: It's time to face the facts. *The Chronicle of Higher Education, 47*(30), B24.

National Council on Measurement in Education. (1985). *Code of professional responsibilities in educational measurement.* Washington, DC: Author.

Nitko, A. J. (2004). *Educational assessment of students* (4th ed.). Upper Saddle River, NJ: Prentice Hall.

Scanlan, J. M., & Care, W. D. (2004). Grade inflation: Should we be concerned? *Journal of Nursing Education, 43,* 475–478.

Steckler, S. L. (1999). Nursing case law update: The nurse with severe hearing disability. *Journal of Nursing Law, 6,* 39–46.

U.S. Department of Education. (n.d.). *Family Educational Rights and Privacy Act (FERPA).* Family Policy Compliance Office, U.S. Department of Education. Washington, DC. Accessed February 27, 2005, from http://www.ed.gov/policy/gen/guid/fpco/ferpa/index.html

Wessling, S. (2003, Winter). Does the NCLEX® pass the test for cultural sensitivity? *Minority Nurse,* 46–50.

Chapter 15

Interpreting Test Scores

As a measurement tool, a test results in a score—a number. A number, however, has no intrinsic meaning and must be compared with something that has meaning in order to interpret it. For a test score to be useful for making decisions about the test, the score has to be interpreted by the teacher. Whether the interpretations are norm- or criterion-referenced, a basic knowledge of statistical concepts is necessary to assess the quality of teacher-made or published tests, understand standardized test scores, summarize assessment results, and explain test scores to others.

TEST SCORE DISTRIBUTIONS

Some information about how a test performed as a measurement instrument can be obtained from computer-generated test- and item-analysis reports. In addition to providing item analysis data such as difficulty and discrimination indexes, such reports often summarize the characteristics of the score distribution. If the teacher does not have access to machine scoring and computer software for test and item analysis, many of these analyses can be done by hand, albeit more slowly.

When a test is scored, the teacher is left with a collection of raw scores. Often these scores are recorded according to the names of the students, in alphabetical order, or by student numbers. As an example, suppose that the scores displayed in Table 15.1 resulted from the administration of a 65-point test to 16 nursing students.

Glancing at this collection of numbers, the teacher would find it difficult to answer such questions as:

1. Did a majority of students obtain high or low scores on the test?
2. Did any individuals score much higher or much lower than the majority of the students?
3. Are the scores widely scattered or grouped together?
4. What was the range of scores obtained by the majority of the students? (Nitko, 2004, p. 480)

To make them easier to visualize, the scores should be arranged in an orderly way, usually from highest to lowest, as in Table 15.2. Ordering the scores in this way makes it obvious that they ranged from 42 to 60, and that one student's score was much lower than those of the other students. But the teacher still

TABLE 15.1   List of Students in a Class and Their Raw Scores on a 65-Point Test

Student	Score		Student	Score
A. Allen	53		I. Ignatius	48
B. Brown	54		J. Jimanez	55
C. Chen	52		K. Kelly	52
D. Dunlap	52		L. Lynch	42
E. Edwards	54		M. Meyer	47
F. Finley	57		N. Nardozzi	60
G. Gunther	54		O. O'Malley	55
H. Hernandez	56		P. Purdy	53

TABLE 15.2   Rank Order of Students from Table 15.1 with Raw Scores Ordered from Highest to Lowest

Student	Score		Student	Score
N. Nardozzi	60		A. Allen	53
F. Finley	57		P. Purdy	53
H. Hernandez	56		C. Chen	52
J. Jimanez	55		K. Kelly	52
O. O'Malley	55		D. Dunlap	52
B. Brown	54		I. Ignatius	48
E. Edwards	54		M. Meyer	47
G. Gunther	54		L. Lynch	42

cannot visualize easily how a typical student performed on the test or the general characteristics of the obtained scores. Removing student names, listing each score once, and tallying how many times each score occurs, results in a frequency distribution, as in Table 15.3. By displaying scores in this way, it is easier for the teacher to identify how well the group of students performed on the exam.

The frequency distribution also can be represented graphically as a histogram. In Figure 15.1, the scores are ordered from lowest to highest along a horizontal line, left to right, and the number of asterisks above each score indicate the frequencies. Frequencies also can be indicated on a histogram by bars, with the height of each bar representing the frequency of the corresponding score, as in Figure 15.2.

A frequency polygon is another way to display a score distribution graphically. A dot is made above each score value to indicate the frequency with which that score occurred; if no one obtained a particular score, the dot is made

TABLE 15.3   Frequency Distribution of Raw Scores From Table 15.1

Raw Score	Frequency
61	0
60	1
59	0
58	0
57	1
56	1
55	2
54	3
53	2
52	3
51	0
50	0
49	0
48	1
47	1
46	0
45	0
44	0
43	0
42	1
41	0

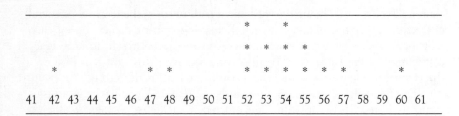

FIGURE 15.1   Histogram depicting frequency distribution of raw scores from Table 15.1.

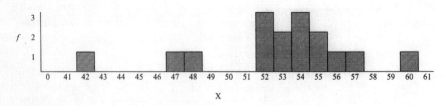

FIGURE 15.2   Bar graph depicting frequency distribution of raw scores from Table 15.1.

Note: X = scores
f = frequencies

on the baseline, at zero. The dots then are connected with straight lines to form a polygon or curve. Figure 15.3 shows a frequency polygon based on the histogram in Figure 15.1. Histograms and frequency polygons thus show general characteristics such as the scores that occurred most frequently, the score distribution shape, and the range of the scores.

The characteristics of a score distribution can be described on the basis of its symmetry, skewness, modality, and kurtosis. These characteristics are illustrated in Figure 15.4. A symmetric distribution or curve is one in which there are two equal halves; the halves are mirror images of each other. Nonsymmetric or asymmetric curves have a cluster of scores or a peak at one end and a tail extending toward the other end. This type of curve is said to be skewed; the direction in which the tail extends indicates whether the distribution is positively or negatively skewed. The tail of a positively skewed curve extends toward the right, in the direction of positive numbers on a scale, and the tail of a negatively skewed curve extends toward the left, in the direction of negative numbers. A positively skewed distribution thus has the largest cluster of scores at the low

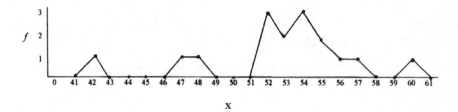

FIGURE 15.3 Frequency polygon depicting frequency distribution of raw scores from Table 15.1.

Note: X = scores
f = frequencies

end of the distribution, which seems counterintuitive. The distribution of test scores from Table 15.1 is nonsymmetric and negatively skewed. Remember that the lowest possible score on this test was zero and the highest possible score was 65; the scores were clustered between 43 and 60.

Frequency polygons and histograms can differ in the number of peaks they contain; this characteristic is called modality, referring to the mode or the most frequently occurring score in the distribution. If a curve has one peak, it is unimodal; if it contains two peaks, it is bimodal. A curve with many peaks is multimodal. The relative flatness or peakedness of the curve is referred to as kurtosis. Flat curves are described as platykurtic, moderate curves are said to be mesokurtic, and sharply peaked curves are referred to as leptokurtic (Krus, 2004). The histogram in Figure 15.1 is a bimodal, platykurtic distribution.

The shape of a score distribution depends on the characteristics of the test as well as the abilities of the students who were tested (Nitko, 2004). Some teachers make grading decisions as if all test score distributions resemble a normal curve, i.e., they attempt to "curve" the grades. An understanding of the characteristics of a normal curve would dispel this notion. A normal distribution is a bell-shaped curve that is symmetric, unimodal, and mesokurtic. Figure 15.5 illustrates a normal distribution.

Many human characteristics such as intelligence, weight, and height are normally distributed; the measurement of any of these attributes in a population would result in more scores in the middle range than at either extreme. However, most score distributions obtained from teacher-made tests do not approximate a normal distribution. This is true for several reasons. The characteristics of a test greatly influence the resulting score distribution; a very difficult test tends to yield a positively skewed curve. Likewise, the abilities of the students influence

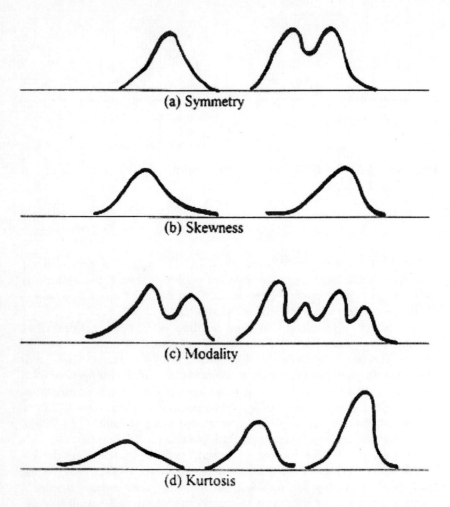

FIGURE 15.4 Characteristics of a score distribution.
Source. Ebel, R. L., & Frisbie, D. A. (1991). *Essentials of educational measurement* (5th ed.). Englewood Cliffs, NJ: Prentice Hall, 1991, p. 58, with permission.

the test score distribution. Regardless of the distribution of the attribute of intelligence among the human population, this characteristic is not likely to be distributed normally among a class of nursing students or a group of newly hired registered nurses (RNs). Since admission and hiring decisions tend to select those individuals who are most likely to succeed in the nursing program or job,

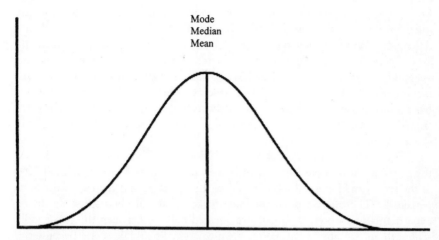

FIGURE 15.5 The normal distribution.

a distribution of IQ scores from a class of 16 nursing students or 16 newly hired RNs would tend to be negatively skewed. Likewise, knowledge of nursing content is not likely to be normally distributed because those who have been admitted to a nursing program or hired as staff nurses are not representative of the population in general. Therefore, grading procedures that attempt to apply the characteristics of the normal curve to a test score distribution are likely to result in unwise and unfair decisions.

Measures of Central Tendency

One of the questions to be answered when interpreting test scores is, "What score is most characteristic or typical of this distribution?" A typical score is likely to be in the middle of a distribution with the other scores clustered around it. Measures of central tendency provide a summary of that score, which is the center around which the scores are grouped (Hopkins, 1998, p. 27). Three measures of central tendency commonly used to interpret test scores are the mode, median, and mean.

The mode, usually abbreviated Mo, is the most frequently occurring score in the distribution; it must be a score actually obtained by a student. It can be identified easily from a frequency distribution or graphic display without mathematical calculation. As such, it provides a rough indication of central tendency. The mode, however, is the least stable measure of central tendency because it tends to fluctuate considerably from one sample to another drawn from the same population (Kubiszyn & Borich, 2003, p. 257). That is, if the same 65-item test that yielded the scores in Table 15.1 was administered to a different group of 16 nursing students in the same school who had taken the same course, the mode might differ considerably. In addition, as in the distribution depicted in Figure 15.1, the mode has two or more values in some distributions, making it difficult to specify one typical score. A uniform distribution of scores has no mode; such distributions are likely to be obtained when the number of students is small, the range of scores is large, and each score is obtained by only one student.

The median, sometimes abbreviated Mdn or Md, is the point that divides the distribution of scores into equal halves. It is a value above which fall 50% of the scores and below which fall 50% of the scores; thus it represents the 50th percentile. The median does not have to be an actual obtained score. In an even number of scores, the median is located halfway between the two middle scores; in an odd number of scores, the median is the middle score. Because the median is an index of location, it is not influenced by the value of each score in the distribution. Thus, it is usually a good indication of a typical score in a skewed distribution containing extremely high or low scores (Nitko, 2004, p. 486).

The mean often is referred to as the "average" score in a distribution, reflecting the mathematical calculation that determines this measure of central tendency. It is usually abbreviated as M or $\overline{X}$. The mean is computed by summing each individual score and dividing by the total number of scores, as in the following formula:

$$M = \frac{\Sigma X}{N} \qquad \text{[Equation 15.1]}$$

where M is the mean, ΣX is the sum of the individual scores, and N is the total number of scores (Kubiszyn & Borich, 2003, p. 252). Thus, the value of the mean is affected by every score in the distribution. This property makes it the preferred index of central tendency when a measure of the total distribution is desired. However, the mean is sensitive to the influence of extremely high or low scores in the distribution, and as such, it may not reflect the typical performance of a group of students (Nitko, 2004, p. 485).

There is a relationship between the shape of a score distribution and the relative locations of these measures of central tendency. In a normal distribution, the mean, median, and mode have the same value, as shown in Figure 15.5. In a positively skewed distribution, the mean will yield the highest measure of central tendency and the mode will give the lowest; in a negatively skewed distribution, the mode will be the highest value and the mean the lowest. Figure

15.6 depicts the relative positions of the three measures of central tendency in skewed distributions.

The mean of the distribution of scores from Table 15.1 is 52.75; the median is 53.5. The fact that the median is slightly higher than the mean confirms that the median is an index of location or position and is insensitive to the actual score values in the distribution. The mean, since it is affected by every score in the distribution, was influenced by the one extreme low score. Because the shape of this score distribution was negatively skewed, it is expected that the median would be higher than the mean because the mean is always pulled in the direction of the tail (Hopkins, 1998, p. 23).

Measures of Variability

It is possible for two score distributions to have similar measures of central tendency and yet be very different. The scores in one distribution may be tightly clustered around the mean, and in the other distribution, the scores may be widely dispersed over a range of values. Measures of variability are used to determine how similar or different the students are with respect to their scores on a test.

The simplest measure of variability is the range, the difference between the highest and lowest scores in the distribution. For the test score distribution in

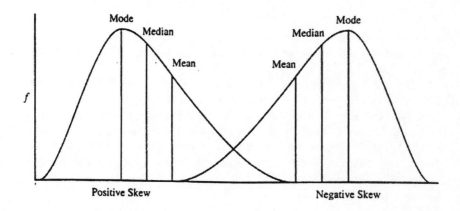

FIGURE 15.6 Measures of central tendency in skewed distributions.

Source. Polit, D. F., & Hungler, B. P. (1999). *Nursing research: Principles and methods* (6th ed.). Philadelphia: Lippincott, p. 450. Reprinted by permission of Lippincott Williams & Wilkins.

Table 15.3, the range is 18 (60 − 42 = 18). The range is sometimes expressed as the highest and lowest scores, rather than a difference score. Because the range is based on only two values, it can be highly unstable. The range also tends to increase with sample size; that is, test scores from a large group of students are likely to be scattered over a wide range because of the likelihood that an extreme score will be obtained (Nitko, 2004, p. 486).

The standard deviation, usually abbreviated as *SD* or *s*, is the most common and useful measure of variability. Like the mean, it takes into consideration every score in the distribution. The standard deviation is based on differences between each score and the mean. Thus, it characterizes the average amount by which the scores differ from the mean. The standard deviation is calculated in four steps:

1. Subtract the mean from each score (X − M) to compute a deviation score (*x*), which can be positive or negative.
2. Square each deviation score (x^2), which eliminates any negative values. Sum all of the squared deviation scores (Σx^2).
3. Divide this sum by the number of test scores to yield the variance.
4. Calculate the square root of the variance.

Although other formulas can be used to calculate the standard deviation, the following definitional formula represents these four steps:

$$SD = \sqrt{\frac{\Sigma x^2}{N}} \qquad \text{[Equation 15.2]}$$

where *SD* is the standard deviation, Σx^2 is the sum of the squared deviation scores, and N is the number of scores (Kubiszyn & Borich, 2003, p. 268; Nitko, 2004, p. 486).

The standard deviation of the distribution of scores from Table 15.1 is 4.1. What does this value mean? A standard deviation of 4.1 represents the average deviation of scores from the mean. On a 65-point test, 4 points is not a large average difference in scores. If the scores cluster tightly around the mean, the standard deviation will be a relatively small number; if they are widely scattered over a large range of scores, the standard deviation will be a larger number (Kubiszyn & Borich, 2003, p. 271).

INTERPRETING AN INDIVIDUAL SCORE

Interpreting the Results of Teacher-Made Tests

The ability to interpret the characteristics of a distribution of scores will assist the teacher to make norm-referenced interpretations of the meaning of any individual score in that distribution. For example, how should the teacher interpret P. Purdy's score of 53 on the test whose results were summarized in Table 15.1? With a median of 53.5, a mean of 52.75, and a standard deviation of 4.1, a score of 53 is about "average." All scores between 49 and 57 fall within one standard deviation of the mean, and thus are not significantly different from one another. On the other hand, N. Nardozzi can rejoice because a score of 60 is almost two standard deviations higher than the mean; thus, this score represents achievement that is much better than that of others in the group. The teacher should probably plan to counsel L. Lynch, because a score of 42 is more than two standard deviations below the mean, much lower than others in the group.

However, most nurse educators need to make criterion-referenced interpretations of individual test scores. A student's score on the test is compared to a pre-set standard or criterion, and the scores of the other students are not considered. The percentage-correct score is a derived score that is often used to report the results of tests that are intended for criterion-referenced interpretation. The percentage correct is a comparison of a student's score with the maximum possible score; it is calculated by dividing the raw score by the total number of items on the test. Although many teachers believe that percentage-correct scores are an objective indication of how much students really know about a subject, in fact they can change significantly with the difficulty of the test items. Since percentage-correct scores are often used as a basis for assigning letter grades according to a predetermined grading system, it is important to recognize that they are determined more by test difficulty than by true quality of performance. For tests that are more difficult than expected to be, the teacher may want to adjust the raw scores before calculating the percent correct on that test.

The percentage-correct score should not be confused with percentile rank, often used to report the results of standardized tests. The percentile rank describes the student's relative standing within a group and therefore is a norm-referenced interpretation. The percentile rank of a given raw score is the percentage of scores in the distribution that occur at or below that score. A percentile rank of 83, therefore, means that the student's score is equal to or higher than the scores made by 83% of the students in that group; one cannot assume, however, that the student answered 83% of the test items correctly. Because there are 99 points that divide a distribution into 100 groups of equal size, the highest percentile rank that can be obtained is the 99th. The median is at the 50th percentile. Differences between percentile ranks mean more at the highest and lowest extremes than they do near the median (Kubiszyn & Borich, 2003).

Interpreting the Results of Standardized Tests

The results of standardized tests usually are intended to be used to make norm-referenced interpretations. Before making such interpretations, the teacher should keep in mind that standardized tests are more relevant to general rather than specific instructional goals. Additionally, the results of standardized tests are more appropriate for evaluations of groups rather than individuals. Consequently, standardized test scores should not be used to determine grades for a specific course or to make a decision to hire, promote, or terminate an employee. Like most educational measures, standardized tests provide gross, not precise, data about achievement. Actual differences in performance and achievement are reflected in large score differences.

Standardized test results usually are reported in derived scores such as percentile ranks, standard scores, and norm group scores. Because all of these derived scores should be interpreted in a norm-referenced way, it is important to specify an appropriate norm group for comparison. The user's manual for any standardized test typically presents norm tables in which each raw score is matched with an equivalent derived score. Standardized test manuals may contain a number of norm tables; the norm group on which each table is based should be fully described. The teacher should take care to select the norm group that most closely matches the group whose scores will be compared to it (Kubiszyn & Borich, 2003, p. 356). For example, when interpreting the results of standardized tests in nursing, the performance of a group of baccalaureate nursing students should be compared with a norm group of baccalaureate nursing students. Norm tables sometimes permit finer distinctions such as size of program, geographical region, and public vs. private affiliation.

SUMMARY

To be meaningful and useful for decision making, test scores must be interpreted in norm-referenced or criterion-referenced ways. Knowledge of basic statistical concepts is necessary to make valid interpretations and to explain test scores to others.

Scoring a test results in a collection of numbers known as raw scores. To make raw scores understandable, they can be arranged in frequency distributions or displayed graphically as histograms or frequency polygons. Score distribution characteristics such as symmetry, skewness, modality, and kurtosis can assist the teacher in understanding how the test performed as a measurement tool as well as to interpret any one score in the distribution.

Measures of central tendency and variability also aid in interpreting individual scores. Measures of central tendency include the mode, median, and mean; each measure has advantages and disadvantages for use. In a normal distribution, these three measures will coincide. Most score distributions from teacher-made tests do not meet the assumptions of a normal curve. The shape of the distribution can determine the most appropriate index of central tendency to use. Variability in a distribution can be described roughly as the range of scores or more precisely as the standard deviation.

Teachers can make criterion-referenced or norm-reference interpretations about individual student scores. Norm-referenced interpretations of any individual score should take into account the characteristics of the score distribution, some index of central tendency, and some index of variability. The teacher thus can use the mean and standard deviation to make judgments about how an individual student's score compares with those of others.

A percentage-correct score is calculated by dividing the raw score by the total possible score; thus it compares the student's score to a pre-set standard or criterion and does not take the scores of other students into consideration. A percentage-correct score is not an objective indication of how much a student really knows about a subject because it is affected by the difficulty of the test items. The percentage-correct score should not be confused with percentile rank, which describes the student's relative standing within a group and therefore is a norm-referenced interpretation. The percentile rank of a given raw score is the percentage of scores in the distribution that occurs at or below that score.

The results of standardized tests usually are reported as percentile ranks or other norm-referenced scores. Teachers should be cautious when interpreting standardized test results so that comparisons with the appropriate norm group are made. Standardized test scores should not be used to determine grades or to make personnel decisions, and results should be interpreted with the understanding that only large differences in scores indicate real differences in achievement levels.

REFERENCES

Hopkins, K. D. (1998). *Educational and psychological measurement and evaluation* (8th ed.). Boston: Allyn & Bacon.

Krus, D. J. (2004). *Visual statistics with multimedia.* Cruise Scientific. Accessed February 24, 2005, from http://www.visualstatistics.net/web%20Visual%20Statistics/Visual%20Statistics%20Multimedia/normalization.htm

Kubiszyn, T., & Borich, G. (2003). *Educational testing and measurement: Classroom application and practice* (7th ed.). New York: John Wiley.

Nitko, A. J. (2004). *Educational assessment of students* (4th ed.). Upper Saddle River, NJ: Prentice Hall.

Chapter 16

Grading

Evaluating students in the classroom and clinical practice provides the basis for assigning a grade for the course. The grade is a symbol reflecting the achievement of students in that course. In addition to grading the course as a whole, grades are given for individual assignments, quizzes, tests, and other learning activities completed by students throughout the course. This chapter examines the uses of grades in nursing programs, problems with grading, grading frameworks, and how to compute grades for nursing courses.

THE PURPOSES OF GRADES

In earlier chapters there was extensive discussion about formative and summative evaluation. Through formative evaluation the teacher provides feedback to the learner on a continuous basis. In contrast, summative evaluation is conducted periodically to indicate the student's achievement at the end of the course or at a point within the course. Summative evaluation provides the basis for arriving at grades in the course. *Grading*, or marking, is defined as the use of symbols, for instance, the letters A through F, for reporting student achievement. Grading is for summative purposes, indicating through the use of symbols how well the student performed in the clinical setting and the course as a whole.

To reflect valid judgments about student achievement, grades need to be based on careful evaluation practices, reliable test results, and multiple evaluation measures. No grade should be determined on one evaluation method or one assignment completed by the students; grades reflect instead a combination of various tests and other evaluation methods. Along a similar line, students may complete assignments that are not included in their grade, particularly if the emphasis is on formative evaluation. Not all of the students' activities in a course, however, need to be graded. Grades serve three broad purposes: (a) instructional, (b) administrative, and (c) guidance and counseling.

Instructional

Grades for instructional purposes indicate the achievement of students in the course. They provide a measure of *what* students have learned and their competencies at the end of the course or at a certain point within it. A "pass" grade in the clinical practicum and a grade of "B" in the nursing course are examples of using grades for instructional purposes.

Administrative

The second purpose that grades serve is administrative. Grades are used for:

- admission of students to entry level and higher degree nursing programs
- progression of students in a nursing program
- decisions about probation and whether students can continue in the program
- decisions about re-entry into a nursing program
- determining students' eligibility for graduation
- awarding scholarships and fellowships
- awarding honors and determining acceptance into honor societies such as Sigma Theta Tau International
- program evaluation studies, and
- reporting to employers.

Guidance and Counseling

The third use of grades is for guidance and counseling. Grades can be used to make decisions about courses to select, including more advanced courses to take or remedial courses that might be helpful. Grades also suggest academic resources that students might benefit from such as reading, study, and test-taking workshops and support. In some situations grades assist students in making career choices including a change in the direction of their careers.

CRITICISMS OF GRADES

Although grades serve varied purposes, there are many criticisms of them. Nitko (2004) identified and responded to a number of these criticisms, which are applicable to grading in nursing programs.

1. Grades are meaningless because of the diversity across nursing education programs, course faculty, clinical teachers, and preceptors.
   - Response: A consistent grading system is needed across sections of nursing courses and for grading clinical practice. It is important that full- and part-time faculty, preceptors, and others involved in the course be oriented as to how to evaluate and grade each of the assignments. Clinical teachers and preceptors should discuss the clinical evaluation process and methods, how to use the clinical evaluation instrument and determine a clinical grade, and grading practices in the course.

2. A single symbol, such as an A or a pass, does not adequately represent the complex details associated with achievement in nursing courses.
   - Response: Grades are not intended to fulfill this need. They do not reflect every detail of the student's learning in a course nor every accomplishment. Instead, grades are a summarization of achievements over a period of time.

3. Grades are not important.
   - Response: Although a grade is only a symbol of achievement, Nitko (2004) emphasized that grades are important. The many ways that grades are used to arrive at educational decisions demonstrate how important they are to students, nursing programs, and others. In addition, grades and overall grade point average (GPA) may predict later achievement such as performance on licensure and certification examinations. Although some may argue that the most valuable outcomes of learning are intangible, grades, nevertheless, are important.

4. Self-evaluations are more important than grades.
   - Response: Developing the ability to evaluate one's own learning outcomes and competencies is essential for continued professional development. Both grades and self-evaluations are needed, not one or the other (Nitko, 2004).

5. Grades are unnecessary.
   - Response: In most educational settings, grades cannot be eliminated because they serve the purposes identified earlier in the chapter. A

certain level of performance is essential for progression in a nursing program and for later educational decisions; grades provide a way of determining whether students are achieving sufficiently to progress through the program.

6. Grades are ineffective motivators.

   • Response: For some students grades are effective motivators although for others this may not be true.

7. Low grades discourage students.

   • Response: While low grades may be discouraging and stressful for students, they are essential for determining progression in a nursing program. Nursing education programs are accountable to the profession and the public for graduating students with knowledge and competencies for safe practice. Not all entering students have the ability to acquire this knowledge and these skills. Low grades are important for counseling students and suggesting remedial instruction; failing grades indicate when students have not met the criteria for continuing in the nursing program.

8. Grades are inflated and thus do not reflect true achievement.

   • Response: Both public and private colleges and universities have undergone considerable grade inflation over the last few decades. Grade inflation has become a national problem (Johnson, 2003). "Grade inflation compresses all grades at the top, making it difficult to discriminate the best from the very good, the very good from the good, the good from the mediocre" (Mansfield, 2001, B24). Students are paying more for their education, and they want a reward of high grades for their "purchase." In one study the most common reason for grade inflation as reported by faculty was pressure from students (McCabe & Powell, 2004). In developing a grading system, it is important for nursing faculty to be clear about the standards for each grade level in that system and to communicate these to students. Scanlan and Care (2004) emphasized that faculty need to develop valid and reliable evaluation methods and learn how to respond to irate nursing students complaining about their grades. Faculty should also periodically review the grades in nursing courses to assess if they are inflated, keeping in mind that nursing students are carefully selected for admission into the program and need to achieve certain grades in courses to progress. For this reason, grades in nursing courses tend to be higher than general education courses in which students are more heterogeneous.

TYPES OF GRADING SYSTEMS

There are different types of grading systems or methods of reporting grades. Most nursing education programs use a letter system for grading (A, B, C, D, E or A, B, C, D, F), which may be combined with "+" and "−". The integers 5, 4, 3, 2, and 1 (or 9 through 1) also may be used. These two systems of grading are convenient to use, yield grades that are able to be averaged within a course and across courses, and present the grade concisely.

Grades also may be indicated by percentages (100, 99, 98, . . .). Most programs use percentages as a basis for assigning letter grades—90 to 100% represents an A, 80 to 89% a B, and so forth. In some nursing programs, the percentages for each letter grade are higher, for example, 92 to 100% for an A, 83 to 91% a B, 75 to 82% a C, 66 to 74% a D, and 65% and below an E or F. It is not uncommon in nursing education programs to specify that students need to achieve at least a C in each nursing course at the undergraduate level and a B or better at the graduate level. Requirements such as these are indicated in the school policies and course syllabi.

Another type of grading system is two-dimensional: pass-fail, satisfactory-unsatisfactory, or credit-no credit. For determining clinical grades, some programs add a third honors category, creating three levels: honors-pass-fail. One advantage of a two-dimensional grading system is that the grade is not calculated in the GPA. This allows students to take new courses and explore different areas of learning without concern about the grades in these courses affecting their overall GPA. This also may be viewed as a disadvantage, however, in that clinical performance in a nursing course graded on a pass-fail basis is not calculated as part of the overall course grade. A pass indicates that students met the clinical objectives or demonstrated satisfactory performance of the clinical competencies. Different systems for grading clinical practice are discussed later in the chapter.

Grade Point Average

One other dimension of a grading system involves converting the letter grade to a grade point system for calculating the grade point average (GPA) or quality point average (QPA). Grades in a 4-point system are typically:

A = 4 points per credit (or unit)
B = 3 points per credit
C = 2 points per credit
D = 1 point per credit
F = 0 points per credit

If a student took two 3-credit courses and one 6-credit nursing course and received an A in one of the 3-credit courses, a C in the other, and a B in the 6-credit course, the grade point average would be:

A　=　4 points/credit　=　4 points × 3 credits　=　12 points
C　=　2 points/credit　=　2 points × 3 credits　=　6 points
B　=　3 points/credit　=　3 points × 6 credits　=　18 points

$$36 \div 12 \text{ (credits)} = 3.0.$$

The letter system for grading also may include plus and minus grades. This is shown in Table 16.1. Bressette (2002) reported on the trend away from grading systems with few categories such as A–F to systems with more categories from adding plus and minus to each grade. Although grade inflation may not decrease when plus and minus are used, these added categories allow for more differentiation for grading and may motivate students who through extra effort can raise their grade (Bressette).

TABLE 16.1　Plus and Minus System

Letter Grade	Grade Points
A	4.00
A–	3.67
B+	3.33
B	3.00
B–	2.67
C+	2.33
C	2.00
C–	1.67
D+	1.33
D	1.00
D–	0.67
F	0.00

ASSIGNING LETTER GRADES

Because most nursing education programs use the letter system for grading nursing courses, this framework will be used for discussing how to assign grades. These principles, however, are applicable to the other grading systems as well. There are two major considerations in assigning letter grades: deciding what to include in the grade and selecting a grading framework.

Deciding What to Include in the Grade

Grades in nursing courses should reflect the student's achievement and not be biased by the teacher's own values, beliefs, and attitudes. If the student did not attend class or appeared to be inattentive during lectures, this behavior should not be incorporated into the course grade unless criteria were established at the outset for class attendance and participation.

The student's grade is based on the tests and evaluation methods developed for the course. The weight given to each of these in the overall grade should reflect the emphasis of the objectives and the content measured by them. Tests and other evaluation methods associated with important content, for which more time was probably spent in the instruction, should receive greater weight in the course grade. For example, a midterm examination in a community health nursing course should be given more weight in the course grade than a paper that students completed about community resources for a family under their care.

How much weight should be given in the course grade to each test and other type of evaluation methods used in the course? The teacher begins by listing the tests, quizzes, papers, presentations, and other evaluation methods in the course that should be included in the course grade. Then the teacher decides on the importance of each of these components in the overall grade for the course. Factors to consider when weighting the components of the course grade are as follows:

1. Components that assess more of the important learning outcomes and competencies should carry more weight in the course grade than those that measure only a few of the outcomes (Nitko, 2004).

2. Components that assess content that was emphasized in the course and for which more time was spent in the instruction should receive the most weight in the course grade (Nitko, 2004).

3. Components that measure the application of concepts and theories to practice and development of higher-level skills should be weighted more heavily than those that focus on recall of content.

4. Components that are more difficult and time consuming for students should receive more weight than those that are easy and require less time to complete.

Selecting a Grading Framework

To give meaning to the grades assigned, the teacher needs a grading framework or frame of reference. There are three grading frameworks used to assign meaning to grades:

1. Criterion-referenced, also referred to as grading with an absolute scale,
2. Norm-referenced or grading with a relative scale, and
3. Self-referenced or grading based on the growth of the student (Nitko, 2004).

Table 16.2 illustrates these grading frameworks. Criterion- and norm-referenced evaluation methods were described in earlier chapters; these same concepts apply to grading frameworks.

CRITERION-REFERENCED GRADING

In criterion-referenced grading, grades are based on students' achievement of the outcomes of the course, the extent of content learned in the course, or how well they performed in the clinical practicum. Students who achieve more of the objectives, acquire more knowledge, and can perform more competencies or with greater proficiency receive higher grades. The meaning assigned to grades, then, is based on these absolute standards without regard to the achievement of other students. Using this frame of reference for grading means that it is possible for all students to achieve an A or a B in a course, if they meet the standards, or a D or F if they do not.

This framework is appropriate for most nursing courses because they focus on outcomes and competencies to be achieved in the course. Criterion-referenced grading indicates how students are progressing toward meeting those outcomes (formative evaluation) and at the end of the course if they have achieved them (summative evaluation). Norm-referenced grading, in contrast, is not appropriate for use in nursing courses that are based on standards or learning outcomes because it focuses on comparing students with one another, not on how they are progressing or on their achievement. For example, formative evaluation in a norm-referenced framework would indicate how each student ranks among the group rather than providing feedback on student progress in meeting the outcomes of the course and strategies for further learning.

Fixed-Percent Method

There are several ways of assigning grades using a criterion-referenced system. One is called the fixed-percent method. This method uses fixed ranges of percent-

TABLE 16.2   Grading Frameworks

Grade	Criterion-referenced	Norm-referenced	Self-referenced
A	All outcomes met. Significant knowledge and cognitive skills gained. Able to perform all clinical competencies at high level.	Achievement/ performance far exceeds average of group (e.g., other students in course, in clinical group).	Made significant progress. Performed significantly higher than expected.
B	All essential outcomes met and at least half of the others. Important content areas learned and able to be applied to new situations. Able to perform most clinical competencies at high level.	Above the average of the group.	Made progress and gained knowledge and skills. Performed higher than expected.
C	All essential outcomes met. Learned essential content. Able to perform most clinical competencies.	Average in comparison with the group.	Made progress in most areas. Met performance level expected by teacher.
D	Only some essential outcomes met. Limited understanding of content. Unable to perform some essential clinical competencies.	Below the average of the group.	Made some gains. Did not meet level of performance for which capable.
F	Most outcomes not achieved. Limited content learned. Most clinical competencies not able to be performed.	Failing achievement/ performance in comparison with the group.	Made no gains. Performance significantly below capability.

Note: Ideas for this table were based on: Nitko, A. J. (2004). *Educational assessment of students* (4th ed.). Upper Saddle River, NJ: Prentice Hall.

correct scores as the basis for assigning grades (Frisbie & Waltman, 1992). A common grading scale is 92 to 100% for an A, 83 to 91% a B, 75 to 82% a C, 66 to 74% a D, and below 65% an E or F. Each component of the course grade—written tests, quizzes, papers, case presentations, and other assign ments—is given a percent-correct score or percent of the total points possible. For example, the student might have a score of 21 out of 25 on a quiz, or 84%. The component grades are then weighted, and the percentages are averaged to get the final grade, which is converted to a letter grade at the end of the course (Kubiszyn & Borich, 2003). With all grading systems, the students need to be informed how the grade will be assigned. If the fixed percent method is used, the students should know the scale for converting percentages to letter grades; this should be in the course syllabus with a clear explanation of how the course grade will be determined.

Computing a Composite (Single) Score for a Course

In using the fixed percent method, the first step, which is an important one, is to assign weights to each of the components of the grade. For example:

Paper on nursing interventions	10%
Papers critiquing issues in clinical practice	20%
Quizzes	10%
Midterm examination	20%
Portfolio	20%
Final examination	20%
	100%

In determining the composite score for the course, the student's percentage for each of the components of the grade is multiplied by the weight and summed; the sum is then divided by the sum of the weights. This procedure is shown in Table 16.3.

Generally, test scores should not be converted to grades for the purpose of later computing a final average grade. Instead, the teacher should record actual test scores and then combine them into a composite score that can be converted to a final grade.

Total-Points Method

The second method of assigning grades in a criterion-referenced system is the total-points method. In this method, each component of the grade is assigned

TABLE 16.3   Fixed-Percent Method for Grading Nursing Courses

Components of Course Grade and Weights

Paper on nursing interventions	10%
Papers critiquing issues in clinical practice	20%
Quizzes	10%
Midterm examination	20%
Portfolio	20%
Final examination	20%

Student	Interven-tion Paper (wt. = 10%)	Issue Papers (wt. = 20%)	Quizzes (wt. = 10%)	Midterm (wt. = 20%)	Portfolio (wt. = 20%)	Final (wt. = 20%)
Mary	85	94	98	92	94	91
Jane	76	78	63	79	70	79
Bob	82	86	89	81	80	83

Composite score for Mary:
$[10(85) + 20(94) + 10(98) + 20(92) + 20(94) + 20(91)] \div 100$ (sum of weights) $= 92.5\%$

Composite score for Jane:
$[10(76) + 20(78) + 10(63) + 20(79) + 20(70) + 20(79)] \div 100 = 75.1\%$

Composite score for Bob:
$[10(82) + 20(86) + 10(89) + 20(81) + 20(80) + 20(83)] \div 100 = 83.1\%$

specific points, for example, a paper may be worth 100 points and midterm examination 200 points. The number of points assigned reflects the weights given to each component within the course, i.e., what each one is "worth." For example:

Paper on nursing interventions	100 points
Papers critiquing issues in clinical practice	200 points
Quizzes	100 points
Midterm examination	200 points
Portfolio	200 points
Final examination	200 points
	1,000 points

The points for each component are not converted to a letter grade; instead the grades are assigned according to the number of total points accumulated at the end of the course. At that time letter grades are assigned based on the points needed for each grade. For example:

Grade	Points
A	900–1,000
B	800–899
C	700–799
D	600–699
F	0–599

One problem with this method is that often the decision about the points to allot to each test and evaluation method in the course is made before the teacher has developed them (Frisbie & Waltman, 1992). For example, to end with 1,000 points for the course, the teacher may need 20 points for each quiz. However, in preparing one of those quizzes, the teacher finds that 10 items adequately cover the content and reflect the emphasis given the content in the instruction. If this were known during the course planning, the teacher could assign 10 fewer points to quizzes and add another assignment worth 10 points, or could alter the points for other components of the course grade. However, when the course is already underway, changes such as these cannot be made in the grading scheme, and the teacher needs to develop a 20-point quiz even if fewer items would have adequately sampled the content. The next time the course is offered, the teacher can modify the points allotted for quizzes in the course grade.

Computing a Composite Score for a Course

In this method the composite score is the total number of points the student accumulates, and no further calculations are needed. Nitko (2004) cautioned teachers to be sure that the weights of the components were reflected in the points given them in the total composite. For example, if the teacher wanted the portfolio to count 20% of the course grade, and the maximum number of points for the course was 1000, then the portfolio would be worth a maximum of 200 points (= 20% of 1000).

NORM-REFERENCED GRADING

In a norm-referenced grading system, using relative standards, grades are assigned by comparing a student's performance with that of others in the class. Students who perform better than their peers receive higher grades (Nitko, 2004). When using a norm-referenced system the teacher decides on the reference group against which to compare student's performance. Should students be compared to others in the course? To students only in their section of the course? Or, to students who completed the course the prior semester or previous year? One issue with norm-referenced grading is that high performance in a particular group may not be indicative of mastery of the content or what students have learned; it reflects instead a student's standing in that group.

Grading on the Curve

Two methods of assigning grades using a norm-referenced system are (a) grading on the curve and (b) by using standard deviations. Grading on the curve refers to the score distribution curve. In this method, students' scores are rank ordered from highest to lowest, and grades are assigned according to the rank order. For example, the teacher may decide on the following framework for grading a test:

Top 20% of students	A
Next 20%	B
Next 40%	C
Next 15%	D
Lowest 5%	F

With this method there would always be failing grades on a test.

After the quotas are set, grades are assigned without considering actual achievement. For example, the top 20% of the students will receive an A even if their scores are close to the next group that gets a B. The students assigned lower grades may in fact have acquired sufficient knowledge in the course but unfortunately had lower scores than the other students. In these two examples, the decisions on the percentages of As, Bs, Cs, and lower grades are made arbitrarily by the teacher. The teacher determines the proportion of grades at each level; this approach is not based on a normal curve.

Another way of grading on the curve is to use the normal or bell curve for determining the percentages of each grade. The assumption of this method is that the grades of the students in the course should reflect a normal distribution. For example:

Top 10% of students	A
Next 20%	B
Next 40%	C
Next 20%	D
Lowest 10%	F

For a norm-referenced system to work correctly, student scores need to be distributed based on the normal curve (Svinicki, 2001). However, nursing students are not heterogeneous and therefore their scores on tests and other evaluation products are not normally distributed. They are carefully selected for admission into the program, and they need to achieve certain grades in courses and minimum GPAs to progress in the program. With grading on the curve, even if most students achieved high grades on a test and mastered the content, some would still be assigned lower grades.

Standard Deviation Method

The second method is based on standard deviations. With this method, the teacher determines the cut-off points for each grade. The grades are based on how far they are from the mean of raw scores for the class instead of on an arbitrary scale (Strashny, 2003). To use the standard deviation method, the teacher first prepares a frequency distribution of the final scores and then calculates the mean score. The cut-off points for a "C" grade range from one-half the standard deviation below the mean to one-half above the mean (University of North Carolina Center for Teaching and Learning, 2001). To identify the "A-B" cut-off scores, the teacher adds one standard deviation to the upper cut-off number of the C range. Subtracting one standard deviation from the lower "C" cut-off provides the range for the "D-F" grades (University of North Carolina Center for Teaching and Learning).

SELF-REFERENCED GRADING

Self-referenced grading is based on standards of growth and change in the student. With this method, grades are assigned by comparing the student's performance with the teacher's perceptions of the student's capabilities (Nitko, 2004). Did the student achieve at a higher level than deemed capable regardless of the knowledge and competencies acquired? Did the student improve performance throughout the course?

Table 16.2 compares self-referencing with criterion- and norm-referenced grading. One major problem with this method is the unreliability of the teacher's perceptions of student capability and growth. A second issue occurs with students who enter the course or clinical practice with a high level of achievement and proficiency in many of the clinical competencies. These students may have the least amount of growth and change but nevertheless exit the course with the highest achievement and clinical competency.

GRADING CLINICAL PRACTICE

Arriving at grades for clinical practice is difficult because of the nature of clinical practice and the need for judgments about performance. Issues in evaluating clinical practice and rating performance were discussed in chapters 12 and 13. Many teachers constantly revise their rating forms for clinical evaluation and seek new ways of grading clinical practice. Although these changes may create a fairer grading system, they will not eliminate the problems inherent in judging clinical performance.

The different types of grading systems described earlier may be used for grading clinical practice. In general these include multidimensional systems such as letter grades, A through F; integers, 5 through 1; and percentages. Grading systems for clinical practice also may be two-dimensional, including the categories pass-fail, satisfactory-unsatisfactory, and met-did not meet the clinical objectives. Some programs add a third category, honors, to acknowledge performance that exceeds the level required. With any of these grading systems, it is not always easy to summarize the multiple types of evaluation data collected on the student's performance in a symbol representing a grade. This is true even in a pass-fail system; it may be difficult to arrive at a judgment as to pass or fail based on the evaluation data and the circumstances associated with the student's clinical and simulated practice.

Regardless of the grading system for clinical practice, there are two criteria to be met: (a) the evaluation methods for collecting data about student performance should reflect the outcomes and clinical competencies for which a grade will be assigned, and (b) the students must understand how their clinical practice will be evaluated and graded.

Decisions about assigning letter grades for clinical practice are the same as grading any course: identifying what to include in the clinical grade and selecting a grading framework. The first consideration relates to the evaluation methods used in the course to provide data for determining the clinical grade. Some of these evaluation methods are for summative evaluation, thereby providing a source of information for including in the clinical grade. Other strategies, though, are used in clinical practice for feedback only and are not incorporated into the grade.

The second consideration is the grading framework. Will achievement in clinical practice be graded from A to F? 5 to 1? Pass-fail? Or variations of these? The related question is, how will the clinical grade be included in the course grade if at all?

Pass-Fail

Categories for grading clinical practice such as pass-fail and satisfactory-unsatisfactory have some advantages over a multidimensional system, although there are disadvantages as well. Pass-fail places greater emphasis on giving feedback to the learner because only two categories of performance need to be determined. With a pass-fail grading system, teachers may be more inclined to provide continual feedback to learners because they do not have to ultimately differentiate performance according to four or five levels of proficiency such as with a letter system. Performance that exceeds the requirements and expectations, however, is not reflected in the grade for clinical practice unless a third category is included—honors-pass-fail. Alfaro-LeFevre (2004) reported from her survey of 79 nursing programs, which were randomly selected, that a pass-fail grading system was used in 59 (75%) of the programs. Fifteen (15%) programs assigned letter grades for the clinical practicum.

A pass-fail system requires only two types of judgment about clinical performance. Do the evaluation data indicate that the student has met the clinical objectives or has demonstrated satisfactory performance of the competencies to indicate a pass? Or, do the data suggest that the performance of those competencies is not at a satisfactory level? Arriving at a judgment as to pass or fail is often easier for the teacher than using the same evaluation information for deciding on multiple levels of performance. A letter system for grading clinical practice, however, acknowledges the different levels of clinical proficiency students may have demonstrated in their clinical practice. Alfaro-LeFevre (2004) questioned whether some clinical nursing courses *should* be assigned pass-fail grades while others are graded using a letter system.

A disadvantage of pass-fail for grading clinical practice is the inability to include a clinical grade into the course grade. One strategy is to separate nursing courses into two components for grading, one for theory and the second for clinical practice (designated as pass-fail), even though the course is considered a whole. Typically, guidelines for the course indicate that the students must pass the clinical component to pass the course. A second mechanism is to offer two separate courses with the clinical course graded on a pass-fail basis.

Once the grading system is determined, there are various ways of using it to arrive at the clinical grade. In one method, the grade is assigned based on the outcomes or competencies achieved by the student. To use this method, the teacher should consider designating some of the outcomes or competencies as critical for achievement. Table 16.2 provides guidelines for converting the clinical competencies into letter grades within a criterion-referenced system. For example, an A might be assigned if all of the competencies were achieved; a B might be assigned if all of the critical ones were achieved and at least half of the others were met.

For pass-fail grading, teachers can indicate that all of the outcomes or competencies must be met to pass the course, or they can designate critical behaviors required for passing the course. In both methods, the clinical evaluation strategies provide the data for determining if the student's performance reflects achievement of the competencies. These evaluation strategies may or may not be graded separately as part of the course grade.

Another way of arriving at the clinical grade is to base it on the evaluation methods. In this system the clinical evaluation methods become the source of data for the grade. For example,

Paper on analysis of clinical practice issue	10%
Analysis of clinical cases	5%
Conference presentation	10%
Community resource paper	10%
Portfolio	25%
Rating scale (of performance)	40%

In this illustration, the clinical grade is computed according to the evaluation methods. Observation of performance, and the rating on the clinical evaluation tool, is only a portion of the clinical grade. An advantage of this approach is that it incorporates into the grade the summative evaluation methods completed by the students.

If pass-fail is used for grading clinical practice, the grade might be computed as follows:

Paper on analysis of clinical practice issue	10%
Analysis of clinical cases	5%
Conference presentation	10%
Community resource paper	10%
Portfolio	25%
Clinical examination, simulations	40%
Rating scale (of performance)	Pass required

This discussion of grading clinical practice suggests a variety of mechanisms that are appropriate. The teacher must make it clear to the students and others how the evaluation and grading will be carried out in clinical practice, through simulations, and in other settings.

Failing Clinical Practice

Teachers will be faced with determining when students have not met the outcomes of the clinical practicum, i.e., have not demonstrated sufficient competence to pass the clinical course. There are principles that should be followed in evaluating and grading clinical practice, which are critical if a student fails a clinical course or has the potential for failing it. These principles are discussed below.

Communicate Evaluation and Grading Methods in Writing

The evaluation methods used in a clinical course, how each will be graded if at all, and how the clinical grade will be assigned should be in writing and communicated to the students. The practices of the teacher in evaluating and grading clinical performance must reflect this written information.

Identify Effect of Failing Clinical Practicum on Course Grade

If failing clinical practice, whether in a pass-fail or a letter system, means failing the nursing course, this should be stated clearly in the course syllabus and policies. By stating it in the syllabus, which all students receive, they have it in writing before clinical learning activities begin. A sample policy statement for pass-fail clinical grading is:

> The clinical component of NUR XXX is evaluated with a Pass or Fail. A Fail in the clinical component results in failure of the course even if the theory grade is 75% or higher.

In a letter grade system, the policy should include the letter grade representing a failure in clinical practice, for example, less than a C grade. A sample policy statement is:

> Students must pass the clinical component of NUR XXX with the grade of "C" or higher. A grade lower than a "C" in the clinical component of the course results in failure of the course even if the theory grade is 75% or higher.

Ask Students to Sign Anecdotal Notes, Rating Forms, and Evaluation Summaries

Students should sign any written clinical evaluation documents—anecdotal notes, rating forms (of clinical practicum, clinical examinations, and performance in simulations), narrative comments about the student's performance, and summaries of conferences in which performance was discussed. Their signatures do not mean they agree with the ratings or comments, only that they have read them. Students should have an opportunity to write in their own comments. These materials are important because they document the student's performance and indicate that the teacher provided feedback and shared concerns about that performance. This is critical in situations in which students may be failing the clinical course because of performance problems.

Identify Performance Problems Early and Develop Learning Plans

Students need continuous feedback on their clinical performance. Observations made by the teacher, the preceptor, and others, and evaluation data from other sources should be shared with the student. Together they should discuss the data. Students may have different perceptions of their performance and in some cases may provide new information that influences the teacher's judgment about clinical competencies.

When the teacher or preceptor identifies performance problems and clinical deficiencies that may affect passing the course, conferences should be held with the student to discuss these areas of concern and develop a plan for remediation. It is critical that these conferences focus on problems in performance combined with specific learning activities for addressing them. The conferences should not be the teacher telling the student everything that is wrong with clinical performance; the student needs an opportunity to respond to the teacher's concerns and identify how to address them.

One of the goals of the conference is to develop a plan with learning activities for the student to correct deficiencies and develop competencies further. The plan should include a statement that one "good" or "poor" performance will not constitute a pass or fail clinical grade and that sustained improvement is needed (Graveley & Stanley, 1993). The plan also should indicate that completing the remedial learning activities does not guarantee that the student will pass the course, and that the student must demonstrate satisfactory performance of the competencies by the end of the course. Faculty should also make it clear that the student is responsible for achievement of the clinical outcomes (Chasens, DePew, Goudreau, & Pierce, 2000).

Any discussions with students at risk of failing clinical practice should focus on the student's inability to meet the clinical objectives and perform the specified competencies, not on the teacher's perceptions of the student's intelligence and overall ability. In addition, opinions about the student's ability in general should not be discussed with others.

Conferences should be held in private, and a summary of the discussion should be prepared. The summary should include the date and time of the conference, who participated, areas of concern about clinical performance, and the learning plan with a timeframe for completion (Gaberson & Oermann, 1999). The summary should be signed by the teacher, the student, and other participants. Faculty members should review related policies of the nursing education program because they might specify other requirements.

Identify Support Services

Students with the potential of failing clinical practice may have other problems affecting their performance. Teachers should refer students to counseling and other support services and not attempt to provide these resources themselves. Attempting to counsel the student and help the student cope with other problems may bias the teacher and influence judgment of the student's clinical performance.

Document Performance

As the clinical course progresses, the teacher should give feedback to the student about performance and continue to guide learning. It is important to document the observations made, other types of evaluation data collected, and the learning activities completed by the student. The documentation should be shared routinely with students, discussions about performance should be summarized, and students should sign these summaries to confirm that they read them.

The teacher cannot observe and document the performance of only the student at risk of failing the course. There should be a minimum number of observations and documentation of other students in the clinical group, or the student failing the course might believe that he or she was treated differently than others in the group. One strategy is to plan the number of observations of performance to be made for each student in the clinical group to avoid focusing only on the student with performance problems. However, teachers may observe students who are believed to be at risk for failure more closely, and document their observations and conferences with those students more thoroughly and frequently than is necessary for the majority of students. When observations result in feedback to students that can be used to improve performance, at-risk students usually do not object to this extra attention.

Follow Policy on Unsafe Clinical Performance

There should be a policy in the nursing program about actions to be taken if the student is unsafe in clinical practice. If the practice is safe even though the student is not meeting the outcomes, the student is allowed to continue in the clinical practicum (Graveley & Stanley, 1993). This is because the outcomes and clinical competencies are identified for achievement at the *end* of the course not during it.

If the student demonstrates performance that is potentially unsafe, however, the teacher can remove the student from the clinical setting, following the policy and procedures of the nursing program. Specific learning activities outside of the clinical setting need to be offered for students to develop the knowledge and skills they lack; practice with simulators is valuable in these situations. A learning plan should be prepared and implemented as described earlier.

Follow Policy for Failure of a Clinical Course

In all instances the teacher must follow the policies of the nursing program. If the student fails the clinical course, the student must be notified of the failure and its consequences as indicated in these policies. In some nursing education programs, students are allowed to repeat only one clinical course, and there may be other requirements to be met. If the student will be dismissed from the program because of the failure, the student must be informed of this in writing. Generally there is a specific time frame for each step in the process, which must be adhered to by the faculty, administrators, and students. The specific set of policies and procedures is not as important as the teacher's knowing what they are and following them with all students (Boley & Whitney, 2003).

GRADING SOFTWARE

A number of the procedures for determining grades are time-consuming, particularly for a large class of students. While a calculator may be used, student grades can be calculated easily with a spreadsheet application such as Microsoft Excel or a course management system such as BlackBoard or WebCT. With a spreadsheet application, teachers can enter individual scores, include the weights of each component of the grade, and compute final grades (Figure 16.1).

Many statistical functions can be performed with a spreadsheet application, which often cannot be computed with a course management system grade book. BlackBoard and other online course management systems provide grade books for teachers to manage all aspects of student grades. The grade book has a spreadsheet view where the course management system loads the students' names, and teachers can easily enter test and other scores (Figure 16.2). The grades can be weighted and a final grade calculated, but usually more advanced statistical analysis cannot be done. One advantage to a course management system grade book is that students usually have online access to their own scores and grades as soon as the teacher has entered them.

There also are a number of grading software programs on the market that include a pre-made spreadsheet for grading purposes, have different grading frameworks that may be used for calculating the grade, and enable the teacher to carry out the tasks needed for grading. With this software the teacher can print out grading reports for the class as a whole and individual students. Some

298

Calculation Sheet

S.No	Name of Students	Exam 1 (Exam) C3	Exam 2 (Exam) D3	Exam 3 (Exam) E3	Exams Total (Exam) F3=SUM(C3:E3)	Exam % G3=(F3/208)*100	Clinical Total Points (Lab) H3	Clinical % I3=(H3/906)*100	Total Points J3=(F3+H3)	Final Course %(Overall) (G3*0.6)+(I3*0.4)	Grade
FORMULAS											
1		32	32	88	152	73.08%	800	88.30%	952	79.17%	
2		27	20	90	137	65.87%	888	98.01%	1025	78.72%	
3		50	27	100	177	85.10%	900	99.34%	1077	90.79%	
4		40	38	76	154	74.04%	850	93.82%	1004	81.95%	
5		42	39	98	179	86.06%	777	85.76%	956	85.94%	
6		47	40	83	170	81.73%	890	98.23%	1060	88.33%	
7		20	40	90	150	72.12%	817	90.18%	967	79.34%	
8		48	40	87	175	84.13%	839	92.60%	1014	87.52%	
9		46	42	101	189	90.87%	856	94.48%	1045	92.31%	
10		40	43	88	171	82.21%	898	99.12%	1069	88.97%	
11		39	46	96	181	87.02%	802	88.52%	983	87.62%	
12		51	47	98	196	94.23%	852	94.04%	1048	94.15%	
13		50	48	100	198	95.19%	889	98.12%	1087	96.36%	
14		48	48	88	184	88.46%	780	86.09%	964	87.51%	
15		50	50	99	199	95.67%	807	89.07%	1006	93.03%	
16		38	50	95	183	87.98%	799	88.19%	982	88.06%	
17		43	50	99	192	92.31%	823	90.84%	1015	91.72%	
18		40	50	85	175	84.13%	856	94.48%	1031	88.27%	
19		50	47	102	199	95.67%	874	96.47%	1073	95.99%	
20		52	39	94	185	88.94%	863	95.25%	1048	91.47%	
Points Possible		52	52	104	208	100.00%	906	100.00%	1114	100.00%	
Weight		0%	0%	0%	60%	0%	40%			100.00%	

FIGURE 16.1 Sample spreadsheet application for grading.

Student Name (Last, First)	clinical practicum Other Pts Possible: 100 Weight: 25%	Casebood summary Assignment Pts Possible: 5 Weight: 0%	Reimbursement presentation Presentation Pts Possible: 100 Weight: 20%	scholarly project Group Project Pts Possible: 100 Weight: 25%	midterm Midterm Exam Pts Possible: 80 Weight: 15%	Final exam Final Exam Pts Possible: 81 Weight: 10%	Total Pts Possible: 466	Weighted Total
	93.4	5	98	91	67	67	421.4	91.53%
	87.63	3	94	91	73	71	419.63	88.91%
	100	5	100	91	67	66	429	93.46%
	100	5	100	97	72	75	449	97.01%
	94.45	5	100	97	71	77	444.45	95.68%
	96.75	5	100	97	73	77	448.75	96.63%
	93.5	5	95	91	64	66	414.5	90.27%
	100	3.5	100	98	69	70	440.5	94.58%
	91.75	5	97	100	69	77	439.75	94.78%
	100	5	100	97	63	69	434	94.58%
	92.5	5	98	98	56	70	419.5	91.37%
	86.5	2	92	91	60	67	398.5	84.3%
	100	5	100	100	76	74	455	98.39%
	91.2	5	95	100	77	75	443.2	95.5%
	97.35	5	100	98	62	71	433.35	94.23%
	94.8	5	100	100	73	81	453.8	97.39%
	100	5	100	97	64	75	441	95.51%
	95.5	5	98	98	74	81	451.5	96.85%

FIGURE 16.2 Sample BlackBoard spreadsheet for grading.

even calculate test statistics. Not all grading software programs are of high quality, however, and should be reviewed prior to purchase.

SUMMARY

Grading is the use of symbols, such as the letters A through F, to report student achievement. Grading is for summative purposes, indicating how well the student met the outcomes of the course and the clinical practicum. Grades need to be based on careful evaluation practices, valid and reliable test results, and multiple evaluation measures. No grade should be determined on one evaluation method or one assignment completed by the students; grades reflect instead a combination of various tests and other evaluation methods.

There are different types of grading systems or methods of reporting grades: the letters A–E or A–F, which may be combined with "+" and "–"; integers 5, 4, 3, 2, and 1 (or 9 through 1); percentages; and categories such as pass-fail and satisfactory-unsatisfactory. Advantages and disadvantages of pass-fail for grading clinical practice were discussed in the chapter.

Two major considerations in assigning letter grades are deciding what to include in the grade and selecting a grading framework. The weight given to each test and the evaluation method in the grade is specified by the teacher according to the emphasis of the objectives and the content measured by them. To give meaning to the grades assigned, the teacher needs a grading framework: criterion-referenced, also referred to as grading with absolute standards; norm-referenced, or grading with relative standards; or self-referenced, grading based on the growth of the student.

One final concept described in the chapter was grading clinical practice and guidelines for working with students who are at risk of failing a clinical course. These guidelines give direction to teachers in establishing sound grading practices and following them when working with students in clinical practice.

REFERENCES

Alfaro-LeFevre, R. (2004). Should clinical courses get a letter grade? *Critical Thinking Indicator*, *1*(1), 1–5. Available at http://www.alfaroteachsmart.com/clinicalgrade newsletter.pdf

Boley, P., & Whitney, K. (2003). Grade disputes: Considerations for nursing faculty. *Journal of Nursing Education, 42*, 198–203.

Bressette, A. (2002). Arguments for plus/minus grading: A case study. *Educational Research Quarterly, 25*(3), 29–42.

Chasens, E. R., DePew, D. D., Goudreau, K. A., & Pierce, C. S. (2000). Legal aspects of grading and student progression. *Journal of Professional Nursing, 16,* 267–272.

Frisbie, D. A., & Waltman, K. K. (1992). Developing a personal grading plan. *Educational Measurement: Issues and Practice, 11*(3), 35–42. Accessed January 30, 2005, from http://depts.washington.edu/grading/plan/frisbie1.htm

Gaberson, K. B., & Oermann, M. H. (1999). *Clinical teaching strategies in nursing education.* New York: Springer.

Graveley, E. A., & Stanley, M. (1993). A clinical failure: What the courts tell us. *Journal of Nursing Education, 32,* 135–137.

Johnson, V. E. (2003). *Grade inflation: A crisis in college education.* New York: Springer-Verlag.

Kubiszyn, T., & Borich, G. (2003). *Educational testing and measurement: Classroom application and practice* (7th ed.). New York: John Wiley.

Mansfield, H. C. (2001, April 6). Grade inflation: It's time to face the facts. *Chronicle of Higher Education, 47*(30), B24.

McCabe, J., & Powell, B. (2004, November). Study reveals faculty attitudes about grade inflation. *The Teaching Professor,* 5–6.

Nitko, A. J. (2004). *Educational assessment of students* (4th ed.). Upper Saddle River, NJ: Prentice Hall.

Scanlan, J. M., & Care, W. D. (2004). Grade inflation: Should we be concerned? *Journal of Nursing Education, 43,* 475–478.

Strashny, A. (2003). *A method for assigning letter grades: Multi-curve grading.* Accessed January 30, 2005, from http://econwpa.wustl.edu:8089/eps/em/papers/0305/0305001.pdf

Svinicki, M. D. (2001). *Evaluating and grading students* (pp. 1–14). Accessed January 30, 2005, from http://www.utexas.edu/academic/cte/sourcebook/grading2.pdf

University of North Carolina Center for Teaching and Learning. (2001, January 30). *Evaluation issues: Grading.* Accessed January 31, 2005, from http://ctl.unc.edu/he2.html

Chapter 17

Program Evaluation

$\mathbf{P}$rogram evaluation is the process of judging the worth or value of an educational program. One purpose of program evaluation is to provide data upon which to base decisions about the educational program. Another purpose is to provide evidence of educational effectiveness in response to internal and external demands for accountability. With the demand for high quality programs, development of newer models for the delivery of higher education such as Web-based instruction, and public calls for accountability, there has been a greater emphasis on systematic and ongoing program evaluation. This chapter presents an overview of program evaluation models and discusses evaluation of selected program components, including curriculum, outcomes, and teaching.

PROGRAM EVALUATION MODELS

A number of models are currently used to guide program evaluation activities in nursing education programs, staff education departments, and patient education programs. These models provide a framework for educators to develop an evaluation plan that includes sources of data and time frames for evaluation. With a planned, systematic evaluation, administrators, faculty members, and others involved in the program have information for quality improvement. There are many evaluation models; a few are described here. Accreditation models such as those used by the National League for Nursing Accrediting Commission (NLNAC), Commission on Collegiate Nursing Education (CCNE), Canadian Association of Schools of Nursing (CASN) for baccalaureate programs in Canada, and Joint Commission on Accreditation of Healthcare Organizations (JCAHO) typically use a combination of self-study and site visits to the institution by a team of peer evaluators. Program evaluation based on an accreditation model is designed to assess whether the program meets external standards of quality.

Another type of model is decision-oriented. With these models, the goal of evaluation is to provide information to decision-makers for program improvement purposes. Sargent and Lewis (2005) indicated that decision models focus more on using evaluation as a tool to improve programs than on accountability. Decision-oriented models usually focus on internal standards of quality, value, and efficacy. Examples of decision-oriented approaches are the Context, Input, Process, Product (CIPP) model (Stufflebeam, 2000, 2002) and the Baldrige Criteria (National Institute of Standards and Technology [NIST], 2005).

The CIPP model asks: What needs to be done? (context); How should it be done? (input); Is it being done? (process); and Did it succeed? (product) (Stufflebeam, 2002). *Context* evaluation assesses the needs, problems, strengths, and weaknesses within a defined environment. Through *input* evaluation, the system capabilities, competing strategies, work plans, and budgets of the selected approach are assessed. Stufflebeam (2002) indicated that input evaluation ensures that the program's strategy is feasible for meeting the needs of the program and its beneficiaries. *Process* evaluation focuses on providing feedback to monitor progress, identify if the plans are being implemented as intended, and make changes as needed. *Product* evaluation measures achievement of the outcomes. Stufflebeam divided product evaluation into (a) impact evaluation (to assess if the program reached the target audience), (b) effectiveness evaluation (to assess the quality and significance of the outcomes), (c) sustainability evaluation (to determine the extent to which a program's contributions are continued over time), and (d) transportability evaluation (to assess the extent to which a program has been or could be applied in other settings) (Stufflebeam, 2002).

The Baldrige Health Care Criteria for Performance Excellence, while developed for health care organizations, provide guidelines that nursing education programs can use for program evaluation. Spath (2005) indicated that the Baldrige Criteria provide an effective framework for evaluating an organization with the goal of performance improvement. There are 19 items to be assessed that are grouped within the following 7 areas:

1. Leadership (e.g., how the organization's leaders guide and sustain the organization; how the organization addresses responsibilities to students, faculty, staff, consumers, partners, and others)
2. Strategic Planning (e.g., how strategic plans are developed and performance is measured)
3. Focus on Students, Stakeholders, and Others (e.g., how the nursing program determines requirements of students and how it builds relationships with students, stakeholders, and others) (Sargent & Lewis, 2005)

4. Measurement, Analysis, and Knowledge Management (e.g., how the organization manages information and performance data; how faculty collect data and use them for program revision and decision making)

5. Faculty and Staff Focus (e.g,, how the program and its leaders develop faculty members to their fullest potential and how well the environment serves the faculty, staff, students, and other stakeholders)

6. Process Management (the organization's processes such as how curricula are reviewed, revised, and delivered), and

7. Organizational Performance Results (e.g., licensure examination results, number of graduates who pass certification examinations, accreditation findings, student and alumni survey results, etc.) (NIST, 2005).

Sargent and Lewis (2005) described how a school of nursing used the Baldrige Criteria as a framework for program evaluation and as a basis for self-assessment.

Other models are systems-oriented. These examine inputs into the program such as characteristics of students, teachers, administrators, and other participants in the program, and program resources. These models also assess the operations and processes of the program as well as the context or environment within which the program is implemented. Finally, systems models examine the outcomes of the program: Are the intended outcomes being achieved? Are students, graduates, their employers, faculty, staff, and others satisfied with the program and how it is implemented? Is the program of high quality and cost effective?

Regardless of the specific model used, the process of program evaluation assists various audiences or stakeholders of an educational program in judging and improving its worth or value. Audiences or stakeholders are those individuals and groups who are affected directly or indirectly by the decisions made. Sargent and Lewis (2005) identified key stakeholders of nursing education programs as students, faculty and staff, partners (health care and community agencies), and consumers. The purpose of the program evaluation determines which audiences should be involved in generating questions or concerns to be answered or addressed. When the focus is formative, that is, to improve the program during its implementation, the primary audiences are students, teachers, and administrators. Summative evaluation leads to decisions about whether a program should be continued, revised, or terminated. Audiences for summative evaluation include program participants, graduates, their employers, prospective students, health care and community agencies, consumers, legislative bodies, funding agencies, and others that might be affected by changes in the program.

When planning a program evaluation, an important decision is whether to use external or internal evaluators. External evaluators are thought to provide objectivity, but they may not know the program or its context well enough to be effective. Program participants may be reluctant to share data and concerns with "outsiders" (Ruegg & Feller, 2003). External evaluators also add expense to the program evaluation. In contrast, an internal evaluator has a better understanding of the operations and environment of the program and can provide continuous feedback to the individuals and groups responsible for the evaluation. However, an internal evaluator may be biased, reducing the credibility of the evaluation (Ruegg & Feller).

CURRICULUM EVALUATION

Curriculum evaluation is not the same as program evaluation. When evaluating the curriculum, the focus is on the course of studies taken by students and is more narrow than program evaluation. A focus on curriculum evaluation leads to generating evaluation questions such as these:

- Are there sufficient resources to support the curriculum as planned?
- Is the planned curriculum congruent with the environment of the program?
- Is the curriculum being implemented as planned?
- What barriers to curriculum implementation exist?
- Are courses optimally sequenced?
- What evidence of instructional quality exists?
- Are students achieving curriculum objectives?
- Are employers satisfied with the competencies of graduates?

While these evaluation questions are important, an educational program involves more than a curriculum. The success of students in meeting the outcomes of courses and the curriculum as a whole may depend as much on the quality of the students admitted to the program or the characteristics of its faculty as it does on the sequence of courses or the instructional strategies used. Similarly, there may be abundant evidence that graduates meet the goals of the curriculum, but those graduates may not be satisfied with the program or may be unable to pass licensure or certification examinations.

Program evaluation is broader than assessing the curriculum. Iwasiw, Goldenberg, and Andrusyszyn (2005), comparing the two, suggested that program evaluation includes all the areas assessed with curriculum evaluation, and in addition, examines how the nursing program relates to the institution, the administrative structure of the nursing program, the multiple roles of faculty (teaching, scholarship/research, clinical practice, and service), student support services, program resources, and other components that influence the effectiveness of the program.

OUTCOMES EVALUATION

Former accreditation criteria that focused on program and curriculum structure often were criticized for inhibiting flexibility, creativity, and the ability of educational programs to respond to the unique needs of their environments. To ensure the quality of nursing education programs and accountability for producing competent graduates, current accreditation criteria emphasize the evaluation of program outcomes. Outcomes evaluation focuses on the educational effectiveness of the program. Outcomes may be specified by accrediting bodies or by the program planners and participants. For example, an accrediting body may require a program to demonstrate evidence that its graduates are able to communicate effectively; the program faculty may specify the satisfaction of students, graduates, employers, and patients as another important outcome.

Keating (2005) recommended developing a master plan for evaluation to provide data for faculty decision making and to meet accreditation criteria and other external review standards. With a master plan, the faculty can systematically collect information about the program to determine if it is meeting the intended outcomes and as a basis for improvement. The master plan specifies the:

- Component or area evaluated,

- Sources of data,

- Tools, instruments, and other evaluation methods for collecting the data,

- Time frame of assessment,

- Who is responsible for each activity associated with the evaluation plan,

- Criteria used to determine whether the intended outcomes have been met,

- Reporting and decision-making mechanisms, and

- Action plans for developing, maintaining, and revising the program.

When data have been collected, analyzed, and used to make decisions about the program, records of these processes should be maintained to document that the master plan has been followed and that the results of program evaluation are being used to maintain and improve program quality.

When considering whether to use teacher-made or standardized assessment tools to evaluate program outcomes, teachers must keep in mind the qualities of effective measurement instruments, as discussed in chapter 2. The availability of a standardized test does not ensure that teachers can make valid and reliable interpretations of the test results. Tools and other strategies for evaluation should be chosen based on the outcomes to be measured.

EVALUATION OF TEACHING

Another area of evaluation involves assessing the effectiveness of the teacher. This evaluation addresses the quality of teaching in the classroom and clinical setting and other dimensions of the teacher's role, depending on the goals and mission of the nursing program. These other roles may include scholarship and research; service to the nursing program, college or university, community, and nursing profession; and clinical practice. It is beyond the scope of this book to examine the multiple dimensions of teacher evaluation in nursing; however, a brief discussion is provided about evaluating the quality of teaching in the classroom and the clinical setting.

The research in nursing education suggests five qualities of effective teaching in nursing: (a) knowledge of the subject matter, (b) clinical competence, (c) teaching skill, (d) interpersonal relationships with students, and (e) personal characteristics. These findings are consistent with studies about teacher effectiveness in other fields.

Knowledge of Subject Matter

An effective teacher is an expert in the content area, has an understanding of theories and concepts relevant to nursing practice, and assists students in applying these to patient care. Teachers need to keep current with nursing and other interventions, new developments in their area of expertise, and research (Oermann, 2004). Knowledge of the subject matter is not sufficient; the teacher must be able to communicate that knowledge to students.

Competence in Clinical Practice

If teaching in the clinical setting, the teacher has to be competent in clinical practice. From a review of the research, Lee, Cholowski, and Williams (2002) concluded that the clinical competence of the teacher was one of the most important characteristics of effective teaching in nursing. The best teachers are expert practitioners who know how to care for patients, can make sound clinical judgments, have expert clinical skills, and can guide students in developing those skills (Gignac-Caille & Oermann, 2001; Prideaux et al., 2000).

Skills in Teaching

The teacher also needs to know how to teach. Berg and Lindseth (2004) found in their study of 171 baccalaureate nursing students that teaching methods, presentation of course materials, and personality were the three main characteristics of an effective teacher according to the students. Competencies in teaching involve the ability to:

- Identify students' learning needs

- Plan instruction

- Present material [or "content"] effectively

- Explain concepts and ideas clearly

- Demonstrate procedures effectively, and

- Use sound evaluation practices.

The research suggests that the teacher's skills in clinical evaluation are particularly important to teaching effectiveness. Evaluating learners fairly, having clear expectations and communicating those to students, correcting mistakes without embarrassing students, and giving immediate feedback are important teacher behaviors (Gignac-Caille & Oermann, 2001).

Positive Relationships with Learners

Another important characteristic is the ability of the teacher to establish positive relationships with students as a group, in the classroom, online environment, and clinical setting, and with students on an individual basis. In a number of studies, the quality of the clinical teacher's interactions with students was an important characteristic of effective teaching (Allison-Jones & Hirt, 2004; Lee et al., 2002). In research by Viverais-Dresler and Kutschke (2001), 56 RN students in a distance education baccalaureate nursing program completed a questionnaire on the importance of varied clinical teacher behaviors. The findings portrayed the best clinical teacher as someone who is approachable, fair, and honest, and a teacher who creates an environment of mutual respect between educator and student. Included in this category of teaching effectiveness is being a role model for students. In the study by Lee et al. (2002), serving as a role model was the top-rated characteristic of an effective clinical teacher from the students' perspective.

Personal Characteristics of Teacher

Effective teaching also depends on the personal characteristics of the teacher. Characteristics in this area include enthusiasm, patience, having a sense of humor, friendliness, and willingness to admit mistakes (Oermann, 2004). In the study by Berg and Lindseth (2004), in which teaching methods, presentation of course materials, and personality were the three primary characteristics of effective teaching, personality was found to be the most important one. This high rating of personal characteristics, though, is not consistent with other studies in nursing education.

HOW TO EVALUATE TEACHING EFFECTIVENESS

Teaching effectiveness data are available from a variety of sources. These include: students, peers, administrators, and others involved in the educational experience such as preceptors.

Student Ratings

Student evaluations are a necessary but insufficient source of information. Because students are the only participants other than the teacher who are consistently present during the teaching-learning process, they have a unique perspective of the teacher's behavior over time. Students can make valid and reliable interpretations about the teacher's use of teaching methods, fairness, interest in students, and enthusiasm for the subject.

There are limitations, though, to the use of student ratings. These ratings can be affected by class size, with smaller classes tending to rate teacher effectiveness higher than larger classes. Ratings by students also can be influenced by the type of course format; for example, discussion courses tend to receive higher ratings than do lecture courses (Davis, 2002). Students have a tendency to rate required and elective courses in their own field of study higher than courses they are required to take outside their majors. Lastly, it is questionable if students can evaluate the accuracy, depth, and scope of the teacher's knowledge since they do not have expertise in the content to make this judgment. Characteristics such as these are best evaluated by peers from one's own nursing education program or other institutions who have expertise in that content area.

Many colleges and universities have a standard form for student evaluation of teaching that is used in all courses across the institution. These forms generally ask students to rate the teacher's performance in areas of: (a) presentation and teaching skills, (b) interactions with students as a group and individually, (c) breadth of coverage of content, and (d) evaluation and grading practices. Students also may be asked to provide a rating of the overall quality of the faculty member's teaching in the course, the extent of their own learning in the course, and the workload and difficulty of the course. Table 17.1 lists typical areas that are assessed by students on these forms. For online courses, some additional questions may be included on the form that relate to the delivery method. Areas that could be evaluated for an online course are listed in Table 17.1.

These general forms, however, do not assess teacher behaviors important in the clinical setting. Faculty members can add to these general forms questions on clinical teaching effectiveness or can develop a separate tool for students to use in assessing teacher performance in clinical courses. Sample questions for evaluating the effectiveness of the clinical teacher are found in Table 17.2.

Students can complete teacher evaluations in class, administered by someone other than the teacher and without the teacher present in the room, or they can be placed online. When establishing an online course evaluation system, it is critical that students' anonymity and confidentiality be protected and that students have the computer capabilities to access the system. Anderson, Cain, and Bird (2005) indicated that the software selected for this purpose needs to guarantee student anonymity but be able to track students for completion. In many institutions, student services can be accessed online, and student evaluation of teaching forms can be made available at those sites. At Oregon State University, for example, students log on, go to the Online Services page, choose Student Records, and then select Course Evaluation. At that point they can select a course to evaluate from the drop-down menu. After completing the rating form, they have an opportunity to make additional comments in the text box (Oregon State University, 2004).

Peer Evaluation

Another source of data for evaluating teacher effectiveness is from peers. Peer review provides feedback to faculty members about their teaching (Appling, Naumann, & Berk, 2001; Center for Instructional Development and Research,

TABLE 17.1 Typical Areas Assessed on Student Evaluation of Teaching Forms

---

Presentation or Teaching Skills

Organized course well
Gave clear explanations
Used examples, illustrations, and other methods to promote understanding of content
Was well prepared for class
Was enthusiastic about content and teaching
Stimulated students' interest in subject
Motivated students to do best work
Used learning activities, readings, and assignments that facilitated understanding of
    course content
Had realistic appreciation of time and effort for students to complete assignments and
    course work

Interactions with Students as Group and Individually

Encouraged student participation and discussion
Showed respect for students' views and opinions
Was readily available to students (e.g., questions after class, by email, by appointment)

Breadth of Coverage of Subject Matter

Demonstrated knowledge of course content
Presented different views and perspectives as appropriate

Evaluation and Grading Practices

Communicated clearly student responsibilities
Explained course assignments, evaluation methods, and grading procedures
Was fair in evaluation and grading
Provided prompt and valuable feedback

Overall Course Evaluation

Course difficulty (e.g., rated on scale of *too difficult* to *too elementary*)
Workload in course (e.g., rated on scale of *too heavy* to *too light*)
Course pace (e.g., rated on scale of *too fast* to *too slow*)
Extent of learning in course (e.g., rated on scale of *a great deal* to *nothing new*)
Overall course rating (e.g., rated on scale of *excellent* to *poor*)

Overall Teacher Evaluation

Overall quality of faculty member's teaching (e.g., rated on scale of *excellent* to *poor*)

TABLE 17.1 *(continued)*

Additional Areas for Evaluation of Online Course

Effectiveness of delivery format, course design, instructional methods, learning activities, and evaluation methods
Quality of online course compared to other course formats (e.g., face-to-face, seminar)
Extent of learning in online course compared to other course formats
Preference for online vs. other course formats

Additional Areas for Evaluation of Teacher in Online Course

Was skilled in using technology
Facilitated online discussion and interactions among students and with faculty member
Encouraged students to express own views
Responded to students' questions and comments in reasonable period of time
Provided timely and valuable feedback on assignments
Posted grades in reasonable period of time

2005). One form of peer evaluation is observing the teacher in the classroom, clinical setting, or laboratory. Observations of teaching performance are best used for formative evaluation because there are too many variables that can influence the reliability of these observations. The faculty member making the observation may not be an expert in that content or clinical practice area and may have limited understanding of how that particular class or practice experience fits into the overall course. Observations can be influenced too easily by personal feelings, positive or negative, about the colleague.

Peer evaluation of teaching can be conducted for Web-based courses as well as in more traditional settings. By reviewing course materials and visiting course Web sites as guest users, peer evaluators of teaching in Web-based courses can look for evidence that teachers demonstrate application of the following principles of effective instruction:

- Providing opportunities for interactions between students and faculty members (e.g., how quickly and thoroughly does the teacher respond to student questions, how does the teacher use course management tools to promote interaction?),

- Promoting interaction and collaboration among students (e.g., does the teacher use group assignments, chat rooms, or peer critique of assignments to enhance student interaction?),

- Providing opportunities for active learning (e.g., does the teacher use simulations, reflective journaling, Web or library searches, and similar

TABLE 17.2   Sample Questions for Measuring Effectiveness of Clinical Teachers

---

Clinical Teacher Evaluation

Purpose: These questions are intended for use in evaluating teacher effectiveness in courses with a clinical component. The questions are to be used in conjunction with the college or university student evaluation of teaching form.

Clinical Teaching Items

Did the teacher

1. Encourage students to ask questions and express diverse views in the clinical setting?
2. Encourage application of theoretical knowledge to clinical practice?
3. Provide feedback on student strengths and weaknesses related to clinical performance?
4. Develop positive relationships with students in the clinical setting?
5. Inform students of their professional responsibilities?
6. Facilitate student collaboration with members of health care teams?
7. Facilitate learning in the clinical setting?
8. Strive to be available in the clinical setting to assist students?

Was the instructor

9. An effective clinical teacher?

---

assignments that require the active involvement of students in their own learning?),

- Giving prompt, meaningful feedback (e.g., does the teacher provide rich feedback on assignments posted to a Web site or submitted via e-mail?),

- Encouraging active engagement and appropriate time spent in course activities (e.g., is there evidence that students spend an appropriate amount of time on course tasks such as assignments and discussions?),

- Communicating appropriate, realistically high expectations of student performance (e.g., does the teacher have reasonably high standards for achievement of course objectives and communicate them effectively to students?),

- Respecting diversity of views, learning styles, and abilities (e.g., does the teacher accommodate a variety of learning modes and preferences, can the learners complete course activities at their own pace?),

- Effective application of instructional design principles (e.g., is the Web-based course well organized, is it easy to locate course materials, are the directions clear?), and

- Effective application of graphic design principles (e.g., is there an inviting Web design for the course, are there web-based sources of technical help, are graphics used appropriately, are the written materials free of errors, is color used in an appealing way?). (Cobb, Billings, Mays, & Canty-Mitchell, 2001)

Peers can review course syllabi, instructional materials, teaching strategies, learning activities, discussion board questions, tests, and other documents developed for courses; materials developed for clinical teaching and clinical learning activities; grants, publications, and similar materials documenting the teacher's scholarship; the teaching portfolio; and other materials. This review can be used for formative purposes, to give suggestions for further development, or for summative purposes, to make decisions about contract renewal, tenure, promotion, and merit pay increases (personnel decisions).

To be most effective, peer review of teaching should take place within a context of continuous improvement of the teaching-learning process. It must be supported by adequate resources for faculty development, mentoring, and modeling of effective teaching by master teachers (Cobb et al., 2001).

Administrator Evaluation

Another source of information for evaluating teaching effectiveness is from administrators. Administrators can review the materials identified earlier, integrate multiple sources of evaluation information, and evaluate the faculty member's progress in meeting professional goals. Evaluation by administrators, though, is most appropriate when used for formative evaluation, not for personnel decisions (Arreola, 2000; Frank-Stromborg & Morgan, 2005).

Teaching Portfolio

Another approach to documenting teaching effectiveness is the use of a teaching portfolio. The portfolio is a collection of teacher-selected materials that describe the faculty member's teaching activities in the classroom, the online environment, clinical practice, the laboratory, and other settings where the instruction took place. The materials selected by the faculty member indicate the scope and quality of his or her teaching beyond student ratings of teaching effectiveness (Oermann, 1999).

There is no one particular format for the portfolio since it should reflect both the purpose of the evaluation, i.e., formative or summative, and the role of the teacher. A portfolio should contain materials related to teaching such as syllabi, teaching strategies, sample tests, student assignments, and online materials, to name a few. The portfolio also includes the faculty member's philosophy of teaching, which should be reflected in the documents in the portfolio. Table 17.3 lists materials typically included in a portfolio for personnel decisions, such as contract renewal, tenure, promotion, and merit pay increases.

Portfolios for instructional improvement (formative evaluation) include these same materials but also identify areas of teaching that need improvement

TABLE 17.3 Suggested Content of a Teaching Portfolio

Material from the Faculty Member

Personal philosophy of teaching

Statement about teaching goals

Description of teaching responsibilities (e.g., classroom instruction, online teaching, clinical instruction)

List of courses taught with dates

Course syllabus; sample teaching strategies, materials, assignments, online activities and discussion board questions, tests, instructional media, and other documents from one or more courses (documents should reflect the types of courses taught, e.g., classroom, online, clinical, laboratory, seminar)

An edited 5-minute videotape of a class or a segment from an online course

Teaching awards and recognition of teaching effectiveness (by alumni, clinical agency personnel, others)

Material from Students

Student ratings of teaching with summaries of ratings over a designated period of time and reflective interpretations of ratings (including reasons why ratings may be low in certain courses and clinical practica)

Samples of student papers, good and poor, with teacher's written comments; other products of student learning

Unsolicited letters from students, alumni, and clinical agency staff who work with students addressing the faculty member's teaching effectiveness (a few that are carefully selected)

Material from Colleagues and Administrators

Peer evaluation of teaching materials

Other Documents

Self-appraisal and teaching goals (short and long term)

Appendices

and efforts to further develop teaching skills such as workshops attended. In this type of teaching portfolio, peer and administrator evaluations of teaching, a self-evaluation of strengths and weaknesses, and other documents that demonstrate areas for improvement and steps taken can be included. However, these are not appropriate for a teaching portfolio that will be used for personnel decisions.

SUMMARY

Program evaluation is the process of judging the worth or value of an educational program for the purposes of making decisions about the program or to provide evidence of its effectiveness in response to demands for accountability. A number of models can be used for program evaluation, including accreditation, decision-oriented and systems-oriented approaches. Accreditation models are designed to determine whether a program meets external standards of quality and typically use a combination of self-study and visits to the institution by a site evaluation team. Decision-oriented models usually focus on internal standards of quality, value, and efficacy to provide information for making decisions about the program. Systems-oriented approaches consider the inputs, processes or operations, and outputs or outcomes of an educational program.

The process of program evaluation assists various audiences or stakeholders of an educational program to judge its worth. Audiences or stakeholders are individuals and groups who are affected directly or indirectly by the decisions made, such as students, teachers, employers, clinical agencies, and the public. An important decision when planning a program evaluation is whether to use external or internal evaluators or both.

Traditional approaches to program evaluation often focused narrowly on the curriculum, and while the curriculum is an important aspect of the program, educational effectiveness may depend as much on the quality of the students selected for the program or the characteristics of the teachers as it does on the sequence of courses or instructional strategies used. Current accreditation criteria reflect the importance of evaluating program outcomes in an effort to ensure quality and increase accountability.

One area of program evaluation involves assessing the quality of teaching in the classroom and clinical setting and other dimensions of the teacher's role, depending on the goals and mission of the nursing program. Research findings suggest five characteristics and qualities of effective teaching in nursing: (a) knowledge of the subject matter, (b) clinical competence, (c) teaching skill, (d) interpersonal relationships with students, and (e) personal characteristics. Teaching effectiveness data are available from a variety of sources, including students, faculty peers, and administrators. The use of a teaching portfolio as a way to document teaching effectiveness is another approach that allows the teacher to select and comment on items that reflect implementation of a personal philosophy of teaching.

REFERENCES

Allison-Jones, L. L., & Hirt, J. B. (2004). Comparing the teaching effectiveness of part-time and full-time clinical nurse faculty. *Nursing Education Perspectives, 25*, 238–243.

Anderson, H. M., Cain, J., & Bird, E. (2005). Online student course evaluations: Review of literature and a pilot study. *American Journal of Pharmaceutical Education, 69*(1): article 5.

Appling, S. E., Naumann, P. L., & Berk, R. A. (2001). Using a faculty evaluation triad to achieve evidence-based teaching. *Nursing & Health Care Perspectives, 22*, 247–251.

Arreola, R. A. (2000). *Developing a comprehensive faculty evaluation system.* Bolton, MA: Anker.

Berg, C. L., & Lindseth, G. (2004). Students' perspectives of effective and ineffective nursing instructors. *Journal of Nursing Education, 43*, 565–568.

Center for Instructional Development and Research. (2005). *Peer review of teaching.* University of Washington, Seattle, WA. Accessed February 18, 2005, from http://depts.washington.edu/cidrweb/PeerColleagueReview.html

Cobb, K. L., Billings, D. M., Mays, R. M., & Canty-Mitchell, J. (2001). Peer review of teaching in web-based courses in nursing. *Nurse Educator, 26*, 274–279.

Davis, B. G. (2002). *Tools for teaching. Student rating forms.* University of California Berkeley. Accessed February 20, 2005, from http://teaching.berkeley.edu/bgd/rating forms.html

Frank-Stromborg, M., & Morgan, B. (2005). Nursing college evaluation systems and their legal implications. In L. Caputi (Ed.), *Teaching nursing: The art and science* (Vol. 3, pp. 423–439). Glen Ellyn, IL: College of DuPage Press.

Gignac-Caille, A. M., & Oermann, M. H. (2001). Student and faculty perceptions of effective clinical instructors in ADN programs. *Journal of Nursing Education, 40*, 347–353.

Iwasiw, C., Goldenberg, D., & Andrusyszyn, M-A. (2005). *Curriculum development in nursing education.* Boston: Jones & Bartlett.

Keating, S. B. (2005). Master planning for program and curriculum evaluation: Systematic assessment and evaluation. In S. B. Keating (Ed.), *Curriculum development and evaluation in nursing* (pp. 260–274). Philadelphia: Lippincott Williams & Wilkins.

Lee, W. S., Cholowski, K., & Williams, A. K. (2002). Nursing students' and clinical educators' perceptions of characteristics of effective clinical educators in an Australian university school of nursing. *Journal of Advanced Nursing, 39*, 412–420.

National Institute of Standards and Technology (NIST). (2005). *Health care criteria for performance excellence.* Gaithersburg, MD: Baldrige National Quality Program, NIST, United States Department of Commerce.

Oermann, M. H. (1999). Developing a teaching portfolio. *Journal of Professional Nursing*, *15*, 224–228.

Oermann, M. H. (2004). Basic skills for teaching and the advanced practice nurse. In L. Joel (Ed.), *Advanced practice nursing: Essentials for role development* (pp. 398–429). Philadelphia: F. A. Davis.

Oregon State University. (2004). Online course evaluations: Student evaluation of teaching. Accessed February 20, 2005, from http://ecampus.oregonstate.edu/soc/start/online-course-evaluation.htm

Prideaux, D., Alexander, H., Bower, A., Dacre, J., Haist, S., Jolly, B., et al. (2000). Clinical teaching: Maintaining an educational role for doctors in the new health care environment. *Medical Education*, *34*(10), 820–826.

Ruegg, R., & Feller, I. (2003). *A toolkit for evaluating public R & D investment models, methods, and findings from ATP's first decade*. Gaithersburg, MD: Economic Assessment Office, Advanced Technology Program, National Institute of Standards and Technology.

Sargent, A. A., & Lewis, E. M. (2005). Application of educational evaluation models to nursing. In S. B. Keating (Ed.), *Curriculum development and evaluation in nursing* (pp. 276–295). Philadelphia: Lippincott Williams & Wilkins.

Spath, P. L. (2005). *Leading your health care organization to excellence: A guide using the Baldrige Criteria*. Chicago: Health Administration.

Stufflebeam, D. L. (2000). The CIPP model for evaluation. In D. L. Stufflebeam, G. F. Madaus, & T. Kellaghan (Eds.), *Evaluation models: Viewpoints on education and human services evaluation* (2nd ed.). Boston: Kluwer.

Stufflebeam, D. L. (2002). CIPP Evaluation Model checklist: A tool for applying the fifth installment of the CIPP Model to assess long-term enterprises. The Evaluation Center, Western Michigan University. Accessed February 18, 2005, from http://www.wmich.edu/evalctr/checklists/cippchecklist.htm#contractual

Viverais-Dresler, G., & Kutschke, M. (2001). RN students' ratings and opinions related to the importance of certain clinical teacher behaviors. *Journal of Continuing Education in Nursing*, *32*, 274–282.

Appendix A

Examples of Rating Forms for Clinical Evaluation

Sample Behaviors from Rating Scale for Formative Evaluation

Maternal-Newborn Nursing
Mid-Term Progress Report

Name_____ Date_____

	OBJECTIVE	Yes	No	Not Obs.
1.	Applies the nursing process to the care of mothers and newborns			
	A. Assesses the individual needs of mothers and newborns			
	B. Plans care to meet the patient's needs			
	C. Implements nursing care plans			
	D. Evaluates the effectiveness of nursing care			
	E. Includes the family in planning and implementing care for the mother and newborn			
2.	Participates in health teaching for maternal-newborn patients and families			
	A. Identifies learning needs of mothers and family			
	B. Utilizes opportunities to do health teaching when giving nursing care			

Note: Not obs. = not observed

Sample Behaviors from Same Rating Scale for Final Evaluation

Maternal-Newborn Nursing
Clinical Performance Evaluation

Name_____ Date_____

	OBJECTIVE	S	U
1.	Applies the nursing process to the care of mothers and newborns		
	A. Assesses the individual needs of mothers and newborns		
	B. Plans care to meet the patient's needs		
	C. Implements nursing care plans		
	D. Evaluates the effectiveness of nursing care		
	E. Includes the family in planning and implementing care for the mother and newborn		
2.	Participates in health teaching for maternal-newborn patients and families		
	A. Identifies learning needs of mothers and family		
	B. Utilizes opportunities to do health teaching when giving nursing care		

Note: S = Satisfactory, U = Unsatisfactory

Clinical Evaluation Instrument Using Satisfactory-Unsatisfactory Scale

Perioperative Nursing
Clinical Performance Evaluation

Name_____   Date_____

OBJECTIVE	S	U
1. Applies principles of aseptic technique		
A. Demonstrates proper technique in scrubbing, gowning, gloving		
B. Prepares and maintains a sterile field		
C. Recognizes and reports breaks in aseptic technique		
2. Plans and implements nursing care consistent with AORN standards and recommended practices for perioperative nursing		
A. Collects physiological and psychosocial assessment data preoperatively		
B. Identifies nursing diagnoses for the perioperative period based on assessment data		
C. Develops a plan of care based on identified nursing diagnoses and assessment data		
D. Provides nursing care according to the plan of care		
E. Evaluates the effectiveness of nursing care provided		
F. Accurately documents perioperative nursing care		
3. Provides a safe environment for the patient		
A. Assesses known allergies and previous anesthetic incidents		
B. Adheres to safety and infection control policies and procedures		
C. Prevents patient injury due to positioning, extraneous objects, or chemical, physical, or electrical hazards		
4. Prepares patient and family for discharge to home		
A. Assesses patient's and family's teaching needs		
B. Teaches patient and family using appropriate strategies based on assessed needs.		
C. Evaluates the effectiveness of patient and family teaching		
D. Identifies needs for home care referral		
5. Protects the patient's rights during the perioperative period		
A. Provides privacy throughout the perioperative period		
B. Identifies and respects the patient's cultural and spiritual beliefs		

Examples of Rating Forms for Clinical Evaluation from Associate Degree Nursing Programs

Chemeketa Community College Nursing Program
NUR 106-209

Clinical Evaluation

Evaluation of student clinical performance is based on data collected by instructor observation. Feedback from staff working with students is another source of data instructors may use in student clinical evaluations. Evaluation focuses on performance-based outcomes (PBOs). PBOs identify specific behaviors that indicate competency in a particular component of the nursing roles.

Clinical PBOs for nursing courses are leveled across the curriculum and are cumulative. It is expected that specific clinical PBOs met satisfactorily in one clinical course will continue to be met satisfactorily in succeeding clinical rotations. Therefore, though clinical PBOs for preceding courses are not always repeated on evaluation tools, they are implied and are included in faculty evaluations of student performance.

Critical elements are simple, discrete, observable behaviors that are mandatory for the specified areas of performance. They are finite units of measurement that are, with few exceptions, the collective basis on which students are passed or failed. Critical elements are the specific indicators that the student is competent to meet the standards of performance established and expected by the faculty.

When a critical element is violated or omitted, patients are actually or potentially endangered, and care being delivered is less than satisfactory. Critical elements are introduced at the beginning of the program and added as the student progresses in the program and skill levels increase.

Student performance that indicates unsafe performance as outlined in the Nursing Program Student Handbook will be reviewed by the Nursing faculty and the director and will be handled individually regarding student's continuation in the program.

Rating Scale for Clinical Evaluation

Satisfactory: Performs at the expected level, verified by direct instructor observation.

Needs Improvement: Inconsistently performs at the expected level.

Unsatisfactory: Performs below expected level.

No Opportunity: Opportunity to achieve is unavailable.

To receive a passing clinical grade, the student must:
- attain a satisfactory rating on all critical elements.
- receive no unsatisfactory ratings on any clinical PBOs.

Guiding Principles

A PBO will reappear on subsequent tools if the level of practice is at a higher level or it becomes a critical element.

- Once a PBO becomes a critical element, it is dropped from subsequent tools.
- Once a PBO is at its highest level, it is dropped from subsequent tools.
- Students are responsible for all PBOs and critical elements from previous terms.
- Skills presented each quarter will be reflected on the clinical evaluation tool.

Chemeketa Community College Nursing Program
NUR 108 Clinical Performance-Based Outcome Tool

Name: _____

Instructor: _____

Absences: _____

S   =   Satisfactory: Performs at the expected level
NI   =   Needs Improvement: Inconsistently performs at the expected level
U   =   Unsatisfactory: Performs below expected level
NO =   No Opportunity: Opportunity to achieve an outcome is unavailable
**   =   **Critical Element**
➤   =   Student provides written description of performance[1]
To receive a passing clinical grade, the student must:
 • attain a satisfactory rating on all critical elements.
 • receive no unsatisfactory ratings on any clinical performance-based outcomes (PBOs).

	Rating	Comments
I. Provider of Care		
A. Nursing Process		
1. **Completes Interactive Worksheets satisfactorily (see Outcome Criteria)		
2. Verbalizes plan of care for assigned patient/s to instructor		
3. **Recognizes alterations in human needs		
B. Human Needs		
1. Neuro/Sensory Function		
** a. **Collects basic data about neurological status**		
2. Oxygenation		
a. Collects data about cardiovascular function, including:		
1) **Locates and palpates pulses		
2) **Auscultates heart sounds at the four locations		
3) **Collects data about tissue perfusion		
b. **Inspects the chest and auscultates breath sounds		
➤c. Reinforces patient teaching in positioning, coughing and deep breathing.		
➤d. Reinforces patient teaching in proper use of devices to improve ventilation		
➤e. Determines appropriate interventions for abnormal pulse oximetry reading		
3. Temperature		
4. Fluid and Electrolyte		

	Rating	Comments
a. Observes for signs of fluid intake and output imbalances		
b. Measures I & O accurately		
c. Validates that the ordered IV solution is infusing		
d. Monitors IV site		
e. Calculates rate and regulates flow of IV solutions (with/without pumps)		
f. Changes IV tubing/bag		
5. Nutrition		
a. Collects data about nutritional status		
b. Assures that patient receives prescribed diet		
c. Administers enteral feedings		
6. Elimination		
** Inspects, auscultates, and lightly palpates abdomen**		
7. Activity ** Provides nursing interventions to promote &/or maintain muscle skeleton function.**		
8. Rest/Sleep ** Organizes care to allow for rest & sleep.**		
9 Comfort		
** a. Collects data about pain using a pain scale**		
** b. Determines appropriate interventions for managing pain.**		
** c. Determines effectiveness of pain management interventions**		
** d. Provides nursing interventions to promote &/or maintain comfort.**		
10. Physiological Safety		
a. Uses transmission-based precaution		
b. Maintains medical and surgical asepsis		
c. Uses standard precautions in the disposal of syringes and needles		
11. Physical Safety		
12. Chemical Safety		
a. Demonstrates knowledge of medications		
b. Prepares and administers medication		
1) Calculates doses accurately		
2) Administers medications by following the six rights		
3) Uses correct technique		
a) Oral		

	Rating	Comments
b) Topical		
➤c) I.M.		
d) S.C.		
c. Collects data about patient response to medication		
13. Security, love, and belonging/self esteem		
➤a. Collects data about family dynamics		
➤b. Identifies risk factors and signs and symptoms of anxiety and stress		
➤c. Provides interventions to decrease patient's stress level		
II. Communicator		
➤A. Adapts communication techniques to patient's own communication patterns and cultural background		
➤B. Adapts communication techniques to patients of varying levels of development		
➤C. Collects data about patient's understanding of previous teaching		
➤D. Reinforces information previously provided by other health professionals		
E. Communicates effectively with patients/ & family		
F. Communicates effectively with health care team, instructors, and peers		
III. Manager of Care		
A. Clarifies plans of care with RN assigned to the patients at the beginning of and throughout the shift		
B. Reports promptly unusual or abnormal patient data to the appropriate person		
C. Completes initial baseline data collection within two hours of care		
➤D. Utilizes worksheet to organize care (attach example)		
E. Completes components of patient care assignment within acceptable time frames for one to two patients		
F. Demonstrates self-direction in providing previously learned nursing care		
➤G. Informs staff nurse of patient's condition whenever leaving the patient care unit and gets report upon returning		
IV. Member Within the Discipline of Nursing		
A. Legal-Ethical Standards		
1. Accepts responsibility for own actions		
2. Documents care in accord with legal standards		

	Rating	Comments
a. Reports and records pertinent data describing nursing care given and patient's responses in a clear, thorough and concise manner according to charting guidelines.		
b. Writes legibly using correct terminology and spelling		
3. Refrains from doing procedures that are beyond level of expertise and /or scope of practice		
B. Personal and Professional Growth		
1. Demonstrates ethical principles and responsibilities		
2. Recognizes personal values that might conflict with professional values		
3. Utilizes procedure/policy manual and available resources to answer questions prior to consulting with other staff members		
4. Identifies own learning needs		
5. Seeks learning opportunities to meet PBOs		

[1]For PBOs marked with a star, student provides a written description of how he/she has met the outcome.

Instructor documents performance on tool for each student in the clinical group. Each student completes the same tool and documents his/her performance in meeting the critical elements and PBOs. Instructor and student review ratings and documentation, and discuss in conference.

Developed by nursing faculty at Chemeketa Community College ADN Program, Salem, Oregon. Reprinted by permission of nursing faculty and Kay Carnegie, 2004.

Student's Name _____

Quarter _____

Instructor _____

COLLEGE OF DuPAGE
ASSOCIATE DEGREE NURSING PROGRAM
CLINICAL EVALUATION TOOL
NURSING 215

This summary is based on specific behaviors listed in the section that follows entitled Criteria for Clinical Evaluation Nursing 215. A student must receive a satisfactory rating in all categories at final evaluation to pass the course. A student who receives unsatisfactory in any category at final evaluation will receive a failing grade for the course.

Code: NO – Not Observed   S – Satisfactory
         NA – Not Applicable   NI – Needs Improvement
                                                   U - Unsatisfactory

CRITERIA FOR EVALUATION	COMMENTS	MIDTERM	FINAL
I. PROFESSIONAL BEHAVIOR			
A. Assumes responsibility for own behavior.		A._____	A._____
B. Demonstrates characteristics of a critical thinker.		B._____	B._____
C. Assumes responsibility for patient care.		C._____	C._____
D. Actively pursues self development.		D._____	D._____
E. Practices within the legal and ethical framework of nursing.		E._____	E._____
II. MANAGING CARE			
A. Sets priorities in giving nursing care.		A._____	A._____
B. Organizes patient care assignments.		B._____	B._____
C. Makes appropriate decisions.		C._____	C._____
D. Demonstrates flexibility.		D._____	D._____
E. Utilizes resources to assist planning and implementing care.		E._____	E._____
F. Identifies tasks to be delegated.		F._____	F._____
III. ASSESSMENT			
A. Collects data.		A._____	A._____
B. Observes patient for normal health.		B._____	B._____
C. Observes patient for alterations in health/status.		C._____	C._____
D. Records patient data.		D._____	D._____
IV. NURSING DIAGNOSIS			
A. Identifies patient problems.		A._____	A._____
B. Develops a list of nursing diagnoses.		B._____	B._____
C. Prioritizes nursing diagnoses.		C._____	C._____
V. PLANNING CARE			
A. Verbalizes a plan of care.		A._____	A._____
B. States appropriate interventions.		B._____	B._____
C. Individualizes patient care.		C._____	C._____
VI. INTERVENTION			
A. Implements planned nursing care.		A._____	A._____
B. Performs basic hygiene care.		B._____	B._____
C. Assesses vital signs.		C._____	C._____
D. Maintains a safe environment for patient and self.		D._____	D._____

E. Administers medications. F. Administers IV fluids. G. Performs other nursing skills introduced in Nursing 100, 104, 111, 112, 213, & 217.		E._____ F._____ G._____	E._____ F._____ G._____

VII. EVALUATION
   A.   Sets patient goals and outcome criteria.
   B.   Collects evaluation data.
   C.   Evaluates data and identifies need for modification of care.
		A._____
		B._____
		C._____
			A._____
			B._____
			C._____

VIII. COMMUNCIATION
   A.   Communicates with patient.
   B.   Communicates with staff.
   C.   Communicates with peers
   D.   Charts patient data.
   E.   Communicates in written assignments.
		A._____
		B._____
		C._____
		D._____
		E._____
			A._____
			B._____
			C._____
			D._____
			E._____

IX. CLIENT/FAMILY TEACHING
   A.   Identifies learning needs.
   B.   Engages in patient/family teaching.
   C.   Constructs a teaching plan.
   D.   Recognizes limitations for teaching.
		A._____
		B._____
		C._____
		D._____
			A._____
			B._____
			C._____
			D._____

X. APPLICATION OF THEORY, CONCEPTS, PRINCIPLES
   A.   Verbalizes knowledge of pathophysiology.
   B.   States principles, concepts, theories.
   C.   Applies principles, concepts, theories.
   D.   Utilizes resources.
		A._____
		B._____
		C._____
		D._____
			A._____
			B._____
			C._____
			D._____

Additional comments:

Faculty signature_____Date_____

Student signature_____Date_____

The student's signature signifies that the student has read and discussed this evaluation with the clinical instructor.

SKILLS PERFORMED _____ COMMENTS

CRITERIA FOR CLINICAL EVALUATION: NURSING 215

(Note from authors: Each category has criteria for clinical evaluation.
An example of the criteria for assessment follows.)

CRITERIA FOR CLINICAL EVALUATION

III.   ASSESSMENT

A.   Collects data.

Satisfactory

Utilizes patient as the primary source of data with minimal supervision.
Utilizes appropriate secondary resources.
Identifies appropriate areas for patient assessment.
Data reflects holistic needs of patient.
Performs assessment techniques appropriately and accurately.
Includes psychosocial as well as physical observations.
Performs priority assessments.

Needs Improvement

Does not utilize the patient as the primary source of data.
Does not utilize appropriate secondary resources.
Inconsistent in identification of appropriate areas for patient assessment.
Holistic needs of patient not reflected in data.
Utilizes incorrect assessment techniques.
Psychosocial components not identified.
Unable to prioritize assessment.

Unsatisfactory

Fails to collect data.
Unable to identify appropriate areas for patient assessment.

B.   Observes patient for normal health.

Satisfactory

Verbalizes how to obtain normal values for common diagnostic tests (i.e., CBC urinalysis).
Verbalizes knowledge of normal physical characteristics.
Conducts a complete nursing assessment, physical and psycho-social.
Identifies normal coping mechanisms of patients.

Needs Improvement

Has difficulty identifying mechanism to obtain lab values.
Has difficulty verbalizing normal physical characteristics.
Needs instructor assistance in conducting a complete nursing assessment.
Has difficulty identifying normal coping mechanisms of assigned patients.

Unsatisfactory

Unable to describe normal physical characteristics in assigned patients.
Unable to conduct a complete nursing assessment.

C.   Observes patient for alterations in health status.

Satisfactory

Verbalizes knowledge of common alterations in health when providing and planning nursing care for patients.

Identifies signs and symptoms of alterations in health for assigned patients.

Identifies changes in patient's health status resulting from altered physiology.

Reports changes in health status of assigned patients to appropriate health team members.

Identifies abnormal diagnostic data on assigned patients and records results in nursing assessments and nursing care plans.

Accurately assesses the patient's developmental levels.

Recognizes inappropriate use of coping mechanisms.

Has difficulty verbalizing common situations in health when providing and planning nursing care for patients.

Needs Improvement

Has difficulty identifying signs and symptoms of alterations in health for assigned patients.

Has difficulty identifying changes in patient's health status resulting from altered physiology.

Reporting changes in health status of assigned patients incomplete or not given to appropriate team member.

Has difficulty identifying abnormal diagnostic test.

Needs assistance in identifying patient's developmental level.

Needs assistance in identifying inappropriate use of coping mechanisms.

Unsatisfactory

Unable to identify alterations in health status when providing nursing care for patients.

Does not report changes in health for assigned patients.

Unable to identify patient's developmental needs.

D.   Records client data.

Satisfactory

Completes appropriate areas of the patient data sheet for each assigned client.

Completes nursing assessments in nursing care plans.

Documents assessment in charting.

Documents alterations in patient's health status in charting.

Needs Improvement

Patient data sheet is incomplete.

Nursing assessment is incomplete.

Has difficulty identifying appropriate data for recording.

Needs instructor assistance to document assessment in charting.

Incomplete documentation of alterations in patient's health status in charting.

Unsatisfactory

Fails to fill out data sheet for each assigned patient.

Fails to include nursing assessment in nursing care plans.

Fails to document assessment observations in charting.

Fails to document alterations in patient's health status in charting.

Developed by College of DuPage, Associate Degree Nursing Program. Reprinted by permission of College of DuPage, Glen Ellyn, Illinois, 2004.

COMMUNITY COLLEGE OF PHILADELPHIA
DEPARTMENT OF NURSING
CLINICAL EVALUATION TOOL

Student Name _____

N101, FALL 200____

ACUTE CARE
Agency:
Unit:
Faculty:

N132, SPRING 200____

ACUTE CARE   **MATERNITY**
Agency: Agency:
Unit: Unit:
Faculty: Faculty:

N231, FALL 200____

ACUTE CARE   **PEDIATRICS**   **COMMUNITY**
Agency: Agency: Agency:
Unit: Unit: Unit:
Faculty: Faculty: Faculty:

N232, SPRING 200____

ACUTE CARE   **LONG TERM CARE**   **COMMUNITY**
Agency: Agency: Agency:
Unit: Unit: Unit:
Faculty: Faculty: Faculty:

End of Semester Assessment

Each student will be evaluated as Satisfactory or Unsatisfactory for each clinical objective required in the nursing course for which the student is enrolled. A student who receives a grade of satisfactory for every required objective receives a satisfactory grade for the clinical portion of the course. A student who receives a grade of unsatisfactory for one or more objectives has not demonstrated the necessary knowledge, skills and abilities for the established level of practice. The student receives an unsatisfactory grade for the clinical portion of the course and, therefore, a grade of "F" for the course.

I. CLIENT NEEDS
A. SAFE, EFFECTIVE CARE ENVIRONMENT

	N101	N132	N231	N232
1. Applies principles of biological, social and nursing sciences	S U	S U	S U	S U
2. Prepares clients for treatments and procedures		S U	S U	S U
3. Coordinates care with appropriate health care personnel			S U	S U
4. Performs treatments and procedures				
a. Oxygen administration				
1. Mask/cannula	S U	S U	S U	S U
2. Other (please list)	S U	S U	S U	S U
b. Monitoring				
1. Intake/output	S U	S U	S U	S U
2. Vital signs	S U	S U	S U	S U
3. Wound drainage	S U	S U	S U	S U
4. Blood glucose	S U	S U	S U	S U
5. Maintains medical asepsis				
a. Maintains universal precautions	S U	S U	S U	S U
b. Maintains infection control principles	S U	S U	S U	S U
6. Maintains surgical asepsis				
a. Changes sterile dressing	S U	S U	S U	S U
b. Maintains venous access lines		S U	S U	S U
c. Change tubing/bag peripheral line		S U	S U	S U
d. Change tubing/bag central line		S U	S U	S U
7. Demonstrates proficiency in math computation	S U	S U	S U	S U
8. Communicates effectively with other health care providers				
a. Documents clients' needs and health care provided appropriately	S U	S U	S U	S U
b. Provides accurate and timely report	S U	S U	S U	S U
9. Seeks help when situation encountered is beyond own knowledge or experience	S U	S U	S U	S U

		N101	N132	N231	N232
10. Provides care for two or more clients		S U	S U	S U	
11. Manages care for a group of clients					
a. Determines appropriate priorities		S U	S U	S U	
b. Delegates tasks to assistive personnel				S U	
c. Manages care provided by assistive personnel				S U	

Comments:

B. PHYSIOLOGICAL INTEGRITY

	N101	N132	N231	N232
1. Administers medication				
a. Oral				
(1) To 1 or 2 client(s)	S U	S U	S U	S U
(2) To 3 or more clients			S U	S U
b. Parenteral	S U	S U	S U	S U
c. Other (please specify)				
2. Identifies drug pharmacokinetics, side effects and interactions	S U	S U	S U	S U
3. Describes client's pathophysiology		S U	S U	S U
4. Maintains good body mechanics	S U	S U	S U	S U
5. Maintains client's activities				
a. Personal hygiene	S U	S U	S U	S U
b. Feeding	S U	S U	S U	S U
c. Mobility	S U	S U	S U	S U
d. Toileting	S U	S U	S U	S U
6. Administers ordered nutritional therapy		S U	S U	S U
7. Administers ordered parenteral fluids		S U	S U	S U
8. Provides comfort measures for client	S U	S U	S U	S U
9. Performs invasive procedures (for example, catheterization insert or remove naso-gastric tube tracheostomy suctioning/ care)			S U	S U
10. Manages emergencies				S U
11. Identifies expected and unexpected responses to therapies		S U	S U	S U

Comments:

C. PSYCHOSOCIAL INTEGRITY

	N101	N132	N231	N232
1. Communicates therapeutically with clients and/or family	S U	S U	S U	S U
2. Assists the client in coping with stress	S U	S U	S U	S U
3. Assesses client's mental status				
4. Describes client's psychopathology		S U	S U	S U

			S U	S U
5. Assesses impact on family dynamics of client's health alteration				

Comments:

D. HEALTH PROMOTION/MAINTENANCE

	N101	N132	N231	N232
1. Maintains health				
a. Teaches client and/or family how to promote and maintain health	S U	S U	S U	S U
b. Prevents complications of immobility	S U	S U	S U	S U
c. Teaches a group how to promote or maintain health			S U	S U
2. Considers client's cultural needs and expectations related to health care	S U	S U	S U	S U
3. Meets developmental needs of assigned clients	S U	S U	S U	S U
4. Assists the client and family to adapt to health alterations		S U	S U	S U
5. Refers client and/or family to appropriate community resources			S U	S U
6. Collaborates with faculty, peers, agency staff, individuals and families to				
a. Assesses targeted community			S U	S U
b. Meets health promotion/disease prevention needs				S U

Comments:

II. PROFESSIONAL BEHAVIOR
A. ATTENDANCE

	N101	N132	N231	N232
1. Attends clinical laboratory (List date of absence) N101 N132 N231 N232	S U	S U	S U	S U
2. Is punctual for clinical laboratory (List date and time of lateness) N101 N132 N231 N232	S U	S U	S U	S U

3. Notifies the instructor and agency prior to any absence or lateness	S U	S U	S U	S U

B. LEGAL-ETHICAL PRACTICE

1. Maintains current CPR certification	S U	S U	S U	S U
2. Maintains current health insurance	S U	S U	S U	S U
3. Maintains liability insurance	S U	S U	S U	S U
4. Adheres to nursing ethical guidelines	S U	S U	S U	S U
5. Functions within legal parameters	S U	S U	S U	S U

Course	Faculty Signature	Date
N101	_____	_____
N132	_____	_____
N231	_____	_____
N232	_____	_____

STUDENT COMMENTS

Student _____ **#** _____

N101 FALL 200__

_____
Signature   **Date**

N132 SPRING 200__

_____
Signature   **Date**

N231 FALL 200__

_____
Signature   **Date**

N232 SPRING 200__

_____

Signature   **Date**

FACULTY COMMENTS

Student _____ **#** _____

N101 FALL 200__

_____

Signature   **Date**

N132 SPRING 200__

_____

Signature   **Date**

N231 FALL 200__

_____

Signature   **Date**

N232 SPRING 200__

_____

Signature   **Date**

Developed by the Community College of Philadelphia Department of Nursing. Reprinted by permission of the Community College of Philadelphia, Philadelphia, Pennsylvania, 2004.

Examples of Rating Forms for Clinical Evaluation from Baccalaureate Nursing Programs

CLINICAL EVALUATION
(Includes LRC)

Student's Name:_____

Faculty's Name: _____

Agency/Unit: _____

Date of Experience: _____

Indicate rating by placing a check mark under Pass or Fail for each objective.

		MIDTERM EVALUATION		FINAL EVALUATION	
		PASS	**FAIL**	**PASS**	**FAIL**
I.	Demonstrates use of supportive nursing care strategies with individuals in the context of the family and/or community.	///////////////////////////////// ///////////////////////////////// /////////////////////////////////		///////////////////////////////// ///////////////////////////////// /////////////////////////////////	
*A.	Demonstrates use of selected physical assessment skills in collection of data.				
*B.	Collects data using the patient, medical record, staff, and other resources.				
C.	Identifies the use of community resources in discharge planning when available.				
II.	Examines the influence of culture on supportive nursing care to individuals and families	///////////////////////////////// /////////////////////////////////		///////////////////////////////// /////////////////////////////////	
*A.	Describes biopsychosocial and cultural needs of individuals with basic health care needs.				
III.	Uses critical thinking in applying the nursing process to supportive care of individuals and families.	///////////////////////////////// ///////////////////////////////// /////////////////////////////////		///////////////////////////////// ///////////////////////////////// /////////////////////////////////	
*A.	Selects from an accepted list of nursing diagnoses based on data.				
*B.	Develops goals related to the nursing diagnosis.				
*C.	Describes measurable outcome criteria related to selected client goals.				
*D.	Develops an individualized plan of action to meet stated goals for individuals with basic needs.				
E.	Identifies revisions of care plan based on evaluation data.				
F.	Shows awareness of educational needs of the client.				
G.	Demonstrates ability to prioritize care.				
IV.	Examines the scientific basis of supportive care.	///////////////////////////////// /////////////////////////////////		///////////////////////////////// /////////////////////////////////	
*A.	Demonstrates ability to correlate pathophysiology with client presentation.				
*B.	Describes scientific rationale to explain biophysical and psychosocial data.				

V. Develops skill implementing a repertoire of supportive measures and technologies.	//////////////////////////////// ////////////////////////////////	/////////////////////////// ///////////////////////////
*A. Carries out/implements proscribed nursing actions/care.		
SELECTED EXAMPLES	////////////////////////////////	///////////////////////////
Accurate calculation, timely administration, and knowledge of medications.	//////////////////////////////// ////////////////////////////	/////////////////////////// ///////////////////////////
Demonstrates proper aseptic technique and use of universal precautions.	//////////////////////////////// ////////////////////////////	/////////////////////////// ///////////////////////////
Demonstrates safety with technical procedures.	////////////////////////////////	///////////////////////////
Is organized.	////////////////////////////////	///////////////////////////
VI. Uses therapeutic communication with individuals and families.	//////////////////////////////// ////////////////////////////	/////////////////////////// ///////////////////////////
*A. Demonstrates use of therapeutic techniques for interaction with ill patients and their families		
VII. Identifies aspects of effective communication in a multidisciplinary care team and faculty.	//////////////////////////////// ////////////////////////////	/////////////////////////// ///////////////////////////
*A. Reports significant changes in patient status to clinical faculty and appropriate personnel.		
B. Denotes ability to obtain report accurately from staff and faculty.		
C. Charting is clear, concise, and accurate according to patients nursing diagnosis.		
D. Demonstrates ability to communicate effectively with staff (physicians nurses, etc.) and faculty.		
VIII. Describes the organizational structure of a clinical practice setting.	//////////////////////////////// ////////////////////////////	/////////////////////////// ///////////////////////////
*A. Responds to individual client needs during hospitalization.		
B. Provides quality care to the hospitalized ill client according to professional standards.		
IX Identifies ethical issues in supportive care of individuals and families.	//////////////////////////////// ////////////////////////////	/////////////////////////// ///////////////////////////
X. Examines progress toward professional learning objectives.	//////////////////////////////// ////////////////////////////	/////////////////////////// ///////////////////////////
*A. Is accountable for own nursing practice (safe, prepared).		
SELECTED EXAMPLES:	//////////////////////////////// ////////////////////////////////	/////////////////////////// ///////////////////////////
Is prepared for clinical assignment.	////////////////////////////////	///////////////////////////
Is on time.	////////////////////////////////	///////////////////////////
Dress is appropriate.	////////////////////////////////	///////////////////////////
Notifies instructor and/or agency in timely manner in case of illness or unavoidable tardiness.	//////////////////////////////// ////////////////////////////	/////////////////////////// ///////////////////////////
Reports off to appropriate staff/faculty.	////////////////////////////////	///////////////////////////
Provides nursing coverage when away from client area.	////////////////////////////////	///////////////////////////
Completes assignments on time.	////////////////////////////////	///////////////////////////
B. Identifies own learning needs, goals in terms of own professional development		
Is on time.	////////////////////////////////	///////////////////////////
Dress is appropriate.	////////////////////////////////	///////////////////////////
Notifies instructor and/or agency in timely manner in case of illness or unavoidable tardiness.	//////////////////////////////// ////////////////////////////	/////////////////////////// ///////////////////////////
Reports off to appropriate staff/faculty.	////////////////////////////////	///////////////////////////
Provides nursing coverage when away from client area.	////////////////////////////////	///////////////////////////
Completes assignments on time.	////////////////////////////////	///////////////////////////
B. Identifies own learning needs, goals in terms of own professional development.		
SELECTED EXAMPLES:	//////////////////////////////// ////////////////////////////////	/////////////////////////// ///////////////////////////
Identifies own strengths and weakness. Uses learning resources.	//////////////////////////////// ////////////////////////////	/////////////////////////// ///////////////////////////

MIDTERM EVALUATION

FACULTY-STUDENT NARRATIVE

SELECT ONE: PASS

FAIL (INCLUDE PLAN FOR IMPROVEMENT)

Faculty Comments:

Student Comments:

Faculty's Signature: _____

Student's Signature: _____

Date: _____

Critical Behaviors

*The following are critical behaviors identified on the Clinical Evaluation Tool for NUR 2050:

Objective I	-	A,B	Objective VI	-	A
Objective II	-	A	Objective VII	-	A
Objective III	-	A, B, C, D	Objective VIII	-	A
Objective IV	-	A, B	Objective IX		A
Objective V	-	A			

Critical behaviors must be passed. A grade of fail in any one of the critical behaviors will indicate unsafe practice and will result in failure of NUR 2050.

FINAL EVALUATION

FACULTY-STUDENT NARRATIVE

SELECT ONE: PASS

FAIL

Faculty Comments:

Student Comments:

Faculty's Signature: _____

Student's Signature: _____

Date: _____

Critical Behaviors

*The following are critical behaviors identified on the Clinical Evaluation Tool for NUR 2050:

Objective I	-	A,B	Objective VI	-	A
Objective II	-	A	Objective VII	-	A
Objective III	-	A, B, C, D	Objective VIII	-	A
Objective IV	-	A, B	Objective IX		A
Objective V	-	A			

Critical behaviors must be passed. A grade of fail in any one of the critical behaviors will indicate unsafe practice and will result in failure of NUR 2050.

Satisfactory completion of the clinical component of the course is dependent upon passing all identified critical behaviors and at least 75% of the remaining items on the clinical evaluation form. Clinical practice is graded as pass or fail. The student must pass the clinical portion of the course to progress in the nursing program.

This tool was developed and modified by Barbara Pieper, PhD, RN, FAAN, CS, CWOCN and Wayne State University College of Nursing faculty. Reprinted by permission of Wayne State University College of Nursing, 2005.

UNIVERSITY OF SOUTHERN INDIANA
N 341: NURSING OF WOMEN AND FAMILIES

Clinical Evaluation Form

Student: _____

Clinical Instructor: _____

Evaluation Completed by: _____

*The student must have a *Pass* in all areas to successfully pass the clinical component of the course. Record a P (Pass) next to each objective if the student met the objective or a F (Fail) if the student did not meet it.

The student is:

1.	**A critical thinker who possesses the knowledge base and communication skills to constructively problem solve, utilize thoughtful decision making, and gather and process meaningful information related to the client, self, healthcare environment, and community at large.**

a.	Collects accurate historical assessment data in orderly, systematic manner utilizing the clinical pathway/care plan.		
b.	Formulates nursing diagnosis statements that are validated by subjective and objective data.		
c.	Identifies priority nursing diagnoses and collaborative problems for assigned clients.		
d.	Evaluates client outcomes and makes appropriate modifications		
e.	Presents findings of relevant nursing research articles to clinical practice.		

2.	**An effective communicator who utilizes verbal, nonverbal, and technological means to communicate appropriately with clients and their families, health professionals, and other members of the community-at-large concerning health-related issues.**

a.	Utilizes appropriate therapeutic verbal and nonverbal communication techniques.		
b.	Individualizes care provided to clients based on individual challenges, socioeconomic and cultural needs.		
c.	Communicates with peers and others within the healthcare setting in a positive and supportive manner.		
d.	Communicates client advocacy concerns to the appropriate person.		
e.	Effectively and accurately documents client information in medical records and weekly student assignments.		

3.		**A safe, competent practitioner who is capable of effectively utilizing resources to provide quality care for clients in diverse environments.**		
	a.	Establishes relevant baseline data, and maintains and interprets ongoing assessment for multiple clients.		
	b.	Implements and evaluates the plan of care for multiple clients.		
	c.	Implements nursing actions safely and effectively following nursing and departmental protocol.		
	d.	Demonstrates competency and safety in medication administration.		
	e.	Performs complete assessments of the laboring, postpartal, and newborn client.		
	f.	Performs various types of initial postpartal assessments.		
	g.	Performs reinforcement of discharge teaching within the home environment.		
	h.	Develops, implements, and evaluates teaching/learning plans for clients with complex healthcare needs.		
4.		**A practitioner who demonstrates role flexibility and leadership in guiding and participating in group and team efforts related to multidisciplinary healthcare.**		
	a.	Communicates and collaborates with client and healthcare team concerning plan of care and expected outcomes while sensitive to client's culture, values, and beliefs.		
	b.	Demonstrates leadership through collaboration and consultation with healthcare team.		
	c.	Participates in discharge planning and implementation.		
5.		**A practitioner who demonstrates professional values and adheres to professional practice standards and ethical codes.**		
	a.	Maintains accountability and responsibility for client care with an open, caring nursing presence.		
	b.	Practices nursing within the legal and ethical framework of the professional nursing value system.		
	c.	Demonstrates advocacy through collaboration and consultation with the healthcare team.		
	d.	Attends and reports on one Professional Learning Activity (PLA).		
	e.	Adheres to USI School of Nursing policies		
	f.	Demonstrates respect for others in all interpersonal interactions including clients, families, healthcare professionals, peers, and faculty.		

COMMENTS:

Date(s) of Clinical Absences:_____

Total Hours of Clinical Absences: _____

Date(s) of Clinical Tardiness:_____

Date(s) of Conference:_____

Instructor's Signature/Initial(s):_____

Student's Signature/Initial(s):_____

Fall 2004

Developed by Gina L. Schaar, RN, MSN. Reprinted by permission of University of Southern Indiana School of Nursing, Evansville, Indiana, 2004.

UNIVERSITY OF ALBERTA FACULTY OF NURSING
NURSING 495
Preceptor Evaluation of Student Clinical Performance

Student: _____   **Unit:** _____

Faculty Tutor: _____   **Hours to date:** _____

Preceptor(s): _____

Report Period: ? Midterm   ? Final   **Rating:** ? Pass   ? Fail

Rating: **3** - Acceptable Standard Exceeded
                             2 - Acceptable Standard Achieved **
                             1 - Acceptable Standard Not Achieved
                             N/A - not Able to Assess

** An Acceptable Standard of nursing practice at the time of the final evaluation is commensurate with that expected of a beginning graduate nurse.

A. Professionalism in Nursing Practice	Examples	Rating
1. Applies legal and ethical standards in nursing practice: • Incorporates client's values, beliefs and rights into care • Prepares for clinical practice • Practices within policies and pro procedures of agency • Integrates knowledge from the discipline of nursing with that of professional standards • Demonstrates an attitude of inquiry. **2. Demonstrates professional behaviours:** • Treats clients, colleagues and faculty with respect • Develops collaborative relationships with clients and health care professionals in the practice environment • Practices professional communication skills with colleagues and faculty • Accepts responsibility for acquiring knowledge necessary for competent nursing practice • Accepts responsibility for own actions • Commits to practising nursing with integrity • Seeks opportunities for professional growth • Strives for and maintains competence in nursing practice • Seeks appropriate opportunities to develop basic leadership and managements skills • Participates in agency activities. **3. Demonstrates personal responsibility and accountability** • Identifies own strengths and limitations • Takes initiative for addressing limitations • Recognizes when help is needed		

	Examples	Rating
• Seeks and responds to feedback in an appropriate and timely manner • Fulfils commitments to others		

B. Competency in Nursing Practice	Examples	Rating
1. Assessment Skills • Uses sound knowledge base upon which to base assessment • Assesses client/family needs in an accurate and comprehensive manner • Demonstrates critical thinking when making assessments **2. Planning Skills** • Uses sound clinical judgment and principles of best practice in planning care • Develops plan for coordination of care of multiple clients • Uses critical thinking when developing plan of care **3. Implementation** • Demonstrates critical thinking when implementing plan of care • Carries out plan for coordination of care of multiple clients • Establishes therapeutic relationships with clients • Practices therapeutic communication skills with clients • Practices psychomotor skills competently • Administers medications competently **4. Evaluation** • Appraises outcomes of nursing interventions • Appraisal of own clinical performance is congruent with that of preceptor and/or faculty **5. Commitment to Continuity of Care** • Communicates verbally relevant information about client response to care • Documents necessary information about client status and nursing interventions in all relevant forums.		

Concluding Comments:

Signatures -
Preceptor: _____   **Date:** _____

Student: _____   **Date:** _____
Note from authors: Students complete same form for self-evaluation.

Reprinted by permission of Faculty of Nursing Collaborative Program, University of Alberta, Alberta, Canada.

University of North Dakota
N 382 Clinical Performance Evaluation Tool

KEY
= Student Rating   Student _____

= Faculty Rating
* = Not observed   Semester/Year _____

Behavioral Objectives	4	3	2	1	0	*	Comments
The student: 1. Assessment Uses assessment skills to determine the health status of the adult client during acute illness.							
1.1. Obtains appropriate and comprehensive data (review of records, texts). Differentiates relevant data from irrelevant.							
1.2. Makes accurate observations and assessments during clinical (eg, V.S., laboratory results. physical assessments, etc.).							
1.3. Correctly identifies physiologic and psychosocial needs.							
2. Planning Uses the nursing process appropriately in planning care for the acutely ill adult client.							
2.1. Selects and appropriately prioritizes nursing diagnoses.							
2.2 Writes short term, measurable, realistic goals when planning nursing care.							
2.3 Plans individualized nursing care using knowledge and nursing supporting sciences.							
3. Implementation Provides appropriate interventions for the acutely ill adult client.							
3.1. Maintains a safe environment.							
3.2 Implements interventions that are specific, realistic, and goal oriented.							

3.3. Sets appropriate priorities during clinical.							
**3.4. Performs therapeutic procedures correctly; administers medications safely and correctly.							
3.5 Incorporates health teaching when planning and providing care for the acutely ill client. Assists client in understanding rationale for care.							
4. Evaluation Evaluates the care provided and makes necessary changes in the plan of care.							
4.1 Evaluates the effectiveness of medications the client receives. Evaluates client responses to therapies and care (eg, IVs, I/O, pain, vitals, etc.)							
4.2. Initiates changes in client care based on evaluation.							
5. Intellectual Inquiry/Problem Solving Utilizes intellectual inquiry and problem solving in caring for adult clients.							
5.1. Demonstrates knowledge of client's health alterations.							
5.2. Explains rationale for diagnostic tests and therapeutic procedures.							
5.3. Provides nursing care that reflects appropriate problem solving.							
6. Communication Communicates effectively with clients, families, and health care professionals.							
6.1. Develops appropriate rapport with clients.							
6.2. Interacts appropriately with the health care team and nursing staff.							
6.3. Provides accurate, meaningful and complete verbal reports; reports deviations promptly.							

6.4. Charts accurately, clearly, concisely and promptly. Uses appropriate terminology.							
6.5 Identifies cultural and spiritual values, beliefs and attitudes (personal and client's) that relate to nursing care of the acutely ill.							
**7. Role Demonstrates accountability for completing assignments and for professional behavior in the preclinical and clinical settings.							
7.1. Is well prepared and on time for clinical experiences. Turns in assignments on time.							
7.2. Initiates self-directed learning. Utilizes time effectively during clinical.							
7.3. Appropriately seeks instructor guidance.							
7.4. Actively participates in pre and post clinical discussions.							
Grade _____						_____	

Faculty Comments:

Student Comments:

Student _____ Faculty _____

Date_____

CRITERIA FOR CLINICAL EVALUATION

PASS

Scale Label	Quality of Performance	Assistance
Always 4 points	Safe and accurate. Proficient, coordinated, confident. Occasional expenditure of excess energy. Within an expedient time period.	Without supporting cues.
Regularly 3 points	Safe and accurate. Efficient, coordinated, confident. Some expenditure of excess energy. Within a reasonable time period.	Occasional supportive cues.
Occasional 2 points	Safe and accurate most of the time. Skillful in parts of behavior. Inefficiency and lack of coordination. Expends excess energy within a delayed time period.	Frequent verbal and occasional physical directive cues in addition to supportive one.
Seldom 1 point	FAIL Safe only with supervision. Unskilled, inefficient and uncoordinated. Considerable expenditure of excess energy. Prolonged time period.	Continuous verbal and frequent physical cues.
Never 0 Points	Unsafe. Unable to demonstrate procedure/behavior. Lacks confidence, coordination, efficiency.	Continuous verbal and physical cues.
X	Not observed.	

**Critical behavior - Failure to meet this objective may result in clinical failure. Seldom or never categories may also result in a failing grade.

Adapted from: Bondy, K. N. (1983). Criterion-referenced definitions for rating scales in clinical evaluation. Journal of Nursing Education, 22(9), 376–382.

Developed by University of North Dakota, College of Nursing Faculty. Reprinted by permission of Roxanne Hurley and University of North Dakota College of Nursing, 2004.

Community Health Nursing (RN section)

CLINICAL EVALUATION FORM

Total Raw Score:_____   Student Name: _____

Mean Score: _____   Faculty Name: _____

Letter Grade: _____   Agency: _____

	4	3	2	1	na
Uses a theoretical framework in care of individuals, families and groups in the community.					
A. Applies concepts and theories in the practice of community health nursing.					
B. Examines multicultural concepts of care as they apply to the community.					
C. Analyzes family theory as a basis for care of clients in a community setting.					
D. Examines relationships of family members within a community setting.					
E. Examines the community as a client through ongoing assessment.					
F. Evaluates health care delivery systems within a community setting.					
Use the nursing process for care of individuals, families and groups in the community and the community as client.					
A. Adapts assessment skills in the collection of data from individuals, families and groups in a community setting.					
B. Uses relevant resources in the collection of data in the community.					
*C. Analyzes client and community data.					
D. Develops nursing diagnoses for individuals, families and groups within the community and the community as client.					
E. Develops measurable outcome criteria and plan of action.					
F. Uses outcome criteria for evaluating plans and effectiveness of interventions.					

	4	3	2	1	na
*G. Assumes accountability for own practice in the community.					
H. Uses research findings and standards for community-based care.					
*I. Accepts differences among clients and communities.					
Is responsible for identifying and meeting own learning needs.					
*A. Evaluates own development as a professional.					
*B. Meets own learning needs in community practice.					
Collaborates with others in providing community care.					
A. Interacts effectively with clients and others in the community.					
B. Uses effectively community resources.					

*Critical behaviors must be passed at 2.0 to pass clinical practicum.

4 = Consistently excels in performance of behavior, independent
3 = Is competent in performance, independent
2 = Performs behavior safely, needs assistance
1 = Unable to perform behavior, requires guidance all the time

FACULTY-STUDENT NARRATIVE

Faculty Comments:

Signature:_____

Date:_____

Student Comments:

Signature:_____

Date:_____

Tool developed by Judith M. Fouladbakhsh, MSN, APRN, BC, AHN-C, CHTP, and Effie Hanchett, PhD, RN. Adapted by permission of J. Fouladbakhsh and E. Hanchett, 2005.

Examples of Rating Forms for Clinical Evaluation from Master's Nursing Programs

UNIVERSITY OF ALABAMA SCHOOL OF NURSING
UNIVERSITY OF ALABAMA AT BIRMINGHAM GRADUATE STUDIES

PRECEPTOR'S EVALUATION OF NURSE PRACTITIONER STUDENT

Student_____Term/Yr_____Course_____#
Hours_____

Clinical Site_____ Preceptor_____

For each item listed below, **CHECK** one block indicating your evaluation of the student.

Scale: 5 = Consistently or Always Demonstrated; 4 = Almost Always Demonstrated; 3 = Occasionally Demonstrated;
2 = Rarely Demonstrated; 1 = Never Demonstrated; 0 = Not Applicable or No Occasion to Observe

I. Professional Characteristics

	5	4	3	2	1	0
1. Performs in a cooperative manner						
2. Demonstrates sensitivity and respect to staff						
3. Uses time productively and is punctual						
4. Identifies own learning needs and takes responsibility for own learning						

II. Clinical Skills

	5	4	3	2	1	0
1. Elicits health histories that are developmentally and age appropriate to the target population, performs physical examinations, and interprets laboratory data based on the client's health status.						
2. Identifies psychosocial and developmental factors that affect the health status of clients and/or their families.						
3. Makes clinical decisions about diagnosis, management, and consultation or referral based on the systematic assessment of clients with common acute or chronic problems.						
4. Implements a plan of care that conforms to theory-based standards of practice.						
5. Demonstrates communication skills with clients and professional colleagues that reflect an accurate perception of both verbal and nonverbal cues.						
6. Demonstrates skill and accuracy in the use of screening and diagnostic tools.						
7. Presents orally to the clinical preceptor an assessment of the client's problems, relevant findings, and plan for management in a concise, organized manner.						
8. Provides anticipatory guidance and health instruction to the client/family in the target population based on assessed risk factors and health maintenance needs.						
9. Demonstrates knowledge of pharmacology through suggestions of appropriate drug choices based on the client's health problem and health history.						
10. Applies knowledge about pharmacological actions of drugs to provide clients with accurate information about the medications prescribed for them.						
11. Provides nutrition counseling consistent with the client's health needs and psychological and cultural characteristics.						
12. Provides for continuity of care through the health record by systematically recording client encounters in the SOAP format.						
13. Identifies conditions in the client or family requiring consultation and/or referral to other health care providers.						
14. Coordinates health care needs of clients with available community resources.						

III. **Overall Clinical Performance**

Above expected (90-100%) ❐
(Demonstrates above average knowledge and performs at a high level of skill.)

Expected (80-89%) ❐
(Demonstrates adequate knowledge and skill to perform in a competent manner.)

Below expected (70-79%) ❐
(Performs with minimal knowledge for safe practice. Requires close supervision. [Please explain below.])

Unacceptable (69% & below) ❐
(Demonstrates inadequate knowledge and skill for safe practice. [Please explain below.])

IV. **Comments**

Please make statements about your overall impression of the student's strengths, weaknesses, and whether you consider the student's clinical performance to be safe. (Use an additional page if necessary.)

Please return this form to:

Jean B. Ivey, DSN, RN, CRNP
Kristen Osborn, MSN, CRNP
1530 3rd Avenue South, Birmingham, AL 35294-1210
FAX: 205-975-6142

Preceptor's Signature and Date

Tool developed by MSN Faculty, Graduate Studies, The University of Alabama School of Nursing, The University of Alabama at Birmingham. Reprinted by permission of The University of Alabama School of Nursing, February 2005.

University of Alabama School of Nursing
University of Alabama at Birmingham Graduate Studies

Preceptor's Evaluation of Nurse Practitioner Student

Student_____ __   Term/Year_____
Course#_____
Clinical Site_____   Preceptor_____
Hours_____

For each item listed below. CHECK one block indicating your evaluation of the student.

Scale: **5** = Consistently or always demonstrated; **4** = Almost always demonstrated; **3** =
Occasionally demonstrated; **2** = Rarely demonstrated; **1** = Never demonstrated; **0** = Not
applicable or no occasion to observe

I. Professional Characteristics

	5	4	3	2	1	0
Performs in cooperative manner						
Applies ethical principles in caring for patients						
Demonstrates sensitivity and respect to staff						
Uses time productively and is punctual						
Identifies own learning needs and takes responsibility for own learning						

II. Clinical Skills

	5	4	3	2	1	0
Elicits health histories that are developmentally & age-appropriate and performs complete or system-focused physical examinations on complex acute, critical, & chronically ill patients						
Distinguishes between normal & abnormal developmental and age-related physiologic & behavioral changes						
Formulates differential diagnosis & prioritizes health problems						
Orders laboratory/diagnostic tests & interprets data to confirm/rule out diagnosis & utilizes data in management of condition						
Utilizes specialty-based technical skills/therapeutic interventions for dx & treatment of health problems (Technical skills check-list on page 2)						
Formulates & implements plan of care addressing health care needs of patients with complex acute, critical, & chronic illness utilizing evidence-based practice						
Manages plan of care through evaluation, modification, & documentation according to patient's response to therapy, changes in condition, & therapeutic interventions to optimize patient outcomes						

Prescribes appropriate pharmacologic & non-pharmacologic treatment modalities						
Demonstrates pharmacological knowledge by choosing appropriate drug therapy & assessing interactive & synergistic effects of pharmacological agents in patients with complex acute, critical, & chronic illnesses						
Provides for health promotion & protection by assessing for risks associated with the care of acutely, chronically, & critically ill patients (i.e. impaired nutrition, immobility, immunocompetence, impaired communication, altered family dynamics, continuity of care)						
Manages pain utilizing pharmacologic & non-pharmacologic interventions & evaluates response to therapy						
Demonstrates effective communication skills with patient, family, staff, & other professionals						
Assesses needs of patient, family, & caregivers						
Develops appropriate educational interventions for patient & family						
Incorporates discharge planning (including home health & hospice therapy) into plan of care & facilitates patient's transition for health care setting to home						
Implements palliative & end of life care in collaboration with family, patient, & other members of multidisciplinary team						

Additional skills for critical care preceptorship:

	5	4	3	2	1	0
Diagnosis of acute & chronic conditions that may result in rapid physiologic deterioration or life-threatening instability & prioritizes health problems						
Implements interventions to support the patient with a rapidly deteriorating physiologic condition						
Utilizes appropriate basic & advanced life support interventions						
Assesses & manages patient's response to life support strategies						
Manages sedation & monitors patient response to sedation						

Therapeutic interventions/skills checklist:

Suturing						
Wound debridement						
CVL insertion & management						
Chest tube insertion						
Lumbar puncture						
Advance life support						
EKG interpretation						

Hemodynamic monitoring						
Radiographic interpretation						
Intubations/airway management						
Ventilator management						
Foreign body removal						
Casting/splinting						
PICC line insertion						
Aseptic technique						

III. Overall Clinical Performance

( )   Above expected (90–100%)

    (Demonstrates above average knowledge and performs at a high level of skill

( )   Expected (80–89%)

    (Demonstrates adequate knowledge and skill to perform in a competent manner)

( )   Below expected (70–79%)

    (Performs with minimal knowledge for safe practice. Requires close supervision. Please explain below.)

( )   Unacceptable (69% & below)

    (Demonstrates inadequate knowledge and skill for safe practice. Please explain below.)

IV. Comments

Please make statements about your overall impression of the student's strength & weaknesses, and whether you would consider the student's clinical performance to be safe. (Use additional page if necessary.)

Preceptor's Signature_____ Date: _____

Please return this form to: UAB School of Nursing, Attn: Jean B. Ivey, DSN, RN, CRNP or Amy Gardner, MSN, CRNP; Phone: 205-996-4193 Fax: 205-975-6142

Developed by Amy C. Gardner, MSN, CRNP, Teaching Staff, Graduate Studies, The University of Alabama School of Nursing, The University of Alabama at Birmingham. Reprinted by permission of A. C. Gardner and The University of Alabama School of Nursing, February 2005.

KENT STATE UNIVERSITY SCHOOL OF NURSING
PRECEPTOR CLINICAL EVALUATION FORM
Graduate Adult Health Psychosocial Interventions

DATE:
STUDENT NAME:_____
CLINICAL SITE/ADDRESS:_____

COURSE OBJECTIVES	COMMENTS
1. Demonstrate clinical reasoning skill for a selected adult/family population with complex health problems; particular focus is on the holistic interrelationship of client's biophysiological health status and health behaviors.	
2. Identify, apply, and evaluate independent nursing psychosocial interventions, demonstrating advanced nursing skills in selected interventions.	
3. Identify, apply, and evaluate independent client education interventions in the areas of health promotion and maintenance, designed to facilitate client (family) learning.	
4. Establish and maintain collaborative relationships with clients, peers, faculty, and other health care professionals.	
5. Participate in appropriate professional consultation with clients, peers, faculty, and other health care professionals, giving and receiving constructive feedback to ensure safe professional practice.	
6. Utilize a personal, professional database of experiences and goals, and self-evaluation of performance to evaluate goals and progress.	

Personal Objectives	Comments
1.	

Personal Objectives	Comments
2.	
3.	
4.	
5.	

Please share comments or recommendations regarding this student's clinical performance.

Please comment on your role and any recommendations for future clinical precepting, e.g., How many hours per week were you able to spend with this student? Did you feel this was an adequate amount of time to meet the students' objectives? Were the expectations of your role clear?

Please review this evaluation with your student and give to student to return to faculty or mail to Harriet Coeling, Kent State University, School of Nursing, Kent, OH 44242-0001. Thank you; your feedback is greatly appreciated.

Signature/Clinical Preceptor:_____ Date: _____
Clinical Site/Address: _____

KENT STATE UNIVERSITY
SCHOOL OF NURSING
CLINICAL SUMMARY EVALUATION FORM
CLINICAL INTERVENTIONS AND HEALTH BEHAVIORS--60056

NAME: _____   STUDENT ID: _____

ADDRESS: _____   DATE: _____

SEMESTER: _____

COURSE OBJECTIVES	MET	NOT MET
1. Demonstrate clinical reasoning skill for a selected adult (and family) client population with complex health problems; with particular focus on the holistic interrelationship of clients' biophysiological health status and health behaviors.		
2. Identify, apply, and evaluate independent nursing interventions in the psychosocial domain, demonstrating advanced nursing skills in selected specific interventions.		
3. Identify, apply, and evaluate independent client education interventions in the areas of health promotion and maintenance designed to facilitate client (family) learning to the selected client population.		
4. Establish and maintain collaborative relationships with clients, peers, faculty, and other health care professionals.		
5. Participate in appropriate professional consultation with clients, peers, faculty, and other health care professionals, giving and receiving constructive feedback to ensure safe professional practice.		
6. Utilize a personal, professional database of experiences and goals, and self-evaluation of performance as an advanced practice professional to evaluate goals and progress.		

Personal Objectives	Met	Not Met

Personal Objectives	Met	Not Met

CLINICAL PLACEMENT

Agency: _____

Agency Preceptor/Supervisor: _____

Hours per week at agency:

Comments:

Faculty: _____
Date: _____

Student: _____
Date: _____

Developed by Faculty in the N60056, Adult Health Nursing: Clinical Interventions and Psychosocial Health Status course at Kent State University, College of Nursing. Reprinted by permission of Faculty at Kent State University, College of Nursing, Kent, OH, 2004

Appendix B

Codes of Ethics in Testing and Educational Measurement

CODE OF FAIR TESTING PRACTICES IN EDUCATION

Prepared by the Joint Committee on Testing Practices

The Code of Fair Testing Practices in Education (*Code*) is a guide for professionals in fulfilling their obligation to provide and use tests that are fair to all test takers regardless of age, gender, disability, race, ethnicity, national origin, religion, sexual orientation, linguistic background, or other personal characteristics. Fairness is a primary consideration in all aspects of testing. Careful standardization of tests and administration conditions helps to ensure that all test takers are given a comparable opportunity to demonstrate what they know and how they can perform in the area being tested. Fairness implies that every test taker has the opportunity to prepare for the test and is informed about the general nature and content of the test, as appropriate to the purpose of the test. Fairness also extends to the accurate reporting of individual and group test results. Fairness is not an isolated concept, but must be considered in all aspects of the testing process.

The *Code* applies broadly to testing in education (admissions, educational assessment, educational diagnosis, and student placement) regardless of the mode of presentation, so it is relevant to conventional paper-and-pencil tests, computer-based tests, and performance tests. It is not designed to cover employment testing, licensure or certification testing, or other types of testing outside the field of education. The *Code* is directed primarily at professionally developed tests used in formally administered testing programs. Although the *Code* is not intended to cover tests made by teachers for use in their own classrooms, teachers are encouraged to use the guidelines to help improve their testing practices.

The *Code* addresses the roles of test developers and test users separately. Test developers are people and organizations that construct tests, as well as those that set policies for testing programs. Test users are people and agencies that select tests, administer tests, commission test development services, or make decisions on the basis of test scores. Test developer and test user roles may overlap, for example, when a state or local education agency commissions test development services, sets policies that control the test development process, and makes decisions on the basis of the test scores.

Many of the statements in the *Code* refer to the selection and use of existing tests. When a new test is developed, when an existing test is modified, or when the administration of a test is modified, the *Code* is intended to provide guidance for this process.

The *Code* is not intended to be mandatory, exhaustive, or definitive, and may not be applicable to every situation. Instead, the *Code* is intended to be aspirational and is not intended to take precedence over the judgment of those who have competence in the subjects addressed.

The *Code* provides guidance separately for test developers and test users in four critical areas:

A.   Developing and Selecting Appropriate Tests
B.   Administering and Scoring Tests
C.   Reporting and Interpreting Test Results
D.   Informing Test Takers

A. Developing and Selecting Appropriate Tests

TEST DEVELOPERS

Test developers should provide the information and supporting evidence that test users need to select appropriate test.

A-1. Provide evidence of what the test measures, the recommended uses, the intended test takers, and the strengths and limitations of the test, including the level of precision of the test scores.

TEST USERS

Test users should select tests that meet the intended purpose and that are appropriate for the intended test takers.

A-1. Define the purpose for testing, the content and skills to be tested, and the intended test takers. Select and use the most appropriate test based on a thorough review of available information.

A-2. Describe how the content and skills to be tested were selected and how the tests were developed.

A-2. Review and select tests based on the appropriateness of test content, skills tested, and content coverage for the intended purpose of testing.

A-3. Communicate information about a test's characteristics at a level of detail appropriate to the intended test users.

A-3. Review materials provided by test developers and select tests for which clear, accurate, and complete information is provided.

A-4. Provide guidance on the levels of skills, knowledge, and training necessary for appropriate review, selection, and administration of tests.

A-4. Select tests through a process that includes persons with appropriate knowledge, skills, and training.

A-5. Provide evidence that the technical quality, including reliability and validity, of the test meets its intended purposes.

A-5. Evaluate evidence of the technical quality of the test provided by the test developer and any independent reviewers.

A-6. Provide to qualified test users representative samples of test questions or practice tests, directions, answer sheets, manuals, and score reports.

A-6. Evaluate representative samples of test questions or practice tests, directions, answer sheets, manuals, and score reports before selecting a test.

A-7. Avoid potentially offensive content or language when developing test questions and related materials.

A-7. Evaluate procedures and materials used by test developers, as well as the resulting test, to ensure that potentially offensive content or language is avoided.

A-8. Make appropriately modified forms of tests or administration procedures available for test takers with disabilities who need special accommodations.

A-8. Select tests with appropriately modified forms or administration procedures for test takers with disabilities who need special accommodations.

A-9. Obtain and provide evidence on the performance of test takers of diverse subgroups, making significant efforts to obtain sample sizes that are adequate for subgroup analyses. Evaluate the evidence to ensure that differences in performance are related to the skills being assessed.

A-9. Evaluate the available evidence on the performance of test takers of diverse subgroups. Determine to the extent feasible which performance differences may have been caused by factors unrelated to the skills being assessed.

B. Administering and Scoring Tests

TEST DEVELOPERS	TEST USERS
Test developers should explain how to administer and score tests correctly and fairly.	Test users should administer and score tests correctly and fairly.
B-1. Provide clear descriptions of detailed procedures for administering tests in a standardized manner.	B-1. Follow established procedures for administering tests in a standardized manner.
B-2. Provide guidelines on reasonable procedures for assessing persons with disabilities who need special accommodations or those with diverse linguistic backgrounds.	B-2. Provide and document appropriate procedures for test takers with disabilities who need special accommodations or those with diverse linguistic backgrounds. Some accommodations may be required by law or regulation.
B-3. Provide information to test takers or test users on test question formats and procedures for answering test questions, including information on the use of any needed materials and equipment.	B-3. Provide test takers with an opportunity to become familiar with test question formats and any materials or equipment that may be used during testing.
B-4. Establish and implement procedures to ensure the security of testing materials during all phases of test development, administration, scoring, and reporting.	B-4. Protect the security of test materials, including respecting copyrights and eliminating opportunities for test takers to obtain scores by fraudulent means.
B-5. Provide procedures, materials and guidelines for scoring the tests, and for monitoring the accuracy of the scoring process. If scoring the test is the responsibility of the test developer, provide adequate training for scorers.	B-5. If test scoring is the responsibility of the test user, provide adequate training to scorers and ensure and monitor the accuracy of the scoring process.
B-6. Correct errors that affect the interpretation of the scores and communicate the corrected results promptly.	B-6. Correct errors that affect the interpretation of the scores and communicate the corrected results promptly.
B-7. Develop and implement procedures for ensuring the confidentiality of scores.	B-7. Develop and implement procedures for ensuring the confidentiality of scores.

C. Reporting and Interpreting Test Results

TEST DEVELOPERS

Test developers should report test results accurately and provide information to help test users interpret test results correctly.

C-1. Provide information to support recommended interpretations of the results, including the nature of the content, norms or comparison groups, and other technical evidence. Advise test users of the benefits and limitations of test results and their interpretation. Warn against assigning greater precision than is warranted.

C-2. Provide guidance regarding the interpretations of results for tests administered with modifications. Inform test users of potential problems in interpreting test results when tests or test administration procedures are modified.

C-3. Specify appropriate uses of test results and warn test users of potential misuses.

C-4. When test developers set standards, provide the rationale, procedures, and evidence for setting performance standards or passing scores. Avoid using stigmatizing labels.

C-5. Encourage test users to base decisions about test takers on multiple sources of appropriate information, not on a single test score.

TEST USERS

Test users should report and interpret test results accurately and clearly.

C-1. Interpret the meaning of the test results, taking into account the nature of the content, norms or comparison groups, other technical evidence, and benefits and limitations of test results.

C-2. Interpret test results from modified test or test administration procedures in view of the impact those modifications may have had on test results.

C-3. Avoid using tests for purposes other than those recommended by the test developer unless there is evidence to support the intended use or interpretation.

C-4. Review the procedures for setting performance standards or passing scores. Avoid using stigmatizing labels.

C-5. Avoid using a single test score as the sole determinant of decisions about test takers. Interpret test scores in conjunction with other information about individuals.

C-6. Provide information to enable test users to accurately interpret and report test results for groups of test takers, including information about who were and who were not included in the different groups being compared, and information about factors that might influence the interpretation of results.

C-6. State the intended interpretation and use of test results for groups of test takers. Avoid grouping test results for purposes not specifically recommended by the test developer unless evidence is obtained to support the intended use. Report procedures that were followed in determining who were and who were not included in the groups being compared and describe factors that might influence the interpretation of results.

C-7. Provide test results in a timely fashion and in a manner that is understood by the test taker.

C-7. Communicate test results in a timely fashion and in a manner that is understood by the test taker.

C-8. Provide guidance to test users about how to monitor the extent to which the test is fulfilling its intended purposes.

C-8. Develop and implement procedures for monitoring test use, including consistency with the intended purposes of the test.

D. Informing Test Takers

Under some circumstances, test developers have direct communication with the test takers and/or control of the tests, testing process, and test results. In other circumstances the test users have these responsibilities.

Test developers or test users should inform test takers about the nature of the test, test taker rights and responsibilities, the appropriate use of scores, and procedures for resolving challenges to scores.

D-1. Inform test takers in advance of the test administration about the coverage of the test, the types of question formats, the directions, and appropriate test-taking strategies. Make such information available to all test takers.

D-2. When a test is optional, provide test takers or their parents/guardians with information to help them judge whether a test should be taken—including indications of any consequences that may result from not taking the test (e.g., not being eligible to compete for a particular scholarship)—and whether there is an available alternative to the test.

D-3. Provide test takers or their parents/guardians with information about rights test takers may have to obtain copies of tests and completed answer sheets, to retake tests, to have tests rescored, or to have scores declared invalid.

D-4. Provide test takers or their parents/guardians with information about responsibilities test takers have, such as being aware of the intended purpose and uses of the test, performing at capacity, following directions, and not disclosing test items or interfering with other test takers.

D-5. Inform test takers or their parents/guardians how long scores will be kept on file and indicate to whom, under what circumstances, and in what manner test scores and related information will or will not be released. Protect test scores from unauthorized release and access.

D-6. Describe procedures for investigating and resolving circumstances that might result in canceling or withholding scores, such as failure to adhere to specified testing procedures.

D-7. Describe procedures that test takers, parents/guardians, and other interested parties may use to obtain more information about the test, register complaints, and have problems resolved.

The *Code* is intended to be consistent with the relevant parts of the *Standards for Educational and Psychological Testing* (American Educational Research Association [AERA], American Psychological Association [APA], and National Council on Measurement in Education [NCME], 1999). The *Code* is not meant to add new principles over and above those in the *Standards* or to change their meaning. Rather, the *Code* is intended to represent the spirit of selected portions of the *Standards* in a way that is relevant and meaningful to developers and users of tests, as well as to test takers and/or their parents or guardians. States, districts, schools, organizations and individual professionals are encouraged to commit themselves to fairness in testing and safeguarding the rights of test takers. The *Code* is intended to assist in carrying out such commitments.

The *Code* has been prepared by the Joint Committee on Testing Practices, a cooperative effort among several professional organizations. The aim of the Joint Committee is to act, in the public interest, to advance the quality of testing practices. Members of the Joint Committee include the American Counseling Association (ACA), the American Educational Research Association (AERA), the American Psychological Association (APA), the American Speech-Language-Hearing Association (ASHA), the National Association of School Psychologists (NASP), the National Association of Test Directors (NATD), and the National Council on Measurement in Education (NCME).

Note: The membership of the Working Group that developed the *Code of Fair Testing Practices in Education* and of the Joint Committee on Testing Practices that guided the Working Group is as follows:

Peter Behuniak, PhD
Lloyd Bond, PhD
Gwyneth M. Boodoo, PhD
Wayne Camara, PhD
Ray Fenton, PhD
John J. Fremer, PhD (Co-Chair)
Sharon M. Goldsmith, PhD
Bert F. Green, PhD
William G. Harris, PhD
Janet E. Helms, PhD

Stephanie H. McConaughy, PhD
Julie P. Noble, PhD
Wayne M. Patience, PhD
Carole L. Perlman, PhD
Douglas K. Smith, PhD (deceased)
Janet E. Wall, EdD (Co-Chair)
Pat Nellor Wickwire, PhD
Mary Yakimowski, PhD

Lara Frumkin, PhD, of the APA served as staff liaison.

CODE OF PROFESSIONAL RESPONSIBILITIES IN EDUCATIONAL MEASUREMENT

Prepared by the NCME Ad Hoc Committee on the Development
of a Code of Ethics:

Cynthia B. Schmeiser, ACT—Chair
Kurt F. Geisinger, State University of New York
Sharon Johnson-Lewis, Detroit Public Schools
Edward D. Roeber, Council of Chief State School Officers
William D. Schafer, University of Maryland

Preamble and General Responsibilities

As an organization dedicated to the improvement of measurement and evaluation practice in education, the National Council on Measurement in Education (NCME) has adopted this Code to promote professionally responsible practice in educational measurement. Professionally responsible practice is conduct that arises from either the professional standards of the field, general ethical principles, or both.

The purpose of the Code of Professional Responsibilities in Educational Measurement, hereinafter referred to as the Code, is to guide the conduct of NCME members who are involved in any type of assessment activity in education. NCME is also providing this Code as a public service for all individuals who are engaged in educational assessment activities in the hope that these activities will be conducted in a professionally responsible manner. Persons who engage in these activities include local educators such as classroom teachers, principals, and superintendents; professionals such as school psychologists and counselors; state and national technical, legislative, and policy staff in education; staff of research, evaluation, and testing organizations; providers of test preparation services; college and university faculty and administrators; and professionals in business and industry who design and implement educational and training programs.

This Code applies to any type of assessment that occurs as part of the educational process, including formal and informal, traditional and alternative techniques for gathering information used in making educational decisions at all levels. These techniques include, but are not limited to, large-scale assessments at the school, district, state, national, and international levels; standardized tests; observational measures; teacher-conducted assessments; assessment support materials; and other achievement, aptitude, interest, and personality measures used in and for education.

Although NCME is promulgating this Code for its members, it strongly encourages other organizations and individuals who engage in educational assessment activities to endorse and abide by the responsibilities relevant to their professions. Because the Code pertains only to uses of assessment in education, it is recognized that uses of assessments outside of educational contexts, such as for employment, certification, or licensure, may involve additional professional responsibilities beyond those detailed in this Code.

The Code is intended to serve an educational function: to inform and remind those involved in educational assessment of their obligations to uphold the integrity of the manner in which assessments are developed, used, evaluated, and marketed. Moreover, it is expected that the Code will stimulate thoughtful discussion of what constitutes professionally responsible assessment practice at all levels in education.

Section 1: Responsibilities of Those Who Develop Assessment Products and Services

Those who develop assessment products and services, such as classroom teachers and other assessment specialists, have a professional responsibility to strive to produce assessments that are of the highest quality. Persons who develop assessments have a professional responsibility to:

1.1   ensure that assessment products and services are developed to meet applicable professional, technical, and legal standards.

1.2   develop assessment products and services that are as free as possible from bias due to characteristics irrelevant to the construct being measured, such as gender, ethnicity, race, socioeconomic status, disability, religion, age, or national origin.

1.3   plan accommodations for groups of test takers with disabilities and other special needs when developing assessments.

1.4   disclose to appropriate parties any actual or potential conflicts of interest that might influence the developers' judgment or performance.

1.5   use copyrighted materials in assessment products and services in accordance with state and federal law.

1.6   make information available to appropriate persons about the steps taken to develop and score the assessment, including up-to-date information used to support the reliability, validity, scoring and reporting processes, and other relevant characteristics of the assessment.

1.7   protect the rights of privacy of those who are assessed as part of the assessment development process.

1.8   caution users, in clear and prominent language, against the most likely misinterpretations and misuses of data that arise out of the assessment development process.

1.9   avoid false or unsubstantiated claims in test preparation and program support materials and services about an assessment or its use and interpretation.

1.10   correct any substantive inaccuracies in assessments or their support materials as soon as feasible.

1.11   develop score reports and support materials that promote the understanding of assessment results.

Section 2: Responsibilities of Those Who Market and Sell Assessment Products and Services

The marketing of assessment products and services, such as tests and other instruments, scoring services, test preparation services, consulting, and test interpretive services, should be based on information that is accurate, complete, and relevant to those considering their use. Persons who market and sell assessment products and services have a professional responsibility to:

2.1   provide accurate information to potential purchasers about assessment products and services and their recommended uses and limitations.

2.2   not knowingly withhold relevant information about assessment products and services that might affect an appropriate selection decision.

2.3   base all claims about assessment products and services on valid interpretations of publicly available information.

2.4   allow qualified users equal opportunity to purchase assessment products and services.

2.5   establish reasonable fees for assessment products and services.

2.6   communicate to potential users, in advance of any purchase or use, all applicable fees associated with assessment products and services.

2.7   strive to ensure that no individuals are denied access to opportunities because of their inability to pay the fees for assessment products and services.

2.8   establish criteria for the sale of assessment products and services, such as limiting the sale of assessment products and services to those individuals who are qualified for recommended uses and from whom proper uses and interpretations are anticipated.

2.9   inform potential users of known inappropriate uses of assessment products and services and provide recommendations about how to avoid such misuses.

2.10   maintain a current understanding about assessment products and services and their appropriate uses in education.

2.11   release information implying endorsement by users of assessment products and services only with the users' permission.

2.12   avoid making claims that assessment products and services have been endorsed by another organization unless an official endorsement has been obtained.

2.13   avoid marketing test preparation products and services that may cause individuals to receive scores that misrepresent their actual levels of attainment.

Section 3: Responsibilities of Those Who Select Assessment Products and Services

Those who select assessment products and services for use in educational settings, or help others do so, have important professional responsibilities to make sure that the assessments are appropriate for their intended use. Persons who select assessment products and services have a professional responsibility to:

3.1   conduct a thorough review and evaluation of available assessment strategies and instruments that might be valid for the intended uses.

3.2   recommend and/or select assessments based on publicly available documented evidence of their technical quality and utility rather than on insubstantial claims or statements.

3.3   disclose any associations or affiliations that they have with the authors, test publishers, or others involved with the assessments under consideration for purchase and refrain from participation if such associations might affect the objectivity of the selection process.

3.4   inform decision makers and prospective users of the appropriateness of the assessment for the intended uses, likely consequences of use, protection of examinee rights, relative costs, materials and services needed to conduct or use the assessment, and known limitations of the assessment, including potential misuses and misinterpretations of assessment information.

3.5   recommend against the use of any prospective assessment that is likely to be administered, scored, and used in an invalid manner for members of various groups in our society for reasons of race, ethnicity, gender, age, disability, language background, socioeconomic status, religion, or national origin.

3.6   comply with all security precautions that may accompany assessments being reviewed.

3.7   immediately disclose any attempts by others to exert undue influence on the assessment selection process.

3.8   avoid recommending, purchasing, or using test preparation products and services that may cause individuals to receive scores that misrepresent their actual levels of attainment.

Section 4: Responsibilities of Those Who Administer Assessments

Those who prepare individuals to take assessments and those who are directly or indirectly involved in the administration of assessments as part of the educational process, including teachers, administrators, and assessment personnel, have an important role in making sure that the assessments are administered in a fair and accurate manner. Persons who prepare others for, and those who administer, assessments have a professional responsibility to:

4.1   inform the examinees about the assessment prior to its administration, including its purposes, uses, and consequences; how the assessment information will be judged or scored; how the results will be distributed; and examinees' rights before, during, and after the assessment.

4.2   administer only those assessments for which they are qualified by education, training, licensure, or certification.

4.3   take appropriate security precautions before, during and after the administration of the assessment.

4.4   understand the procedures needed to administer the assessment prior to administration.

4.5   administer standardized assessments according to prescribed procedures and conditions and notify appropriate persons if any nonstandard or delimiting conditions occur.

4.6   not exclude any eligible student from the assessment.

4.7   avoid any conditions in the conduct of the assessment that might invalidate the results.

4.8   provide for and document all reasonable and allowable accommodations for the administration of the assessment to persons with disabilities or special needs.

4.9   provide reasonable opportunities for individuals to ask questions about the assessment procedures or directions prior to and at prescribed times during the administration of the assessment.

4.10   protect the rights to privacy and due process of those who are assessed.

4.11   avoid actions or conditions that would permit or encourage individuals or groups to receive scores that misrepresent their actual levels of attainment.

Section 5: Responsibilities of Those Who Score Assessments

The scoring of educational assessments should be conducted properly and efficiently so that the results are reported accurately and in a timely manner. Persons who score and prepare reports of assessments have a professional responsibility to:

5.1   provide complete and accurate information to users about how the assessment is scored, such as the reporting schedule, scoring process to be used, rationale for the scoring approach, technical characteristics, quality control procedures, reporting formats, and the fees, if any, for these services.

5.2 ensure the accuracy of the assessment results by conducting reasonable quality control procedures before, during, and after scoring.

5.3 minimize the effect on scoring of factors irrelevant to the purposes of the assessment.

5.4 inform users promptly of any deviation in the planned scoring and reporting service or schedule and negotiate a solution with users.

5.5 provide corrected score results to the examinee or the client as quickly as practicable should errors be found that may affect the inferences made on the basis of the scores.

5.6 protect the confidentiality of information that identifies individuals as prescribed by state and federal law.

5.7 release summary results of the assessment only to those persons entitled to such information by state or federal law or those who are designated by the party contracting for the scoring services.

5.8 establish, where feasible, a fair and reasonable process for appeal and rescoring the assessment.

Section 6: Responsibilities of Those Who Interpret, Use, and Communicate Assessment Results

The interpretation, use, and communication of assessment results should promote valid inferences and minimize invalid ones. Persons who interpret, use, and communicate assessment results have a professional responsibility to:

6.1 conduct these activities in an informed, objective, and fair manner within the context of the assessment's limitations and with an understanding of the potential consequences of use.

6.2 provide to those who receive assessment results information about the assessment, its purposes, its limitations, and its uses necessary for the proper interpretation of the results.

6.3 provide to those who receive score reports an understandable written description of all reported scores, including proper interpretations and likely misinterpretations.

6.4 communicate to appropriate audiences the results of the assessment in an understandable and timely manner, including proper interpretations and likely misinterpretations.

6.5 evaluate and communicate the adequacy and appropriateness of any norms or standards used in the interpretation of assessment results.

6.6   inform parties involved in the assessment process how assessment results may affect them.

6.7   use multiple sources and types of relevant information about persons or programs whenever possible in making educational decisions.

6.8   avoid making, and actively discourage others from making, inaccurate reports, unsubstantiated claims, inappropriate interpretations, or otherwise false and misleading statements about assessment results.

6.9   disclose to examinees and others whether and how long the results of the assessment will be kept on file, procedures for appeal and rescoring, rights examinees and others have to the assessment information, and how those rights may be exercised.

6.10   report any apparent misuses of assessment information to those responsible for the assessment process.

6.11   protect the rights to privacy of individuals and institutions involved in the assessment process.

Section 7: Responsibilities of Those Who Educate Others About Assessment

The process of educating others about educational assessment, whether as part of higher education, professional development, public policy discussions, or job training, should prepare individuals to understand and engage in sound measurement practice and to become discerning users of tests and test results. Persons who educate or inform others about assessment have a professional responsibility to:

7.1   remain competent and current in the areas in which they teach and reflect that in their instruction.

7.2   provide fair and balanced perspectives when teaching about assessment.

7.3   differentiate clearly between expressions of opinion and substantiated knowledge when educating others about any specific assessment method, product, or service.

7.4   disclose any financial interests that might be perceived to influence the evaluation of a particular assessment product or service that is the subject of instruction.

7.5   avoid administering any assessment that is not part of the evaluation of student performance in a course if the administration of that assessment is likely to harm any student.

7.6   avoid using or reporting the results of any assessment that is not part of the evaluation of student performance in a course if the use or reporting of results is likely to harm any student.

7.7   protect all secure assessments and materials used in the instructional process.

7.8   model responsible assessment practice and help those receiving instruction to learn about their professional responsibilities in educational measurement.

7.9   provide fair and balanced perspectives on assessment issues being discussed by policymakers, parents, and other citizens.

Section 8: Responsibilities of Those Who Evaluate Educational Programs and Conduct Research on Assessments

Conducting research on or about assessments or educational programs is a key activity in helping to improve the understanding and use of assessments and educational programs. Persons who engage in the evaluation of educational programs or conduct research on assessments have a professional responsibility to:

8.1   conduct evaluation and research activities in an informed, objective, and fair manner.

8.2   disclose any associations that they have with authors, test publishers, or others involved with the assessment and refrain from participation if such associations might affect the objectivity of the research or evaluation.

8.3   preserve the security of all assessments throughout the research process as appropriate.

8.4   take appropriate steps to minimize potential sources of invalidity in the research and disclose known factors that may bias the results of the study.

8.5   present the results of research, both intended and unintended, in a fair, complete, and objective manner.

8.6   attribute completely and appropriately the work and ideas of others.

8.7   qualify the conclusions of the research within the limitations of the study.

8.8   use multiple sources of relevant information in conducting evaluation and research activities whenever possible.

8.9   comply with applicable standards for protecting the rights of participants in an evaluation or research study, including the rights to privacy and informed consent.

Afterword

As stated at the outset, the purpose of the *Code of Professional Responsibilities in Educational Measurement* is to serve as a guide to the conduct of NCME members who are engaged in any type of assessment activity in education. Given the broad scope of the field of educational assessment as well as the variety of activities in which professionals may engage, it is unlikely that any code will cover the professional responsibilities involved in every situation or activity in which assessment is used in education. Ultimately, it is hoped that this Code will serve as the basis for ongoing discussions about what constitutes professionally responsible practice. Moreover, these discussions will undoubtedly identify areas of practice that need further analysis and clarification in subsequent editions of the Code. To the extent that these discussions occur, the Code will have served its purpose.

To assist in the ongoing refinement of the Code, comments on this document are most welcome. Please send your comments and inquiries to:

Dr. William J. Russell
Executive Officer
National Council on
Measurement in Education
1230 Seventeenth Street, NW
Washington, D.C. 20036-3078

Appendix C

9 Principles of Good Practice
for Assessing Student Learning

The assessment of student learning begins with educational values. Assessment is not an end in itself but a vehicle for educational improvement. Its effective practice, then, begins with and enacts a vision of the kinds of learning we most value for students and strive to help them achieve. Educational values should drive not only *what* we choose to assess but also *how* we do so. Where questions about educational mission and values are skipped over, assessment threatens to be an exercise in measuring what's easy, rather than a process of improving what we really care about.

1. **Assessment is most effective when it reflects an understanding of learning as multidimensional, integrated, and revealed in performance over time.** Learning is a complex process. It entails not only what students know but what they can do with what they know; it involves not only knowledge and abilities but values, attitudes, and habits of mind that affect both academic success and performance beyond the classroom. Assessment should reflect these understandings by employing a diverse array of methods, including those that call for actual performance, using them over time so as to reveal change, growth, and increasing degrees of integration. Such an approach aims for a more complete and accurate picture of learning, and therefore firmer bases for improving our students' educational experience.

2. **Assessment works best when the programs it seeks to improve have clear, explicitly stated purposes. Assessment is a goal-oriented process.** It entails comparing educational performance with educational purposes and expectations—those derived from the institution's mission, from faculty intentions in program and course design, and from knowledge of students' own goals. Where program purposes lack specificity or agreement, assessment as a pro-

cess pushes a campus toward clarity about where to aim and what standards to apply; assessment also prompts attention to where and how program goals will be taught and learned. Clear, shared, implementable goals are the cornerstone for assessment that is focused and useful.

3. **Assessment requires attention to outcomes but also and equally to the experiences that lead to those outcomes.** Information about outcomes is of high importance; where students "end up" matters greatly. But to improve outcomes, we need to know about student experience along the way—about the curricula, teaching, and kind of student effort that lead to particular outcomes. Assessment can help us understand which students learn best under what conditions; with such knowledge comes the capacity to improve the whole of their learning.

4. **Assessment works best when it is ongoing not episodic.** Assessment is a process whose power is cumulative. Though isolated, "one-shot" assessment can be better than none, improvement is best fostered when assessment entails a linked series of activities undertaken over time. This may mean tracking the process of individual students, or of cohorts of students; it may mean collecting the same examples of student performance or using the same instrument semester after semester. The point is to monitor progress toward intended goals in a spirit of continuous improvement. Along the way, the assessment process itself should be evaluated and refined in light of emerging insights.

5. **Assessment fosters wider improvement when representatives from across the educational community are involved.** Student learning is a campus-wide responsibility, and assessment is a way of enacting that responsibility. Thus, while assessment efforts may start small, the aim over time is to involve people from across the educational community. Faculty play an especially important role, but assessment's questions can't be fully addressed without participation by student-affairs educators, librarians, administrators, and students. Assessment may also involve individuals from beyond the campus (alumni/ae, trustees, employers) whose experience can enrich the sense of appropriate aims and standards for learning. Thus understood, assessment is not a task for small groups of experts but a collaborative activity; its aim is wider, better-informed attention to student learning by all parties with a stake in its improvement.

6. **Assessment makes a difference when it begins with issues of use and illuminates questions that people really care about.** Assessment recognizes the value of information in the process of improvement. But to be useful, information must be connected to issues or questions that people really care about. This implies assessment approaches that produce evidence that

relevant parties will find credible, suggestive, and applicable to decisions that need to be made. It means thinking in advance about how the information will be used, and by whom. The point of assessment is not to gather data and return "results"; it is a process that starts with the questions of decision-makers, that involves them in the gathering and interpreting of data, and that informs and helps guide continuous improvement.

7. **Assessment is most likely to lead to improvement when it is part of a larger set of conditions that promote change.** Assessment alone changes little. Its greatest contribution comes on campuses where the quality of teaching and learning is visibly valued and worked at. On such campuses, the push to improve educational performance is a visible and primary goal of leadership; improving the quality of undergraduate education is central to the institution's planning, budgeting, and personnel decisions. On such campuses, information about learning outcomes is seen as an integral part of decision making, and avidly sought.

8. **Through assessment, educators meet responsibilities to students and to the public.** There is a compelling public stake in education. As educators, we have a responsibility to the publics that support or depend on us to provide information about the ways in which our students meet goals and expectations. But that responsibility goes beyond the reporting of such information; our deeper obligation—to ourselves, our students, and society—is to improve. Those to whom educators are accountable have a corresponding obligation to support such attempts at improvement.

Authors: Alexander W. Astin; Trudy W. Banta; K. Patricia Cross; Elaine El-Khawas; Peter T. Ewell; Pat Hutchings; Theodore J. Marchese; Kay M. McClenney; Marcia Mentkowski; Margaret A. Miller; E. Thomas Moran; Barbara D. Wright. This document was developed under the auspices of the AAHE Assessment Forum with support from the Fund for the Improvement of Postsecondary Education with additional support for publication and dissemination from the Exxon Education Foundation. Copies may be made without restriction.

Source. American Association for Higher Education. (2003). 9 Principles of Good Practice for Assessing Student Learning. Accessed February 6, 2005, from http://www.aahe.org/assessment/principl.htm
Reprinted by permission of the American Association for Higher Education, 2005.

Index

Springer Series on the Teaching of Nursing

Diane O. McGivern, RN, PhD, FAAN, Series Editor
New York University

Advisory Board: Ellen Baer, PhD, RN, FAAN; Carla Mariano, EdD, RN, AHN-C, FAAIM, Janet A. Rodgers, PhD, RN, FAAN; Alice Adam Young, PhD, RN

Annual Review of Nursing Education Series

Marilyn H. Oermann, PhD, RN, FAAN, Editor
Kathleen T. Heinrich, PhD, RN, Associate Editor

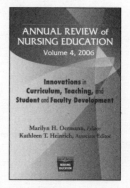

Volume 4: Innovations in Curriculum, Teaching, and Student and Faculty Development

This is "must" reading for anyone teaching nursing, at any level, in any program or institution. It covers trends and innovative strategies to help you develop a curriculum and be more effective in using it. Educators describe problems—such as students who cannot write or high NCLEX failure rates—and how they tackled and solved them. Each chapter contains common sense approaches to every educator's questions. This is a resource no nursing education program can afford to be without!

Partial Contents:

- Genetics Interdisciplinary Faculty Training (GIFT): Integrating Genetics into Graduate Nursing Curricula, *B.S. Turner, J. Strand,* and *M.C. Speer*
- Designing a Course for Educating Baccalaureate Nursing Students as Public Policy Advocates, *D. Faulk* and *M.P. Ternus*
- Introducing and Using Handheld Technology in Nursing Education, *F. Cornelius* and *M.G. Gordon*
- Developing Emotional Competence through Service Learning, *R. Hunt*
- Use of Progression Testing Throughout Nursing Programs: How Two Colleges Promote Success on the NCLEX-RN®, *N.R. Mosser, J. Williams,* and *C. Wood*

Dec. 2005 392pp softcover 0-8261-2447-X

Also Available

Volume 1: 2003 392pp hardcover 0-8261-2444-5
Volume 2: 2004 400pp hardcover 0-8261-2445-3
Volume 3: 2005 440pp softcover 0-8261-2446-1

11 West 42nd Street, New York, NY 10036-8002 • Fax: 212-941-7842
Order Toll-Free: 877-687-7476 • Order On-line: www.springerpub.com

SPRINGER PUBLISHING COMPANY

Educating Nurses for Leadership

Harriet R. Feldman, PhD, RN, FAAN
Martha J. Greenberg, PhD, RN, Editors

This book provides tools for nurse educators and administrators to prepare nurses to be effective leaders so that they may advance health care practice and the profession of nursing. Part I describes a Leadership Education Model and its six modules of leader as achiever, communicator, critical thinker, expert, mentor, and visionary. Part II presents proven strategies from schools across the United States for integrating leadership into the nursing curriculum. Part III discusses strategies that can be used in the clinical setting by administrators and staff developers. The annotated bibliography at the back of the book offers important additional resources on leadership development in nursing.

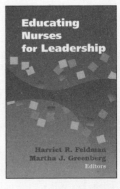

Partial Contents:

Part I: A Model for Educating Future Leaders • Preparing Nurse Leaders: A Leadership Education Model, *J.A. Lemire* • Leader as Visionary, *J. Aroian* • Leader as Expert, *B. Frank* • Leader as Achiever, *J. Dienemann* • Leader as Critical Thinker, *J.A. Lemire* • Leader as Communicator, *P.A. Haynor* • Leader as Mentor, *C. Vance*

Part II: Using Nursing History to Educate for Leadership, *S.B. Lewenson* • Reflective Journaling: Bridging the Theory-Practice Gap, *D. Morgan, J. Johnson,* and *D. Garrison* • Using Group Process to Develop Caring Leaders, *L. Wagner* • Using Parse's Theory to Educate for Leadership, *S. Ramey* and *S. Bunkers*

Part III: Leadership Education in the Clinical Setting • Practice-Oriented Leadership Education, *J. Aroian* and *J. Dienemann* • Using Shift Coordinators to Teach Leadership Skills Needed for NCLEX-RN, *J. Aucoin* and *S. Letvak* • Teaching the Value of Evidence-Based Practice, *B. Frank* • Developing Evidence-Based Practice Skills Through Experiential Learning, *K. Sackett* and *J. Jones*

2004   352pp   hardcover   0-8261-2664-2

11 West 42nd Street, New York, NY 10036-8002 • **Fax: 212-941-7842**
Order Toll-Free: 877-687-7476 • **Order On-line: www.springerpub.com**

Best Practices in Nursing Education
Stories of Exemplary Teachers

Mary Jane Smith, PhD, RN
Joyce J. Fitzpatrick, PhD, RN, FAAN

"What is teaching and how does one go about doing it are the questions that are answered in this book...[it] will become a classic in the field and is a tribute to the individuals who told their stories..."
—from the Foreword, **Jeanne M. Novotny**

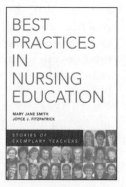

"Teaching is a gift we give to each other, and learning is a gift that we give to ourselves."
—from the Introduction, **Mary Jane Smith and Joyce J. Fitzpatrick**

Who better to learn from about teaching than teachers themselves?

Written by teachers and about teachers, this book is for graduate students in nursing education as well as mid-career nurse educators. Contained in this volume are narratives based on interviews with twenty-one distinguished teachers of nursing. The contributors to this volume provide multiple role models for career development and offer their wisdom, including:

Contents:

- Deciding on a career in teaching nursing
- Preparing and mentoring in teaching
- Maintaining excellence
- Embarrassing teaching moments
- Most and least rewarding times
- Significant challenges
- Advice for new teachers
- Balancing professional and personal life

2005   232pp   0-8261-3235-9   softcover

11 West 42nd Street, New York, NY 10036-8002 • Fax: 212-941-7842
Order Toll-Free: 877-687-7476 • Order On-line: www.springerpub.com

Distance Education in Nursing
Second Edition

Jeanne M. Novotny, PhD, RN, FAAN
Robert H. Davis, BSN, RN, Editors

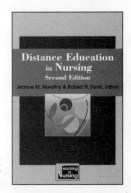

"Provides the educator interested in distance education with realistic advice on the field. The topic is timely, includes a comprehensive overview, the information is accessible."
—**American Journal of Nursing**
praise for previous edition

This second edition of the award-winning **Distance Education in Nursing** offers basic introductory information on distance teaching and learning in nursing and also brings the application of newly developed computer technology to this environment. It is written for every nurse educator, from novice to expert, by such distinguished contributors as Diane Billings, Suzanne Hetzel Campbell, and Marilyn Oermann.

Each chapter begins with stories of real-life distance education moments from both teachers and students, their experiences, and ways in which distance education has improved their quality of life.

Partial Contents:

Part I: Teaching and Learning Strategies for Distance Education • Teaching a Web-Based Course, *M.L. McHugh* • Supporting Learner Success, *C.L. Mueller* and *D.M. Billings* • Faculty Preparation for Teaching Online, *A.E. Johnson*

Part II: Experiences of Specific Programs • Teaching Online Pathophysiology, *H. Lee, N. Holloway,* and *L. Field* • A Distance Learning Master's Degree Program for Nurse-Midwives and Nurse Practitioners, *S. Stone*

Part III: Where Are We Going with Distance Education? • Program Innovations and Technology in Nursing Education: Are We Moving Too Quickly?, *M.H. Oermann* • Attitudes Toward Distance Education, *R.H. Davis*

Teaching of Nursing
September 2005   280pp   softcover   0-8261-4694-5

11 West 42nd Street, New York, NY 10036-8002 • Fax: 212-941-7842
Order Toll-Free: 877-687-7476 • Order On-line: www.springerpub.com